EVIDENCE-BASED PRACTICE
OF COGNITIVE-BEHAVIORAL THERAPY

Evidence-Based Practice of Cognitive-Behavioral Therapy

DEBORAH DOBSON
KEITH S. DOBSON

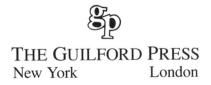

THE GUILFORD PRESS
New York   London

Library of Congress Cataloging-in-Publication Data

Dobson, Deborah J. G. (Deborah June Gora), 1954–
  Evidence-based practice of cognitive-behavioral therapy / Deborah Dobson
and Keith S. Dobson.
      p. ; cm.
  Includes bibliographical references and index.
  ISBN 978-1-60623-020-6 (hardcover : alk. paper)
1. Cognitive therapy.   2. Evidence-based psychiatry.   I. Dobson, Keith S.
II. Title.
  [DNLM: 1. Cognitive Therapy—methods.   2. Evidence-Based Medicine—
methods.   3. Mental Disorders—therapy.   WM 425.5.C6 D635e 2009]
  RC489.C63D63 2009
  616.89´1425—dc22

                                                            2008050373

About the Authors

Deborah Dobson, PhD, is a psychologist with the Calgary Health Region and Adjunct Associate Professor in the Departments of Psychology and Psychiatry at the University of Calgary. She also maintains a private practice, where she provides assessments and cognitive-behavioral therapy for adult clients, and is Director of Clinical Training for the Calgary Consortium in Clinical Psychology. Dr. Dobson is the President of the Board of the Canadian Mental Health Association–Calgary Division and was the Chair of the Clinical Section for the Canadian Psychological Association from 2007 to 2008. Her professional interests include client access to empirically supported treatments, clinical training, consumer advocacy, and cognitive-behavioral therapies.

Keith S. Dobson, PhD, is Professor of Clinical Psychology at the University of Calgary, where he has served in various roles, including past Director of Clinical Psychology and current Head of Psychology and Co-Leader of the Hotchkiss Brain Institute Depression Research Program. Dr. Dobson's research has focused on cognitive models and mechanisms in depression and the treatment of depression, particularly using cognitive-behavioral therapies. His research has resulted in over 150 published articles and chapters, 8 books, and numerous conference and workshop presentations in many countries. In addition to his research in depression, Dr. Dobson has written about developments in professional psychology and ethics, and he has been actively involved in organized psychology in Canada, including a term as President of the Canadian Psychological Association. He was a member of the University of Calgary Research Ethics Board for many years and is President of the Academy of Cognitive Therapy as well as President-Elect of the International Association for Cognitive Psychotherapy. Dr. Dobson is a recipient of the Canadian Psychological Association's Award for Distinguished Contributions to the Profession of Psychology.

Preface

Health care systems around the world are demanding that practitioners utilize effective and efficient treatments for mental health problems. Publicly funded systems often face severe constraints in the range and amount of service they can provide, whereas private insurance companies and managed care corporations seek to control costs to maximize shareholder profits. The drive to identify and to implement effective, time-limited treatments, as well as the strong emphasis on empirical outcomes, has led to the development of practice guidelines that favor such approaches.

These practice guidelines now highlight cognitive-behavioral therapy as a psychological treatment of choice for problems ranging from depression, anxiety, and personality disorders to chronic pain, addictions, and relationship distress. As a result, many students and practitioners seek to learn about the basics of cognitive-behavioral therapy to supplement their clinical training and supervision. They also want to understand how to apply the results of psychotherapy outcome and process research to practice. If a treatment has empirical support, how does that support translate into what is done in the clinic or therapy office? What specifics of practice are supported by research findings? Conversely, what are the limits of our knowledge and of clinical judgment and sound ethical conduct that guide clinicians' behavior? This volume is intended to answer these questions and to bridge the gap between practice and research.

Although many texts have been written on cognitive-behavioral therapy, very few have taken the perspectives of practice, science, and the systems within which they are embedded. The trend within the field has been to focus on specific problem areas, such as social phobia (Heimberg & Becker, 2002) or other phobic disorders (Antony & Swinson, 2000), and/or specialized types of therapy (Segal, Williams, & Teasdale, 2002;

Young, Klosko, & Weishaar, 2003). Increasingly, we know which inter-ventions work for which problems, and numerous treatment manuals have been written for clinicians and their clients. Yet little has been writ-ten about applications of cognitive-behavioral therapy that cut across problems, report on empirical support, and provide practical advice for the clinician. This book does just that.

Much is similar about various applications of cognitive-behavioral therapy, and this book describes the "common factors" of assessment, interventions, and consultation. Many aspects of the practice of cognitive-behavioral therapy have become commonplace and are assumed to be "best practice." In this book we explore these practices and the empiri-cal support behind them. We also identify areas in which the evidence lags behind common practice, both to make readers aware of these areas and to stimulate further research. We also discuss some common myths about cognitive-behavioral therapy (both critical and unduly positive) to provide readers with a sense of our perspective on the field.

All clinicians work within larger systems such as hospitals, clinics, or private settings. Those clinicians who ignore the larger system do so at their peril, because practice is ultimately dependent on promotion and funding of evidence-based services. Little has been written to date on implementing and promoting cognitive-behavioral therapy within sys-tems. Therefore, this book also addresses the important topic of how to translate evidence related to cognitive-behavioral therapy into enhanced funding. We also discuss training, the politics of publicly funded health care and managed care, and working within interdisciplinary teams.

We believe this book will be of most use to people who are in the pro-cess of discovering cognitive-behavioral therapy. This audience includes graduate students and interns in clinical and counseling psychology, resi-dents in psychiatry, and new practitioners in other mental health pro-grams. We also hope that seasoned professionals and psychotherapists in independent practice find their ideas reinforced throughout this book, or that they find a few "nuggets" to integrate into their practice. As the title suggests, our effort is to be as practical as possible, and base links to practice on the available evidence.

This book reflects an attempt to marry the best of science with the realities of clinical practice. We have tried to be practical in our sugges-tions and realistic about what cognitive-behavioral therapy can provide. With this practical focus in mind, we structured the book in such a way that chapters related to the conduct of therapy occur earlier, followed by some of the contextual issues that surround the field, and how to advance training in the field. Many of the chapters provide not only dis-cussion of their respective topics but also case materials to illustrate these ideas. We regularly make reference to "him" or "her" to discuss clients illustrated in the cases. We also provide examples of particular concepts or techniques in each chapter and use the fictitious case of "Anna C" as a running illustration of how a cognitive-behavioral therapy case might evolve. None of the cases in this book depicts a real person; rather, cases are drawn from edited, amalgamated, and fictionalized clients and representations of situations we have encountered over the years.

In contrast to the more practical earlier chapters of the book, the final few chapters take a step back from the application of cognitive-behavioral therapy with individuals to examine some of the issues surrounding this psychotherapeutic approach. Thus, we discuss some of the challenges with implementation, the myths that surround the approach, and the outcome research base. We conclude with some additional ideas about how to obtain cognitive-behavioral therapy training, as well as how to start and maintain a cognitive-behavioral therapy practice.

Most books more or less directly reflect the backgrounds of their authors. This book is no exception in this regard. Our own training was very much driven by the scientist-practitioner model, and we both value both the science and the practice of cognitive-behavioral therapy. Our focus in this book is on cognitive-behavioral therapy with adults, since that is the work we do and the dimension of the field we know best. At the same time, we each bring complementary skills sets to this book—one with a more academic and research focus, and the other with a broader practice and professional skills set. But we both have participated in research, conducted workshops, taught formal courses, supervised trainees, seen our own clients, and worked in various health and educational systems, so our common experiences are considerable. We also attend conferences on a regular basis to stay abreast of advances in the field. Notably, we are both members of the Academy of Cognitive Therapy (*www.academyofct.org*). Whereas our own models of therapy have a decided emphasis to them, we have written this book from a somewhat broader perspective and discuss issues related to the process of psychotherapy that are not often discussed in books on cognitive-behavioral therapy.

No book comes into print without the support of a number of people. We want to acknowledge the large number of people who have touched our lives and supported our own development in this field. Some of the major personal influences for us, both together and separately, include Aaron Beck, Judith Beck, Brian Shaw, Neil Jacobson, Steven Hollon, Zindel Segal, John Teasdale, Robert Wilson, Robert Leahy, Leslie Sokol, Robert DeRubeis, Maureen Leahey, Kerry Mothersill, Gayle Belsher, David Hodgins, James Nieuwenhuis, and Nik Kazantzis. We have had the chance to work with a large number of extremely talented graduate students, trainees, interns, and residents over the years, and we have been rewarded by both their struggles and achievements, some of which now include scientific contributions to the field. We also acknowledge that some aspects of Chapter 12, in fact, originated in discussions between one of us (D. D.) and Gina DiGiulio, while she was working on her pre-doctoral internship. This book was encouraged by Jim Nageotte, Senior Editor at The Guilford Press, and we particularly want to acknowledge his support and help, as well as that of Guilford's other editorial staff. We also wish to note the ongoing love and support we both receive from and give to our children, Kit, Beth, and Aubrey, and our granddaughters, Alexandra and Clementine. We hope that this book contributes to the field and that, ultimately, clients are the major beneficiaries of the ideas within its covers. Our work is predicated on a desire to help people who struggle with mental health problems, and we hope that this book can be a useful part of the growing library in the field of cognitive-behavioral therapy.

Contents

Chapter 1   Introduction and Context of Cognitive-Behavioral   1
              Interventions
              Principles of Cognitive-Behavioral Therapy, 4
              Current Context: Where Are We Now?, 5
              Social and Cultural Factors in Cognitive-Behavioral Therapy, 8
              In Summary, 11

Chapter 2   Assessment for Cognitive-Behavioral Therapy   13
              Know Your Evidence Base: Empirically Based
                Assessment, 14
              Tools for Cognitive-Behavioral Assessment, 16
              Assessment as an Ongoing Process, 29

Chapter 3   Integration and Case Formulation   32
              Case Formulation, 33
              Steps in Case Formulation, 39

Chapter 4   Beginning Treatment: Planning for Therapy   55
              and Building Alliance
              Treatment Planning, Goal Setting, and the
                Therapeutic Contract, 56
              Relationship Factors within Cognitive-Behavioral
                Therapy, 65

Chapter 5   Beginning Treatment: Basic Skills   74
              Sequencing and Length of Treatment, 75
              Orientation and Session Structure, 76
              Psychoeducation, 78
              Homework Assignment, 80
              Problem-Solving Interventions, 82

Chapter 6   Behavior Change Elements in   90
              Cognitive-Behavioral Therapy
              *Behavioral Interventions to Increase Skills and to
                  Plan Action, 91*
              Behavioral Interventions to Decrease Avoidance, 103
              Behavioral Activation, 112
              A Final Comment Regarding Social Context, 113

Chapter 7   Cognitive Restructuring Interventions   116
              Identification of Negative Thoughts, 117
              Methods for Collecting Negative Thoughts, 124
              Interventions for Negative Thinking, 127

Chapter 8   Assessing and Modifying Core Beliefs and Schemas 149
              Defining Schemas, 151
              Discovering Beliefs and Schemas, 153
              Changing Schemas, 158
              Schema Change Methods, 160
              Acceptance-Based Interventions, 171

Chapter 9   Completion of Treatment and Prevention of Relapse 175
              *Concepts and System Factors Related to
                  Therapy Completion, 176*
              Completion of Therapy, 183
              Relapse Prevention, 190

Chapter 10 Challenges in Conducting Cognitive-Behavioral   197
              Therapy
              Challenges That Originate with the Client, 198
              Challenges That Originate with the Therapist, 216
              *Challenges That Originate with the
                  Therapeutic Relationship, 221*
              Challenges That Originate Outside of Therapy, 223

Chapter 11 The Research Context of Cognitive-Behavioral   224
              Therapy
              A Global Perspective on Outcome, 225
              Treatments That Work, 234
              A Review of the Literature, 237

Chapter 12 Myths about Cognitive-Behavioral Therapy   244
              Negative Beliefs, 246
              Positive (but Distorted) Beliefs, 262

Chapter 13 Starting and Maintaining a Cognitive-Behavioral   265
              Practice
              Obtaining and Accepting Referrals, 266
              Communicating Specialties, Limits, and Exclusion Criteria
                 to Potential Clients, 270
              Communicating to Your "Marketplace," 273
              Ways to Increase Your Cognitive-Behavioral Practice, 273
              Further Training and Supervision in Cognitive-Behavioral
                 Therapy, 276
              Coming Full Circle: The Context Matters, 282

Appendix A The Cognitive Therapy Scale   285

Appendix B Review Articles Regarding the Efficacy
              of Cognitive-Behavioral Therapy   291

              References   297

              Index   313

Chapter 1

ཚ

Introduction and Context of Cognitive-Behavioral Interventions

Cognitive-behavioral therapy has broad evidence as a powerful intervention for mental health problems in adults. Many books have been published in the field of cognitive-behavioral therapy, both from research and practical perspectives. Cognitive-behavioral treatments have an empirical base and the majority of practitioners, at least in North America, are trained in a scientist-practitioner model.

Given the wide support for and training in cognitive-behavioral therapy, why are we writing another book on a type of treatment that has been widely described in both the academic and popular press? We believe that the bridge between science and practice requires more traffic. Many books are written from either a science or a practice base, and few travel in both directions across that bridge. While the cognitive-behavioral model may provide an underlying value system toward practice that uses the most up-to-date research findings, it is exceedingly difficult for most practitioners to be aware of the research literature in all the areas in which they provide treatment. As a practitioner in a busy setting, you may wonder how to keep up with the literature.

We are in a unique position to provide a bridge between science and practice, because we bring experience from both sides of the discipline. Consequently, we work to build a stronger bridge that we hope will be useful in your practices as clinicians. We hope that information about empirical outcomes and the methods to translate this knowledge into practice will help you in day-to-day work with not only clients but also the systems within which you practice. Understanding and using empirical research to bring the art of psychotherapy into the scientific realm are desirable goals for the provision of optimal services to clients.

It is important to underpin the scientific bases of cognitive-behavioral interventions with clinical observations. We believe that science and practice can be happily married as equal partners. In this book, our first goal is to bridge science and practice in a bidirectional fashion. Where we can, we present what scientific evidence there is regarding the use of cognitive-behavioral therapy for various problems, and in various settings. We also identify gaps in our knowledge from clinical practice. We hope that interested readers and future researchers will pursue these knowledge gaps in the field. As cognitive-behavioral therapy becomes more widely practiced, it is critical that research-based adaptations of the model integrate the approach into various cultures around the world or within our own communities.

A second goal for this volume is to distill the principles of cognitive-behavioral interventions from the literature and to provide practical guidelines for their applications in a wide variety of contexts. Many cognitive-behavioral treatment manuals have been written, often for increasingly specific diagnostic categories of the *Diagnostic and Statistical Manual of Mental Disorders* of the American Psychiatric Association (2000). Typically, these manuals have been developed in a rigorous way and tested on carefully selected clients in specialty clinics. There is a great deal of overlap among cognitive-behavioral treatments for different diagnostic disorders. Yet, in practice, the majority of clients have multiple problems or comorbidities, which may or may not respond fully to the treatments offered in the manuals. Which manual, if any, should be used first? What should a clinician do if the client chooses not to work on any of the diagnosable problems? These problems may include subclinical or nondiagnosable problems such as low self-esteem, sleep disturbance, problems of daily adjustment, and interpersonal difficulties. They may also include contextual problems, such as inadequate access to health care, poverty, and family violence. Consequently, although diagnosis may offer an important understanding of a set of symptoms, a client may be more concerned about other aspects of his or her life.

Given these considerations, we offer a broad perspective on cognitive-behavioral therapy that is not tied to diagnosis or even to a particular set of problems. Diagnosis is not necessarily a critical feature of either cognitive-behavioral assessment or case conceptualization. Whereas diagnostic categories may not be used to treat clients in some settings, their use may be common to the diagnosis of clients in other settings. As clinicians, it is difficult for us to know how to apply manuals. Most practitioners do not work in specialty clinics, and most clients want help with multiple problems. We hope that it will be helpful to many clinicians to have the current distillation and description of the essential features of cognitive-behavioral treatments for adults.

Cognitive-behavioral treatments have a number of common elements that are adapted for use with different problems. It is useful for clinicians to learn these common elements in their practice and to adapt them to more challenging situations or clients, as needed. As such, our view about the treatment of mental health problems is broad. This book is primarily oriented toward the use of cognitive-behavioral therapy with individual adults. Although we appreciate the strong results that some forms of group, couple, or family cognitive-behavioral therapy have attained, the practice of cognitive-behavioral therapy is largely one of individual treatments. Consequently, our focus is on individual treatment for adults.

We aim to provide guidelines for cognitive-behavioral practitioners in different settings with "typical clients." These clients may have problems with anxiety, depression, relationships, or adjustment to change, or simply with living. They may use too many substances and have self-destructive habits or poor lifestyle balance. They may struggle to make decisions about marriage, their careers, or whether to have children. They may report being dissatisfied with their jobs or very unhappy. They are likely to be worried and to be looking for relief from their concerns. These are the types of problems that clients present to their therapists. Cognitive-behavioral interventions can be very helpful for a wide variety of problems. It is important for clinicians to be flexible in their application of treatments to maximize client outcomes and satisfaction. Therefore, another goal is to help clinicians learn to assess and understand their client's problems using clinical case formulation to make decisions about interventions.

Finally, we believe that context is crucial to our practices. Our clients' problems develop in the contexts of their lives and the social systems in which they interact. We also practice within certain contexts or systems, and these factors make a huge difference in how we treat our clients. If funding is limited treatment is likely to be brief, even for people with severe problems. If our system does not support cognitive-behavioral interventions, we may be less likely to deliver them. Similarly, the time and the culture within which we practice make a difference. It is no coincidence that cognitive-behavioral therapy originated in Western cultures, and in particular, in those with a positive orientation toward science, a belief in logical positivism, and a general conviction that science can solve most of humankind's problems. Just as it is important to understand how our client's learning history led to problem development, it is also important to have a perspective on the historical and cultural context of the therapy. Various histories of cognitive-behavioral therapy exist (e.g., Dobson & Dozois, 2001), so we do not provide the historical perspective in this volume. This chapter now turns to a brief review of the principles of cognitive-behavioral therapy, then considers some of the social and cultural factors that influenced its development and continue to influence our practices.

PRINCIPLES OF COGNITIVE-BEHAVIORAL THERAPY

Therapists often wonder what the relationships are among such various approaches including "cognitive-behavioral therapy," "cognitive therapy," "problem-solving therapy," "rational-emotive (behavior) therapy," "interpersonal cognitive therapy," "schema therapy," and the variety of other titles that have become associated with this broad approach to treatment. By way of a brief overview, and consistent with Dobson and Dozois (2001), we see the following three basic propositions, or principles, that cut across all the treatments in the cognitive-behavioral therapy movement:

1. *The access hypothesis*, which states that the content and process of our thinking is knowable. Thoughts are not "unconscious" or "preconscious," or somehow unavailable to awareness. Rather, cognitive-behavioral approaches endorse the idea that, with appropriate training and attention, people can become aware of their own thinking.

2. *The mediation hypothesis*, which states that our thoughts mediate our emotional responses to the various situations in which we find ourselves. The cognitive-behavioral model does not endorse the idea that people simply have an emotional response to an event or situation, but rather, the way that we construe or think about the event is pivotal to the way we feel. Similarly, it is our cognitions or thoughts that strongly influence our behavioral patterns in various life situations. For example, we feel anxious only when we view a situation as threatening. When we have a "threat cognition," we also are likely be motivated to escape the situation or to avoid it in the future, if possible. These thoughts, as well as the corresponding emotional responses and behavioral reactions, may all become routine and automatic over time. Cognitive-behavioral theorists argue that there is cognitive mediation between the event and the person's typical responses in that situation.

3. *The change hypothesis*, which is a corollary of the two previous ideas, states that because cognitions are knowable and mediate the responses to different situations, we can intentionally modify the way we respond to events around us. We can become more functional and more

adaptive by understanding our emotional and behavioral reactions, as well as using cognitive strategies systematically.

In addition to these principles, the cognitive-behavioral movement also endorses a general philosophical perspective termed the *realist assumption* (Dobson & Dozois, 2001; Held, 1995). Although there are variations on this theme within the cognitive-behavioral therapy movement, the general idea of the realist assumption is that a "real-world" or an objective reality exists independently of our awareness of it. As such, people can come to know the world more accurately and operate within its principles. Generally speaking, we argue that a more accurate appraisal of the world, and a closer adaptation to its demands, is one of the indicators of good mental health. Conversely, an individual may misperceive the situation around him or her, causing the person to act out of concert with his or her social environment. As a result, the individual is likely to experience negative emotional and interpersonal consequences. Although no one can know his or her world perfectly, and to some extent we are all "out of step" with our environment, an individual who distorts the world around him- or herself, or fails to see situations for what they are, is likely to have more problems than someone who is more realistic.

The cognitive-behavioral model considers the *usefulness* of different thoughts, in addition to the *accuracy* of situation-specific thoughts. We recognize that patterns of thinking, including general ideas, assumptions, and schemas, are derived over time from our experiences with the social environment. These assumptions and schemas also affect how we view the world. Furthermore, because they potentially limit the types of situations into which we put ourselves, or the possible range of activities in which we can imagine ourselves engaged, they predispose us to certain ways of thinking that may become self-fulfilling. Thus, once schemas become established, they not only affect our memories of the experiences we have had but also dictate our future development and range of activity. In this sense, people "create," as well as react to their own reality.

CURRENT CONTEXT: WHERE ARE WE NOW?

The development of evidence-based medicine and, in particular, evidence-based psychotherapy has been helpful to cognitive-behavioral therapy. In the 1990s, there was a movement toward the identification of empirically supported treatments (Chambless & Ollendick, 2001). Mental health disciplines within North America have also endorsed the need for training and practice in empirically supported therapies. For example, the psychiatric residency standards of the American Psychiatric Association, as well as the accreditation standards for the training of clinical and counseling psychologists of the American and Canadian Psychological Associations, require that trainees at least be exposed to empirically supported treatments.

Cognitive-behavioral therapy has been used in the treatment of a wide variety of disorders and problems. It has been broadly disseminated through treatment manuals and books to members of the mental health community, and increasing knowledge about this approach is disseminated to the public through the media and websites (e.g., *www.academyofct. org*). The public is increasingly requesting cognitive-behavioral therapy as a broad approach to treatment. As clinicians who value research, we must be cautious to ensure that the popularity of cognitive-behavioral therapy does not surpass the evidence for its efficacy (see Chapter 11, this volume). It is certainly more in demand in Western society than a number of the available provider services. Indeed, there is an acute shortage of qualified cognitive-behavioral therapists in many countries relative to demand and the therapy's potential value to society.

To take the example of depression, we know that at any given point in time approximately 3% of the population is experiencing a major depressive episode (Kessler, 2002). The population of the United States is approximately 300 million people, so this translates into approximately 9 million cases of clinical depression today. Clinical trials of cognitive-behavioral therapy for depression often use a 20-session treatment protocol. If all of these cases of depression were treated adequately (and solely) with cognitive-behavioral therapy, approximately 180 million treatment sessions would be required! And this is for depression alone; the point prevalence of all treatable mental disorders is obviously a much larger number. Any cursory review of the number of available providers and programs makes it clear that this quantity of cognitive-behavioral therapy sessions is simply not available. Some health care systems, such as the National Health Service in the United Kingdom, have been recommending a "stepped approach" whereby minimal interventions are used for mild problems. These interventions can include bibliotherapy, psychoeducation, and cognitive-behavioral self-help groups. One of the purposes of these new approaches is to extend available resources. Most clinicians in busy practices are looking for treatment "extenders," such as self-help groups or community programs.

Given the dramatic imbalance between demand and supply of cognitive-behavioral services, what is happening? The demand for evidence-based therapy has prompted training programs to incorporate more of these treatments into their curricula. It is likely that more service providers will be available to deliver evidence-based practice over the long term. In the shorter term, we also note the development of a large market for postdegree continuous learning certificate programs, continuing education activities, the publication of treatment manuals, and other diverse forms of education. Many practitioners are taking advantage of these activities. Another positive development has been the growth of services devoted to or that at least include cognitive-behavioral therapy. Cognitive-behavioral therapy clinics now exist in a variety of settings, ranging from private practice to outpatient clinics, tertiary and specialty care clinics, and community-based programs. Health maintenance organizations (HMOs) in the United States particularly have moved toward the inclusion of cognitive-behavioral therapy programs within their range of offered services. This emphasis on cognitive-behavioral therapy in HMOs is no doubt partly predicated on shorter-term treatments and consequent lower costs relative to alternative treatments. It is also a result of the increased success of these approaches relative to other, typically longer-term approaches. Reduced time to recovery reflects improved overall functioning on the part of the client, and reduced costs translate into lower overall health care costs.

Notwithstanding the previously mentioned positive features of the emphasis on cognitive-behavioral therapy, there also are some difficulties and challenges. Many practitioners are interested in obtaining more training and supervision. When can a clinician state that he or she has expertise in cognitive-behavioral therapy? In the absence of a "gold standard" to train therapists in this approach, it is likely that a great deal of variability in the quality of cognitive-behavioral therapy exists, and what is being described as "cognitive-behavioral therapy" has different meaning in different settings.

For example, it is common for clinicians to use cognitive-behavioral techniques in the context of another type of treatment, or to use a hybrid approach. Practitioners may add cognitive-behavioral therapy to other approaches and use techniques in an "eclectic" practice, but without an overall cognitive-behavioral case formulation. Another common misconception is that because cognitive-behavioral therapy is "technique" driven, it is relatively easy to learn and apply in practice. As we argue later in this book, our general position is that if there is an evidence-based, manualized treatment for a particular problem, and a client with that same problem, then the clinician should adhere closely to the manual and forgo his or her clinical judgment, unless there is strong reason to do otherwise.

Another downside of the public demand for cognitive-behavioral therapy is that clinicians are tempted to use it to treat problems for which there is little or no evidence of its success. This temptation is natural, because clinicians generally try to mitigate the distress of their clients, and other effective treatments may not exist. Unfortunately, if a treatment fails in an area in which it has not been developed or validated, the outcome might be taken as evidence that the treatment model is at fault. The overzealous application of the principles of cognitive-behavioral therapy in problem areas in which it is less likely to work represents a challenge, because the reputation of the approach will suffer in the long run.

It is important to recall that the evidence base for many of the cognitive-behavioral therapies was first gathered in research clinics. Such clinics provide an excellent first test of the clinical efficacy of treatments, but they often employ strict inclusion and exclusion criteria for participants, and closely supervise therapists and the extra services located within them. In contrast, clients with multiple problems often present to a clinical practice, where it may not be possible to screen for inclusion and exclusion criteria. These clients are generally more difficult to treat than clients seen in research clinics. Given these differences in clientele, it should not be surprising to learn that outcomes in clinical settings are often not as strong as those in the first research trials. Thus, although cognitive-behavioral therapy may well have strong clinical utility, the context of the mental health clinic may delimit those benefits in comparison to the trials that led to the development and dissemination of the treatments in the first place.

These points bring us back to one of our reasons for writing this book: to provide an overview of effective treatments, and to help you understand ways to approach and treat mental health problems using the principles of cognitive-behavioral treatments in practical but evidence-based ways.

SOCIAL AND CULTURAL FACTORS IN COGNITIVE-BEHAVIORAL THERAPY

The development of any psychological treatment does not take place in a vacuum but is inextricably linked to societal beliefs and practices at the time of its inception. Cognitive-behavioral therapy has developed within the context of a number of different societal and cultural trends. As cognitive-behavioral therapists, it is important to understand the context of what we do, because this knowledge provides a backdrop to our practices. This understanding places our approach to clients' problems within the social and cultural context within which we all live. Considering these factors will lead to an appreciation of the limits to cognitive-behavioral therapy and knowledge about when to vary the standard practices to meet the needs of particular clients. Just as psychodynamic therapy grew out of late-19th- and early-20th-century values, and the intellectual climate at that time, cognitive-behavioral therapy has grown from the more recent culture within North America, Europe, South Africa, and other parts of the world.

We live in a society that places an emphasis on individualism, that values independence, personal choice, and the ability to determine and to have control over the future. Many individuals within Western society believe that they can control many, if not most, aspects of their lives. This perception of personal control, theoretically, can lead people to take more responsibility for their physical and mental health. Conversely, with this sense that they *should* have control, individuals who feel helpless and who lack choices can experience negative affect and anxiety in such a society.

Distressed people are likely to become more easily isolated in a society that places more emphasis on individualism. Family, work, and community social groups may take less responsibility in looking after these individuals' needs. Consequently, people may be more likely to feel isolated, with a lack of a sense of community. Rather than look to social supports for help to fulfill these needs, people may seek therapy, especially if it might help them learn needed skills to meet their own emotional and social needs. The originators and practitioners of cognitive-behavioral therapy also value setting goals, making choices, and taking action and control where realistic. These aspects of cognitive-behavioral therapy make it an ideal approach for the type of society within which it developed.

We also live in a world with burgeoning, easily accessed information that has led to a veritable explosion of available information to the average person. One of the by-products of the enormous change in availability of information has been a certain "demystification" of psychotherapy. Technologically savvy clients can scan international journals and university libraries around the world for current and well-reputed evidence about treatments. Clients frequently have information about self-diagnosed problems and request specific types of help. It is not uncommon for clients to have done preliminary research and reading, and to come to an outpatient mental health service requesting cognitive-behavioral therapy by name.

With an increase in accessibility of information, there may be a greater openness toward people with mental health problems. Along with greater openness comes decreased stigma regarding mental health problems. Many organizations, such as the National Alliance for Mental Illness and the Canadian Mental Health Association, have had public awareness campaigns. Mental health literacy surveys have been completed, and the results have been surprising. For example, in Alberta, Canada, approximately 85% of people randomly surveyed by telephone in 2006 were able to identify accurately a depressed person in a standardized scenario (Wang, 2007). Although stigma still exists, the same survey Australia showed a 10% increase in awareness over a decade (Wang, 2007).

In addition to increased public awareness, it is becoming more socially acceptable to seek treatment for mental health problems. Psychotherapy satisfaction surveys have been completed in popular and widely read magazines, such as *Consumer Reports*. It has become more acceptable for the average person to seek out psychotherapy services, and many more public figures have come forward to talk openly about their mental disorders. Examples of these courageous individuals include Margaret Trudeau, Jane Pauley, and J. K. Rowling. When inspired by public figures to seek treatment, people commonly request practical and effective therapies, such as cognitive-behavioral treatments.

People often receive the message that they are "consumers" of health care, and that they need to purchase a good "product." Popular magazine articles instruct the reader on questions to ask of their health care providers. Therapists receive demands from potential and actual clients with specific service requests, including cognitive-behavioral therapy. Consumers of mental health services have also become strong lobbyists for themselves and their families. The advocacy groups that have developed help to hold the health care "industry" accountable for its practices. In general, the consumer movement has been helpful to empirically supported and short-term treatments. Consumerism also supports treatments that take an active collaborative and egalitarian stance with clients. Transparency in therapy is also likely to be desirable to consumers, with the goals, rationale, and methods of the approach clearly described. These activities are typical of cognitive-behavioral therapy.

Related to consumerism is the issue of cost containment in health care. Health care costs in most developed countries have escalated dramatically within the past few decades for a number of reasons, including advances in technology and an aging population. Cost containment provides a justification for the use of short-term, practical treatments. Because of the combination of increased requests for mental health services and increased openness, as discussed earlier, combined with the limited availability of treatments, there have been pressures for short-term treatments, "caps" on services, or limits on the access to services. Health authorities, hospital governing boards, HMOs, and insurance companies regularly monitor economically related parameters such as hospital length of stay, numbers of treatment sessions, client satisfaction, and health care outcomes. Most health care systems must be accountable to the *bottom line*, which is the cost of providing services in comparison to the outcomes of those same services. All of these factors make cognitive-behavioral therapy desirable, because it is relatively inexpensive to provide, it demonstrates measurable and observable positive outcomes, and it tends to lead to lower relapse rates.

The emphasis on economic factors has influenced research and development, as well as direct service delivery. In broad terms, research dollars flow from either public or private interests. Increasingly, public availability of research and development funds has been limited, and increasingly the focus of these sources of funding is on the solution of public problems, social issues, or perceived health care system needs. With a relative decrease in public funds for research, lobby groups, foundations, and private research agencies have increased their influence in the research enterprise. In general, the research and development funding groups' focus on short-term, evidence-based interventions has been conducive to further research and the development of cognitive-behavioral theories and therapies.

The final general factor that has spurred the development of cognitive-behavioral therapy is our faster paced society, with the attendant perception of limited time and an emphasis on efficiency and effectiveness. This time pressure has led to a focus on practical and short-term solutions to problems. A number of interrelated factors have led to a preference for short-term and practical solutions to problems. Many people report increased stress in their lives and feel pressed for time. Most families in North America have two income earners, leading to a "time crunch" relative to self-care and other types of personal activities. There is an increased demand for quick, commonsensical, and practical advice that is accessible and helpful. These attributes may be found in cognitive-behavioral therapy.

IN SUMMARY

Each of the previously mentioned factors has contributed in its own way to the growth and development of short-term, evidence-based, outcome-focused psychotherapies. The evidence base for cognitive-behavioral therapy has risen dramatically over the past 20 years, and increasing numbers of people are aware of the research findings. Agencies that fund these therapies, such as public health care systems, private insurance companies, HMOs, and foundations, are increasingly aware of, and committed to, positive and measurable treatment outcomes. If two therapy outcomes are equivalent, but one is quicker and less costly, most people are likely to choose the more rapid and cheaper option.

Why should the average clinician care about these factors? It is important to understand these contextual factors and help to alleviate system pressures. The knowledge base regarding cognitive-behavioral therapies far outstrips their availability as a health service. The challenge for the next generation of researchers, mental health planners, and clinicians will be to learn how to disseminate effective mental health treatments to the largest number of people possible. One conclusion from this discussion is that cognitive-behavioral therapy has become a very suitable type of psychological treatment for this time in our history. Cognitive-behavioral therapy can be viewed as a "therapy whose time is now."

The following chapters not only provide practical suggestions for applications within your practice but also review specific research findings for the common elements of cognitive-behavioral therapy. We hope to provide practical guidelines for assessment and case formulation, as well as the major behavioral, cognitive, and schema-focused interventions. Ending treatment can be difficult for many practitioners, and we provide a discussion of this step, including relapse prevention. Many challenges can and do occur in practice, and we cover some of these and provide suggestions for ways to manage them.

It is crucial as we increase our practice of cognitive-behavioral therapy that we continue to question its components. We also need to be open to other effective approaches as they become available. Just because a cognitive-behavioral treatment has been shown in clinical research trials to be effective compared to a waiting-list control group or a medication treatment does not necessarily mean that the same treatment will be effective in your practice. As therapists, we must retain not only our humanity (McWilliams, 2005) but also our humility and curiosity regarding the various elements of cognitive-behavioral therapy.

Chapter 2

ဢ

Assessment for Cognitive-Behavioral Therapy

In this chapter, we review the assessment processes in cognitive-behavioral therapy, with the intent of providing practical tools for your practice. Where they exist, we also present the empirical base for making clinical decisions, consistent with the overall goal of this text of bridging the gap between science and practice. Although many texts have reviewed psychological and psychiatric assessments in detail, few have reviewed the practical aspects of this process. Even fewer have differentiated the useful tools for a cognitive-behavioral clinician.

There are many volumes related to psychological assessment (e.g., Groth-Marnat, 2003; Antony & Barlow, 2002) and diagnostic interviewing (e.g., Othmer & Othmer, 1994). These texts are excellent sources for the conceptual issues involved in assessment and provide resources for the range of assessment measures that exist, as well as their psychometric properties. Given the existence of these resources, we do not provide general information regarding diagnostic or psychological assessment. Most clinicians are well versed in DSM-IV (American Psychiatric Association, 2000), and the basic principles and practices for conducting psychological assessment, such as the administration and interpretation of psychological tests. Good case conceptualization and treatment planning rest on a foundation of valid and appropriate assessment, so if you are interested in further training in these areas, we recommend the previously mentioned references as a starting point.

Psychological assessment can serve a number of purposes, including intellectual or cognitive assessment, assessment of learning disabilities or personality functioning, and the diagnosis of psychological disorders. The assessment tools and practices discussed in this chapter are intended for assessment in cognitive-behavioral therapy, not other types of psychological assessment. The goals of assessment for cognitive-behavioral treatment include gathering information about the diagnoses and problems that the client may be bringing into therapy, determining the strengths and weaknesses of the client related to treatment planning, beginning to orient the client to the model, and engaging the client in the early steps of treatment. The initial interviews also help you begin to develop interpersonal rapport with the client, to develop the problem list jointly, and to begin the cognitive-behavioral case formulation. This chapter reviews assessment practices, and provides tips and tools for assessment in a cognitive-behavioral clinical practice. Prior to discussion regarding assessment itself, we turn briefly to a review of the evidence base for empirically based assessment, particularly within cognitive-behavioral therapy.

KNOW YOUR EVIDENCE BASE:
EMPIRICALLY BASED ASSESSMENT

Empirically based assessment has lagged behind the field's emphasis on empirically based treatments and relationships despite the fact that all therapy treatments and relationships begin with assessment (Hunsley, Crabb, & Mash, 2004). It is also surprising that this lag has occurred given the long history of psychometric research in assessment. Empirically based assessment, however, includes not only the reliability and validity of the interview, self-report, and other types of measures used in an assessment but also diagnostic and treatment utility of these measures, improvements in decision making for clinicians, and practical considerations, such as cost and ease of administration (Hunsley & Mash, 2005). Meyer et al. (2001) and Hunsley (2002) have differentiated psychological testing from psychological assessment. *Psychological assessment* is a broader concept than testing, and typically relies upon multiple sources of information, integration of that information, and the use of clinical judgment and decision making. Thus, whereas psychological testing is generally done in support of assessment and is typically an essential component of it, it is only one part of an empirically based assessment.

The Psychological Assessment Work Group (PAWG) was commissioned by the Board of Professional Affairs of the American Psychological Association in 1996. Their report (Meyer et al., 2001) concluded that (1) psychological test validity is strong and compelling; (2) psychological test validity is comparable to medical test validity; (3) distinct assessment methods provide unique sources of information; and (4) clinicians who rely exclusively on interviews are prone to inadequate or incomplete assessment understanding.

One notable finding of the Meyer et al. (2001) report was that the predictive validity coefficients for various psychological tests are comparable to and sometimes surpass those for medical tests. For example, the use of routine ultrasound examinations was unrelated to a successful pregnancy outcome ($r = .01$), as was the relationship between the Beck Hopelessness Scale and subsequent suicide ($r = .08$). In contrast, expressed emotion was moderately and significantly related to subsequent relapse for individuals with schizophrenia and mood disorders ($r = .32$). Consequently, psychological tests can enhance our ability to make predictions.

Unfortunately, the Meyer et al. (2001) report did not examine any scales that might predict outcomes for cognitive-behavioral interventions; nor was there any specific measure of cognitive distortions or any other factor unique to cognitive-behavioral therapy. One reason that cognitive-behavioral measures and their relationship to outcomes are not included is the historic divide between the practices of assessment and treatment. A single measure may have good psychometric properties, but empirically based assessments are intended to consider the scientific validity of the assessment process itself, not just the properties of a single measure. Instruments are only parts of the overall assessment process, and the process itself needs to be empirically supported.

Hunsley and Mash (2005) include both diagnostic and treatment utility in their definition of empirically based assessment. *Diagnostic utility* is defined as the degree to which assessment data help to formulate a diagnosis. *Treatment utility* was defined by Hayes, Nelson, and Jarrett (1987) as the degree to which assessment contributes to beneficial treatment outcome. Essentially, Hayes et al. asked whether assessment contributes to a successful treatment outcome. Nelson-Gray (2003) also raised the issue of treatment utility of psychological assessment. She described standardized diagnostic interviews and noted that although the incremental validity of these tools could be examined in terms of outcomes, such research has generally not take place. Thus, although most clinicians establish a diagnosis for their clients, Nelson-Gray argues, this process is primarily useful in choosing a treatment rather than in predicting outcome of the treatment. There has been little research on diagnostic utility. Research in this area would involve assessing outcomes for clients by using the same treatment in which diagnosis was determined using a standardized diagnostic interview as opposed to an unstandardized interview or other tools, such as a functional analysis.

In contrast to diagnostic assessment, functional analysis has been the traditional strategy linking behavioral assessment and treatment. In a traditional behavioral functional analysis, environmental variables that are hypothesized to control the target or problem behavior are identified in the assessment, then targeted for change in the treatment. Several studies have demonstrated the treatment utility of the functional analysis, particularly with more severe problems (e.g., Carr & Durand, 1985).

In summary, it is clear that the movement toward evidence-based or empirically supported assessment is in its infancy. Achenbach (2005) described the promotion of evidence-based treatments without attention to evidence-based assessment as being similar to building a magnificent house without constructing the foundation. It is important to remain aware of the initiative toward evidence-based assessment, particularly once assessment guidelines and recommended processes have been developed. In the future, we may have greater ability to link assessment results to treatment outcomes within cognitive-behavioral practice.

TOOLS FOR COGNITIVE-BEHAVIORAL ASSESSMENT

A large numbers of specific tests, tools, and measures have been developed for psychological assessment. It can be difficult to keep up with the literature in choosing the most useful and empirically supported tools and methods for our practices. Many popular measures do not have good psychometric properties (Hunsley et al., 2004), and most are not specific to cognitive-behavioral practice. For example, a psychological test that assesses personality traits is not likely to be useful when traits are not the focus of intervention. A measure of general symptoms, such as the Symptom Checklist-90—Revised (SCL-90-R; Derogatis, 1994), can identify distress and specific symptoms in a number of areas but may not add useful information to a cognitive-behavioral assessment, over and above a simple problem list from the client.

It is good practice to use multiple methods and measures to maximize validity in all assessments. It is also important that these multiple methods have good psychometric properties and add sufficient new information to the assessment to be useful. Simply adding more measures does not necessarily improve validity. A diagnostic interview is often the starting point for cognitive-behavioral assessment, but successful treatment planning likely hinges upon a more comprehensive assessment of cognitive and behavioral variables. There are several compendia of empirically supported measures for different problems, such as anxiety (Antony, Orsillo, & Roemer, 2001) and depression (Nezu, Ronan, Meadows, & McClure, 2000). The measures included in these texts have sound psychometric properties, are easily available for clinical use, and are intended for use in cognitive-behavioral therapy. Most were developed in research settings, however, so the treatment utility or the applicability to different settings or populations has not necessarily been established. In the sections that follow, we review some of the more commonly employed, psychometrically sound assessment methods used in cognitive-behavioral therapy.

The Interview

Assessments begin with an interview. Of the many types of assessment interviews, numerous structured and semistructured interviews have been developed. Some of these are commercially available to qualified professionals. Most structured interviews are intended to help the interviewer determine the *diagnosis* with which the client is presenting rather than the *problems* he or she may want to focus on in therapy. Examples of diagnostic interviews include the Structured Clinical Interview for DSM-IV Axis I Disorders (SCID; First, Spitzer, Gibbon, & Williams, 1997), the Schedule for Affective Disorders and Schizophrenia (SADS; Endicott & Spitzer, 1978), the Primary Care Evaluation of Mental Disorders (PRIME-MD; Spitzer et al., 1994), the Diagnostic Interview Schedule (DIS; Robins, Cottler, Bucholz, & Compton, 1995), and the Anxiety Disorders Interview Schedule for DSM-IV (ADIS-IV; Brown, DiNardo, & Barlow, 1994).

These diagnostic instruments range from semistructured to highly structured interviews. With the exception of the PRIME-MD, which takes only 10–20 minutes to administer, they take from 45 to 120 minutes to administer. The PRIME-MD was developed as a screening tool for primary care physicians' use for clients with suspected, but not yet identified, psychiatric problems. As such, it is a good first screen for diagnostic purposes, but it falls far short of the others in comprehensiveness and thoroughness. Of all of these interviews, the ADIS-IV may best identify situations and reactions that are useful for cognitive-behavioral therapy, particularly if the major problem appears to be an anxiety or mood disorder. For example, it lists potential feared situations for the various anxiety disorders and can help you begin to conceptualize the problem rather than simply develop a diagnosis.

If diagnostic screening is important in your practice, consider the Mini-International Neuropsychiatric Interview (MINI), version 5.0 (Sheehan et al., 1998). This tool is a clinician-administered, structured diagnostic interview with reasonably good breadth of coverage, despite being shorter than many other structured interviews (approximately 15 minutes). The MINI is also available in over 30 languages and can be downloaded at *www.medical-outcomes.com*. It is available at no cost to qualified professionals.

Structured and semistructured interviews require extensive training and may not be practical or useful in all clinical settings. In addition to focusing on a diagnosis, most were developed for research, and have been used primarily in research settings. Diagnostic interviews focus on symptoms and their development, and tend to be reliable and valid methods to ensure that presenting symptoms meet DSM-IV criteria for certain diagnoses. Although these interviews are very useful for diagnostic purposes, they are less helpful for ascertaining useful information for the initial stages of cognitive-behavioral therapy, because that is not their purpose. They do not help in identifying thought patterns, nor in conducting a functional analysis of behavior. If provision of a formal diagnosis is important for your practice, consider how to incorporate diagnostic questions within the overall assessment (see Figure 2.1). In addition to determination of diagnoses, other information is necessary to assess the appropriateness of cognitive-behavioral therapy and begin to conceptualize a client's problems.

As suggested earlier, cognitive-behavioral therapy requires considerable information in addition to a diagnostic assessment. Unfortunately, no standardized format or structured interview is available for cognitive-behavioral assessment. This information, however, is necessary to understand the client's problems from a cognitive-behavioral conceptualization. Obtaining this information typically begins in the first interview, although assessment continues throughout the case and may be supplemented at any time. From our perspective, a comprehensive assessment to begin cognitive-behavioral therapy includes the following information:

• The *problem*(s) that bring the client into therapy at this point in time. The major problem named by most clients is usually related to the diagnosis, but creating a Problem List is not the same as simply listing the symptoms related to the client's diagnosis (if he or she has one). For example, a male client with major depression may be unemployed. His problems may include depressed mood, low energy, sleep disturbance, and loss of motivation that interferes with a job search. However, his Problem List may include both financial concerns and family conflict, which are not symptoms of depression per se.

• The *triggers* (antecedents) and *consequences* of the problem(s). This process usually requires careful questioning on the part of the interviewer to determine the hypothesized antecedents that control or trigger problem behaviors and emotions. It is helpful to be as specific as possible in the questioning—for example, "What situations lead you to feel _____?," "Please describe each situation in detail," "Describe your mood over the course of a typical day," "Describe exactly what happened and how your mood was yesterday," "Who do you feel the worst/best around?," "What occurred after your mood dropped?," "How did you

FIGURE 2.1. Sample initial interview for cognitive-behavioral therapy.

Name: _____ Date: _____

Discuss consent for assessment, confidentiality, and limits to confidentiality; purpose of assessment; reporting system; and any training purposes for the assessment and observation. Obtain consent. Mention that you will be taking notes during the interview.

General information

1. Age and date of birth.
2. Marital status (if single, recent relationships). Any children? Names and ages, if appropriate.
3. Current living situation. With whom do you live? What is the accommodation?
4. How are you currently supporting yourself?
5. Brief employment history.
6. What is your education level/last grade completed and when?
7. Reason for referral and description of current problem(s).
   - Situations when the problem occurs (obtain detailed list).
   - Situations that are avoided because of the problem.
   - Rating of current functioning (from 1 = best ever to 10 = worst ever).
   - Impact of the problem upon current functioning (0–100% affected).
   - Which area(s) of your life are most affected (e.g., school, work, friendships, family)? Least affected?
   - What is the most difficult thing for you to do because of the problem(s)?
   - What are your typical reactions when you are experiencing this problem(s)?
   - Physical reactions (include panic attacks).
   - Emotional reactions.
   - What are your thoughts before, during, and after the situation? (Primer questions include "What do you imagine happening if … ?" It is helpful to have specific examples or images to identify thoughts.)
   - What do you typically do when this happens?
   - Have you noticed any patterns to these reactions (e.g., times when things get better or worse; times of day, days of the week, seasons)?
   - What other factors affect how you feel in these situations (e.g., other people, environmental factors, duration of situation, your own or others' expectations)?
   - What have you found that helps to reduce the problem(s) (e.g., can be divided into negative and positive coping, use of medications, strategies learned in previous therapy, self-help methods)?
   - Are there ways that you try to protect yourself when you are experiencing these problem(s)? Are there small things that you do to help yourself "get through" situations (e.g., making preparations, taking medications, relying on other people, avoiding certain aspects of the situation)?
   - Can you think of any skills that you might develop that would decrease the problem(s) (e.g., social skills, conflict resolution, job skills)?
8. Aside from the problem(s) we have just discussed, are there other current stressors in your life right now? What are they?
9. How would you describe your current mood? Rating is from 1 to 10 (worst)
   - If you feel low or depressed, how long have your been feeling this way?
   - Have you lost interest in things that you previously enjoyed?
   - How do you feel about the future?

(continued)

FIGURE 2.1. (*continued*)

- How have you been sleeping recently? How is your appetite?
- Have you ever thought about harming yourself (differentiate suicidal behavior from self-harm behavior)?
- If yes, assess when, the frequency, the method, history of attempts, and family suicide history.
- What holds you back from hurting yourself?
- Have you had treatments for depression? If yes, when? How effective were they?

10. Do you have any other current psychological concerns?
11. Current physical health—any concerns? Current medications (type and dose)?
12. Current drug and alcohol use, including caffeine. Have you had any past problems with substance abuse? Any treatment history for substance use?
13. Are you currently involved in any community programs or volunteer work?
14. What do you like to do in your free time?
15. History of current problems—When did your problems begin? Can you remember a specific incident that you believe caused the problem?
    - What were you like as a child and adolescent? Do you remember any developmental problems? What were your school and family experiences like growing up?
    - Did you have any family problems growing up? Do you have any history of abuse?
    - Have you ever sought help for any psychological or psychiatric problems in the past?
    - Is there anyone in your family with a history of anxiety disorders, depression, substance abuse, and so forth? Is there anyone in your family that you consider to have problems similar to your own? Is there any family psychiatric history?
16. Who is in your family of origin? Provide the first names of your parents and siblings; provide their current ages and where they live.
17. Who are you closest and least close to in your family? Who would you approach for support? Who would you approach in the event of a crisis or emergency?
18. Have I missed anything?
19. Use three or four adjectives to describe yourself as a person (including strengths and weaknesses). (If client is unable to describe him- or herself, ask how someone who knows the client very well would describe him or her.)
20. What are some of your hopes and goals for being here? What are one or two things you would like to change about the problem(s) we have discussed?
21. Do you have any questions? (Explain to the client what will happen next.)

respond to that change in your mood?," "What happened next?" These questions help to describe the topography of the problem, as well as help the interviewer begin to understand the triggers and consequences in the client's daily life. The goal of these questions is to develop a map of the functional relationship between the client and the many events that are happening in his or her life.

- The client's *reactions* when experiencing the symptoms. It is useful to distinguish among these reactions the *affect* (feelings or emotions and physiological reactions), *cognitions* (thoughts, ideas, images), and *behaviors* (actions or action tendencies). On the one hand, most clients can differentiate among feelings, thoughts, and actions, and these distinctions start to orient them to a cognitive-behavioral model of therapy. On the other hand, in these three areas of assessment, whereas it is relatively easy for clients to notice their feelings and what they are doing (or not doing), it can be more difficult for them to "catch" their thoughts. In such cases, it is helpful to ask clients to identify a specific, recent, difficult situation to help them to slow the process down, and to attend to their various reactions in all three areas. It is also possible to construct hypothetical situations in the assessment interview to see whether clients can use imagery and to suggest what their likely reactions would be. Some clients initially struggle to differentiate thoughts from feelings. Some clients who lack a sufficient vocabulary for emotional terms benefit from instruction on how to talk about feelings or lists feeling words they can use to distinguish between thoughts and feelings. By helping clients understand these differences in the initial interviews, the therapist orients clients to the model used in therapy.

• Current *coping and approach–avoidance patterns*. Coping can be positive, such as approaching a problem situation or talking to someone about a problem, or negative, such as avoiding certain situations or using substances (e.g., alcohol or drugs) to cope. The assessment of approach–avoidance patterns involves understanding the ways clients "manage" their symptoms and problems. For example, an anxious client might avoid anxiety by staying away from situations in which he or she previously experienced anxiety. Examples of avoidance include being overly passive or conflict avoidant when anxious, withdrawing from people when depressed, or avoiding challenging situations when one's self-efficacy is low. Avoidance can also take the form of safety behaviors (e.g., doing things to keep oneself "safe"), avoidance of negative emotions, protecting oneself from arousal (e.g., avoidance of exertion or excitement), minimizing stimulation, or compulsively checking circumstances about which one is fearful. These patterns tend to be both unique to the client and to his or her patterns of avoidance. Assessment of these patterns requires sensitivity, awareness, and careful questioning on the part of the clinician.

• *Skills deficits, lack of knowledge*, or other issues that may be associated with the problem. Not all clients exhibit skills deficits or lack knowledge. Also, even if it appears that the client lacks skills, it is important to distinguish these apparent deficits from the distress expressed by the client. For example, a depressed and avoidant client may appear to lack social skills, but his or her low mood and anxious avoidance may be masking adequate skills. It is instructive to note that some apparent deficits may not be psychological in nature. For example, one of us

(D. D.) treated a client with a height phobia, but whose job included building bridges across large expanses of water. He was experiencing numerous symptoms of anxiety, coupled with vertigo. A visual assessment, however, revealed that the client completely lacked depth perception, and that his phobia likely developed in response to his visual problem. Under the circumstances, he would not have been safe working on the bridge. Rather than overcome his phobia, he needed to talk to his employer about minimizing risk on the job. Finally, some clients do have skills deficits or lack knowledge. In our experience, many of these clients come from socially, emotionally, or intellectually impoverished family backgrounds. For example, a client with low self-esteem and a history of abuse may lack information about social relationships, or what is "normal" and "abnormal" behavior in families. In such cases, it may be necessary to include in the treatment plan an educational and skills practice focus to ensure successful problem resolution. After all, a client with a driving phobia needs to have driving skills to be a safe driver, regardless of whether he or she is fearful.

• Current *social support, family concerns, or interpersonal or sexual problems*. It is well recognized that whereas the provision of adequate social support can mitigate problems, the presence of family, interpersonal, or sexual problems can exacerbate them. Our orientation toward this area of assessment is to deal with it as we deal with any other area, and to openly ask about these areas of functioning. Questions that we would ask in this area include "Who would you turn to if you had a serious problem?," "Who are you closest to in your family?," "How often do you spend time with _____?" "How often do you talk to _____?," "Is there anyone you often get into arguments with?," or "Do you have any worries about sex?"

• *Other current problems*. Regardless of the presenting problem, it is always a good idea to ask about certain common problems. Although it is fairly uncommon to have these problems and not mention them, sometimes clients do not connect their presenting problems with these other issues going on in their lives. Possible factors to assess include common psychological problems, such as anxiety, depression, hopelessness, and suicide risk. If the person is in any kind of joint living arrangement, psychological, sexual, and domestic abuse should be considered. Medical conditions should be reviewed, especially those that are chronic or persistent. Alcohol and drug use (including prescription drugs and nonprescription psychoactive drugs) should also be assessed, with a view toward determining substance abuse or dependence. Finally, practical life issues, such as financial or legal concerns, should be considered.

• The *development and course of the problems*. Having established the broad spectrum of possible problems that the client is experiencing, it is worthwhile to try to establish the time lines associated with the problems. Our sense is that it is not usually worth the time to do a detailed time line for every problem, but to determine the onset and course of the major problems likely is worthwhile. We try to determine whether any discrete events appeared to trigger the symptoms. A helpful set of questions to ask regarding client knowledge is "What was happening in your life when these problems began?," "Do you make any connection between these events and your problems?," or "What is your idea about the development of this problem?" Clients' answers help guide you to determine whether they already have formed a theory, and how conducive the model is to cognitive-behavioral interventions. Because many clients have heard, for example, that their depressive symptoms are "caused by a biochemical imbalance," some reorientation work on your part may be required. On the other hand, if clients already have a rudimentary idea that their problems are the result of some personal vulnerability and life stressors, then you can use this knowledge to underscore how this way of thinking is very compatible with how you work in therapy.

• *History of treatment*, including past efforts to self-manage the problems, past treatments (both pharmacological and psychotherapeutic), knowledge about the problem, and response to treatment. Included in useful information are questions such as how often the client has received treatment, the type and likely adequacy of the treatment(s), and who the service providers were (or are; sometimes it is necessary to communicate with other therapists to coordinate treatment). It is very helpful to assess the client's efforts to deal with his or her problems. This latter information tells you about the client's model of the problem, his or her ability to problem-solve and implement solutions, determination and consistency in problem solution, and how he or she likely dealt with the lack of success of these strategies.

Figure 2.1 provides a sample structured interview, with a specific sequence and possible questions. This interview can easily be adapted for use in different practices or with different populations. Other questions can be added for specific purposes. The interview is not intended to replace a diagnostic assessment, but it may be sufficient for many cognitive-behavioral practices in which a very detailed and accurate diagnosis is not required or helpful. Table 2.1 provides a list of other questions to consider in developing a semistructured interview for your practice.

For your practice, it may be helpful to purchase one or two structured interviews, then adapt them to client problems with which you often deal. Although the reliability and validity of the interview is likely to suffer with such an adaptation, the result is generally a more comprehensive and clinically appropriate assessment than an unstructured

TABLE 2.1. Favorite Assessment Questions of Clinicians

Before starting the interview

- Do you have any concerns or questions about _____ observing the session (in addition to the consent form)?
- Do you have any concerns about a report being sent to _____ (in addition to usual consent form)?

When starting the interview

- What brings you here today? Why have you come now?
- Why are you seeking help at this particular time?
- What brings you in?
- What types of difficulties have you been experiencing?
- Are you experiencing any increased or unusual stress at this time?

For problem assessment

- Please describe the problems that bring you in today.
- It can be helpful to break problems down into thoughts, feelings, and behaviors. When you experience _____, what are you thinking? Feeling? Doing?
- How much control (on a scale of 1 to 10, with 10 being *total control* and 1 being *no control at all*) do you have over this problem?

For current functioning

- How have you been sleeping and eating recently? How many hours a night do you sleep? What have you eaten so far today? How about on a usual day?
- Please describe a typical day in detail, starting from when you get up in the morning?
- What is your source of income? Do you have any financial problems?
- Are you on any regular medication? What is it? Do you know the dose?
- Do you drink alcohol or take any drugs? Which ones and how much?

For risk assessment and instillation of hope

- On bad days, do you sometimes think that life is not worth living?
- What keeps you going on bad days? Are there people that you think of when you are having thoughts of harming yourself?
- Do you ever hurt yourself separately from thoughts of suicide? (Use examples.)

For assessing self-concept and self-esteem

- How would you describe yourself as a person?
- How would a person who knows you well (e.g., _____) describe you?
- How would you describe yourself to someone else (e.g., someone who has never met you before, a potential employer, a friend).

For assessing family history and social support

- Are you like anybody else in your family? Does anyone else in your family have the same or similar problems?
- Is there any family history of _____?
- How would you describe your partner? Your mother? Your father?
- Who are you closest to (in the world)? If you had an emergency, who would you call?
- How often do you talk to or see the people you are close to? (Get specifics.)
- What support system do you have in place at this time?

(continued)

TABLE 2.1. (*continued*)

For assessing habits, substance use, and abuse

- Do you use rewards when you are struggling with problems? Do they include
  _____ ? (drugs, activities, foods, alcohol, gambling, shopping)
- What purpose does this behavior serve for you?
- Have you noticed that using alcohol or other drugs helps you cope with this situation, or have they hindered your ability to cope?

For assessing past attempts at change and treatments

- What interventions/treatments have you had in the past?
- What was helpful and not helpful about each of them?
- What have you already tried to manage your problems? How did that work for you?
- Have you overcome problems in the past? How?

For ending the interview and instilling hope for change

- What would you be doing differently if you no longer had this problem in your life?
- Is there anything else we should talk about today that was not covered?
- Is there anything we have missed?
- What else do I need to know to understand you and your concerns?
- Tell me something important that you'd like me to know about yourself that we have not yet had a chance to talk about today?
- Do you have any questions for me?
- Is there anything else you would like to know about this process?
- What would you like to get out of these sessions?
- What are your hopes for this process?
- What are your hopes and goals for therapy?
- Do you have any specific goals for change?

Note. These questions were developed and modified from participant responses during two clinical assessment workshops sponsored by the Psychologists' Association of Alberta (November 2004 and January 2005).

interview. Typically, the result also is more practical and shorter than the more comprehensive version, making it easier to use and more client-friendly. We recommend the MINI for screening purposes. We would also recommend having copies of a semistructured cognitive-behavioral interview, such as that found in Figure 2.1, available as you conduct your intake interview. If you see many clients with similar problems, this interview can be adapted for your purposes, listing the typical situations with which your clients present. Many clinicians incorporate a diagnostic and a cognitive-behavioral assessment into the same interview. Whereas there are differences between the two, there is also considerable overlap.

Self-Report Measures

Although a large range of self-report tests exist, the most useful ones for cognitive behavioral practice can be divided into symptom measures, and cognitive and behavioral measures. Many of these tests were developed for research rather than for clinical purposes.

Many useful measures of symptom severity exist, and some are widely used in clinical practice. It can be difficult to sort through the most useful measures for your purposes, because so many different ones exist. Two very useful and comprehensive reviews assess empirically supported and accessible measures for adults with anxiety (Antony et al., 2001) and depressive disorders (Nezu et al., 2000). Antony and Barlow (2002) also review in detail assessment approaches for many different psychological problems. A complete list of psychological tests in all assessment areas, along with references for relevant research, may be found in *The Sixteenth Mental Measurements Yearbook* (Spies & Plake, 2005; *www.unl. edu/buros/bimm/index.html*).

Many measures in these texts are available for clinical use at no cost. Some measures, however, such as the Beck Anxiety Inventory (BAI; A. T. Beck & Steer, 1993) or the Beck Depression Inventory–II (BDI-II; A. T. Beck, Steer, & Brown, 1996), must be purchased through a psychological testing company. For further information on some of these tools, see *harcourtassessment.com*.

It is very useful to keep several different empirically supported measures on hand for problems that you typically see in your practice. The many general measures of anxiety include the BAI (A. T. Beck & Steer, 1993) and the State–Trait Anxiety Inventory (STAI; Spielberger, Gorsuch, Lushene, Vagg, & Jacobs, 1983), although these tend to be quite global. More specific anxiety symptom measures, such as the Yale–Brown Obsessive–Compulsive Scale (Y-BOCS; Goodman et al., 1989a, 1989b) or the Social Phobia Scale (Mattick & Clarke, 1998), can be considered if you work with specific forms of anxiety disorders. Useful scales for working with depression include the BDI-II (A. T. Beck et al., 1996) and the Beck Hopelessness Scale (BHS; A. T. Beck & Steer, 1988). All of these measures are suitable for repeated assessment, so they may be employed as an index of treatment success. Although some measures must be purchased through a commercial testing center, many scales are reprinted for clinical use in the Antony et al. (2001) and Nezu et al. (2000) texts.

Whereas the previously mentioned scales primarily measure symptoms and can be used to evaluate changes in symptoms over time, it is also helpful to employ behavioral and cognitive measures related to your work. For example, the Mobility Inventory for Agoraphobia (Chambless, Caputo, Gracely, Jasin, & Williams, 1985) is a quick and easy-to-use scale related to a client's ability to get out of the house and his or her range of mobility outside of the home. The Fear Questionnaire (Marks & Mathews, 1979) evaluates several different types of phobias and clients' potential avoidance of different situations or stimuli. The Cognitive-

Behavioral Avoidance Scale (Ottenbreit & Dobson, 2004) can be used to assess tendencies to avoid social and nonsocial situations. The Young Schema Questionnaire (YSQ; Young & Brown, 2001) is a comprehensive scale of potential maladaptive schemas that might underlie more symptomatic expressions of problems. All of these measures, with the possible exception of the YSQ, are suitable for repeat assessment; which of these might be applicable to your practice depends on your clients and the types of problems they present.

Observational Aids

The clinician is trained to observe the client, beginning with the initial telephone call or contact. Very useful data are obtained through careful observation of the client, including verbal and nonverbal communication skills, and both the content and nonverbal aspects of responses to the questions and measures used in the assessment. Traditionally, behavior during the assessment is seen as a "sample" of the client's overall behavior and may be hypothesized to generalize to similar situations. It is helpful to jot down observations about client behavior, as well as select quotes during and immediately following the interview. Noting the length of time the client takes to complete questionnaires and test behavior is useful.

In addition to the observational skills, measures of skills deficits and interpersonal difficulties, such as the Inventory of Interpersonal Problems (Horowitz, Rosenberg, Baer, Ureno, & Villasenor, 1988), may be considered for integration into the assessment process. We particularly encourage consideration of practical tools, such as a stopwatch (to measure the duration of behaviors), a golf counter (to measure the frequency of behaviors), a one-way mirror (for observation by other clinicians or students), and audio- or videotaping equipment, so that interviews can be observed following the assessment. Although audiotape is simpler to set up, it is far easier to complete and do reliability checks with videotaped sessions, if any behavior rating scales are used by observers.

More formal observation can be built in as part of a behavioral skills or avoidance assessment. For example, consider keeping copies of standardized situations for role plays to assess communication skills. Behavioral avoidance tests can be completed to assess specific or social phobias.

Self-Monitoring

"Self-monitoring involves the systematic self-observation and recording of the occurrences (or nonoccurrences) of specified behaviors and events"

(Haynes, 1984, p. 381). Numerous methods exist for self-monitoring. Generally, it is most useful to adapt self-monitoring methods to the specific client and specific problems he or she brings to the assessment. It is useful to have several different, standard self-monitoring forms that can then be adapted for use with different problems and clients during the assessment. Basic forms include a Behavioral Activity Schedule for clients to record their daily activities over a week, a Panic Attack Log, a Dysfunctional Thoughts Record, and a Simple Frequency Record form for clients to track different behaviors, including discrete activities such as hair pulling, eating, smoking, arguments, or initiation of conversations. It is typical to modify these forms for individual clients: For example, a client presenting with trichotillomania may monitor the number of hairs pulled in response to different triggers or the length of time spent pulling hair, or sample activity in different portions of each day. It may be useful to develop templates for forms that can easily be modified. It is often necessary to be creative about how to obtain self-monitoring information. Possible methods include free-form records, adapted forms, or even downloadable Palm pilot programs that help to examine the relationship among triggers, mood, and thoughts. Ask about and respect the client's preference for self-monitoring to increase chances of the client's successful adherence to the self-monitoring plan.

Other Sources of Information

Family and Significant Others

It is often useful to obtain information from family members or significant others, particularly if they live with the client and have been able to observe changes across time. Of course, it is necessary to obtain the client's consent to talk to other people, and often it is wise to interview these people in the presence of the client. The client's reaction to the interview, as well as communication patterns among the individuals in the interview, can be observed. In certain situations, particularly when the primary problems are work-related, it can be helpful to interview the client's employer, direct supervisor, or a colleague, again with client consent and presence, if possible. A semistructured format can easily be used to interview significant others to obtain information similar to that obtained from the client, but from an alternative point of view.

Prior Documentation

Prior documentation can be very useful for establishing past assessment results, diagnoses, and treatments or recommendations, if available. Some clients have difficulty recalling details of treatments and may report having had a particular type of treatment, when there is no evidence to support this claim. Clients sometimes also report past counseling or therapy but are not able to describe specific aspects of the approach. A review of past records may clarify the treatments provided and also prevent repetition of assessment procedures or allow longitudinal assessment of clients who have had long-term problems. The range of documentation that can be considered for examination includes past psychological and psychiatric reports, and progress notes; and hospital, school, and employment records. In some cases, there may also be client-generated records, such as personal notes, diaries, or self-monitoring that can be used as part of the assessment plan.

Other Considerations in Selecting Tools for Your Library

In addition to the empirical status of assessment tools, there are a number of considerations in selecting such instruments. These considerations include the cost, availability, ease of administration, language level and readability, and acceptability to your clients. The most psychometrically sound and sensitive tool is likely to remain in the filing cabinet if it is overly lengthy, tedious, and complicated to use and score. If clients complain when they complete it, or if they struggle to understand the measure, its then accuracy is compromised. Reading levels, language, and cultural appropriateness of the assessment tools are important considerations. Another consideration in choice of assessment is whether the system within which you work supports use of the measures you select. Ideally, other practitioners will be using the same or similar tools, and the data can be pooled across clients and over time to assess patterns and outcomes in the setting. The tools are more likely to be used if enthusiasm develops within a group of practitioners.

ASSESSMENT AS AN ONGOING PROCESS

All clinicians conduct some type of initial assessment for all clients, but it is much less common to complete ongoing or outcome measurement on a routine basis. Indeed, many settings place a premium on the initial assessment but ignore the importance of repeated or exit evaluations. Because assessment is an ongoing process in cognitive-behavioral therapy rather than a static or one-time process, another important consideration is to have some measures that are suitable for repeat across time. Repeated assessment tools typically are shorter in length than other measures and tend to focus on more specific problems that are the focus of treatment.

Sensitivity to change is an important factor in the choice of these measures, because some measures assess variables that take a long time to change (e.g., the YSQ quality-of-life measures). The purpose of ongoing assessment is to evaluate progress and outcomes.

Different types of ongoing assessment can be very useful not only to assess outcomes, but also to influence the process or course of therapy. We discuss in other chapters the ongoing measurement during the course of treatment, but these assessments include the following.

Within-Session Evaluations

These often informal evaluations, such as asking the client's response to the initial interview, occur at the end of a treatment session. Evaluations include asking for verbal or written ratings of various experiences or ideas (e.g., "How strongly do you feel anger on a scale of 1–10?"; "How much do you believe a certain thought on a scale of 0–100%?"; or "How anxious do you feel using a Subjective Units of Distress Scale?"), or having the client complete a Session Satisfaction form or a Symptom Checklist.

Periodic Reevaluation of Goals

When setting goals during the initial sessions of therapy, it is useful to reevaluate them at a certain point (e.g., after six or eight sessions of treatment). This evaluation can be formal or informal. One method for doing this type of evaluation is Goal Attainment Scaling (GAS; Hurn, Kneebone, & Cropley, 2006; Kiresuk, Stelmachers, & Schultz, 1982), which consists of naming the client's problem(s) in the first session and getting a rating of the severity of the problems (e.g., on a 0–100% scale). This baseline rating can then be compared to subsequent ratings of the severity of the same problems, to see whether the goal of reducing these problems is being met. It should be noted that the GAS method can also be used to rate how much certain goals have been met in therapy; their repeated assessment on a percentage rating scale may be used as an index of specific improvement in treatment, and may even figure into decisions to terminate or to continue treatment.

Ongoing Outcome Measures

It may be helpful to use symptom, behavioral, or cognitive measures at certain points in treatment, such as after the 6th, 10th, or 15th session, depending on the length of treatment. Outcome measures can include client self-monitoring records or ratings that can then be graphed as feedback for the client. Our general perspective is to share the results of repeated assessments with the client, unless there is some reason not to do this. Such a feedback process can stimulate discussion about the speed of progress, roadblocks to successful treatment, and the need for ongoing treatment. This feedback also involves the client more in the process, because his or her perception of change can be compared to the formal assessment methods, and his or her ideas about why therapy is or is not proceeding well can be discussed. It is often very reinforcing of the client's efforts to see actual outcome data signifying change.

Completion of Treatment and Follow-Up Assessment

It is common to evaluate progress toward goals set at the beginning and during treatment. A reassessment of the problems that brought the client to therapy is very appropriate, as well as a discussion of other resources or treatment, should they require further help. It is very helpful and reinforcing of client change to provide clear feedback about the results of any measures that have been completed. Clients are often surprised at the amount of progress that they have made. Consider giving clients a summary of their test results. If it is appropriate, consider sending a copy of the assessment results to a client's family physician or other caregivers. Although follow-up assessment is perhaps less common in psychotherapy than it should be (see Chapter 9, this volume), such assessment might include a telephone call, or symptom or other checklists sent by mail.

The next chapter reviews the integration of assessment results and the development of the Problem List into an initial case formulation. It also reviews how to communicate the assessment results to clients, referral sources, and other participants in the process of treatment.

Chapter 3

Integration and
Case Formulation

Once you have completed the initial assessment, you need to integrate, understand, and formulate the array of information into a coherent set of hypotheses regarding the client and his or her problems. Ideally, these hypotheses not only describe relationships among the client's current problems but also begin to suggest relationships between underlying beliefs, current automatic thoughts, and resulting emotional reactions and behaviors. The case formulation also leads to intervention planning, with respect to both what interventions are likely to be used and their sequencing.

Depending on your own practices and needs in your work setting, you may develop a case formulation immediately following the assessment, or after the first few sessions. Our own perspective is that the case formulation should be developed from the first session, even though the formulation will evolve over time, as you understand the client better with ongoing contact and treatment. Following the development of the case formulation, the results are typically communicated to the client(s) and the referral source, either verbally or in writing, or both.

The case formulation is the bridge from assessment to treatment. Goal setting and treatment planning follow logically and naturally from the case formulation, which has been described as "a hypothesis about the nature of the psychological difficulty (or difficulties) underlying the problems on the patient's problem list" (Persons, 1989, p. 37). Kuyken, Fothergill, Musa, and Chadwick (2005) state that individualized cognitive case formulation is the *heart* of evidence-based practice in cognitive-behavioral therapy. Your comprehensive assessment, which has used reliable and valid measures, including a cognitive-behavioral interview, provides the necessary information to build a case formulation. In this chapter, we discuss the evidence base for cognitive case formulation. Having done so, we then discuss how to develop a problem list and an initial case formulation, how to communicate these results, and how to set initial treatment goals and conduct treatment planning.

CASE FORMULATION

Background of Case Formulation

Clinical case formulation is a broad concept that has been applied and used in many types of individualized or idiographic psychotherapy, including cognitive-behavioral therapy. Case formulation, a central tool for virtually all psychotherapies (Eells, 1997), is the way in which assessment leads to intervention, incorporating the theoretical principles of the approach into practice. As noted earlier, case formulation provides the explanatory link between practice, theory, and research for any given client (Kuyken et al., 2005). It should lead to the selection and use of the most appropriate, theoretically sound, and empirically based interventions for the client's problems. Ideally, it can also guide the timing and sequencing of the interventions, and predict difficulties with implementing therapy. It also takes the individual differences of the client into account to maximize the effects of therapy.

One of the questions asked about cognitive-behavioral therapy is whether every client requires an individualized case conceptualization, or whether treatment manuals can be applied to future cases that are similar to those of the clients on whom the treatment was empirically evaluated. Cognitive-behavioral therapy has sometimes been criticized for providing a "one-size-fits-all" manual-based therapy for clients who meet criteria for a given diagnosis. This criticism is unfounded for several reasons. Although the initial assessment in many research trials primarily serves the purpose of ensuring that the clients meet diagnostic criteria for the study and do *not* meet exclusion criteria, and although this assessment further "gets the client into" the treatment, it does not necessarily help the treating clinician plan all aspects of treatment. Once a client has been entered the study, the initial interview provides the information by which the clinician formulates the case, and the interventions that follow from that formulation.[1]

It is true that relatively more structured, manual-based treatments do not necessarily use a highly individualized case formulation approach. However, all treatment manuals are based on a theoretical conceptualization of the clinical problem(s) commonly seen in that client group, and so provide interventions with a high probability of success. The concern about standardized treatments is perhaps greatest in group interventions, where there may be even less individualization of interventions than in individual cognitive-behavioral treatment. In cognitive-behavioral groups, the needs of the individual client are less apparent, and there is limited time and opportunity to focus on each individual. But even in these instances, clients are encouraged to adapt the general interventions to their own unique circumstances. In summary, there is a great deal of variability in the treatment manuals included in empirically supported cognitive-behavioral treatments, ranging from those that leave considerable discretion to the treating clinician to those that provide session-by-session plans that are followed carefully.

Case formulation has been a feature of cognitive-behavioral therapy for a long time, and a number of variations on case formulation have been developed (e.g., Nezu, Nezu, & Lombardo, 2004). Two commonly discussed methods for case formulation in cognitive-behavioral therapy are those developed by Persons (1989) and J. S. Beck (1995). These methods are described in more detail below. In addition, other types of formulations can be included in cognitive-behavioral therapy: a behavioral or functional-analytic formulation (Haynes & O'Brien, 2000; Martell, Addis, & Jacobson, 2001), or an interpersonal formulation (Mumma & Smith, 2001). The behavioral formulation focuses on variability across situations rather than on stability, whereas the interpersonal formulation focuses on causal relationship factors between the client's cognitions and recurring interpersonal patterns.

As a clinician, you probably treat a range of clients and cannot decide as easily whom to include or exclude in your practice as you might within a clinical trial. This type of practice likely means that you have a greater responsibility to develop individualized treatment plans to meet the unique needs of your clients. Also, regardless of the extent of the use of case formulation in outcome studies, most clinical practice requires

---

[1]A classic example of this reality is in the first major treatment manual for cognitive-behavioral therapy, which was *Cognitive Therapy of Depression* (A. T. Beck, Rush, Shaw, & Emery, 1979). This book has been used as the "standard" treatment manual in many studies in cognitive-behavioral therapy. The interventions used for an individual client rest, however, on an idiographic case formulation.

more individualized case formulation, because the typical client present-ing for treatment is more complex and has more problems than the aver-age subject in an outcome study. It is because of these complexities and issues that most clients require careful assessment, case conceptualiza-tion, and treatment planning. Consequently, it is crucial for you as a cognitive-behavioral therapist to develop and practice good case formu-lation skills.

Knowing the Evidence Base

The case formulation is "the place" where clinicians take assessment results, and apply their inferences and interpretations to the facts of the case; in essence, it is the conduit between the descriptive results of the assessment and the treatment plan. As such, case formulation is the most likely place where errors can be made. Given the pivotal role of case for-mulations, the amount of research directed toward this topic is remark-ably small.

Is case formulation an art or a science, or as Bieling and Kuyken (2003) asked the question, "Is cognitive case formulation science or sci-ence fiction?" In two of the few studies done, Persons and her colleagues (Persons, Mooney, & Padesky, 1995; Persons & Bertagnolli, 1999) found that when asked to review sample clinical cases, clinicians were able reli-ably to identify between 60 and 70% of clients' maladaptive overt behav-iors (e.g., agree on the Problem List) but were less able to agree on the underlying beliefs or attitudes leading to these overt behaviors. If this result is valid, then it suggests that whereas the treatment planning to solve current problems will likely be fairly consistent across cognitive-behavioral therapists, the consistency of the case formulations of the cause of the problems, and the preventive work to prevent future prob-lems, may be more variable.

Bieling and Kuyken (2003) have also suggested that good reliability between raters can be attained for the descriptive, but not for the inferen-tial, components of the case formulation. They have suggested, however, that the reliability of case formulation can be improved through training and the use of more systematic and structured methods of determining the case formulation. In support of this suggestion, Kuyken et al. (2005) taught practitioners who attended workshops to develop a case formu-lation, then tested the reliability and quality of participants' work. A "benchmark" case formulation provided by J. S. Beck was used for the comparison. These results showed that participants in this study agreed on both the descriptive features and the theoretically inferred compo-nents of the case formulation (although reliability was lower for the latter than for the former). Prior training and accreditation with a cognitive-behavioral organization was associated with higher quality outcomes. Overall, these results suggest that reliability of case formulations can be improved with training and practice. These results are also supported by the work of Kendjelic and Eells (2007), who demonstrated that the quality of generic case formulations can be improved with training.

The existing literature on case formulation suggests that although the basic informational aspects of the case formulation may be obtained reliably, it is more difficult for raters or clinicians to agree on the hypothesized relationships between these elements. These findings are not surprising given that descriptive components of a case include demographic data, measurable symptoms, and interpersonal and other behaviors. Inferential components include the underlying maintaining and causative factors, which often are not measured using reliable and valid tools, and which rely on clinical judgment and experience. At this point in time, it is not clear what the optimal training methods are to develop the skill of case formulation in cognitive-behavioral therapy.

Despite the relative lack of understanding of how best to train case conceptualization in cognitive-behavioral therapy, it appears that there are ways in which the reliability of therapy case formulation can be improved. For example, Luborsky and Crits-Christoph (1998) have completed numerous studies on a case formulation method called core conflictual relationship theme (CCRT), albeit in the context of brief psychodynamic psychotherapy. In this method, core themes in relationship conflicts are inferred by the therapist from clients' descriptions of their relationships. A systematic scoring method has been developed to rate these core themes, which in turn are related to the underlying psychodynamic theory. Studies have found that raters, particularly more skilled and systematic judges, can agree quite reliably on these themes. These themes have been shown to have a modest relationship with symptom changes during brief psychodynamic therapy. Consequently, CCRT appears to be a method that meets the criteria of reliability, validity, and improvement of outcomes. According to Bieling and Kuyken (2003), an accurate case formulation derived with this method can lead to improved outcomes by helping to choose the best interventions and/or enhance the therapeutic relationship. Consequently, it appears that case formulation can have a scientific basis, beyond its descriptive components. Cognitive-behavioral case formulation does not have as long a history as the work done on the CCRT, however, and cognitive-behavioral researchers and practitioners could learn from this body of research.

Few studies have assessed the validity of the cognitive-behavioral case formulation, or determined its treatment utility. Mumma (2004) developed a process that can be used to validate case formulation for work with individual clients; however, the process is complex and relies heavily on cooperation from the client to provide large amounts of data. Unfortunately, although it seems inherently important to individualize the treatment according to unique client needs, there is also no *known* relationship between case formulation and improved outcomes for clients. In contrast, several studies indicate that treatment utility can be improved with a functional-analytic assessment, leading to a functional-analytic formulation, in clients with severe behavior disorders. These findings are likely due to the fact that fewer inferences tend to be required in functional analysis (e.g., Carr & Durand, 1985).

Several studies suggest that clinical outcomes may be better for manual-based, highly structured approaches compared to individualized treatments for more routine clinical problems (Kuyken et al., 2005). It is possible that future research may support the use of an idiographic case formulation, primarily for clients with more complex and/or multiple problems. In support of this idea, Persons, Roberts, Zalecki, and Brechwald (2006) described a naturalistic outcome study in which case formulation–driven cognitive-behavioral therapy was used for clients presenting with both anxiety and depression. The clients showed improvement with this approach. Unfortunately, from a research perspective, there was no comparison to clients treated with either another type of formulation or a cognitive-behavioral therapy approach without case formulation. Kuyken et al. (2005) stated: "Research is needed to examine the vital question of whether formulation is linked to improved outcomes through the selection of better targeted interventions as has been shown with brief psychodynamic psychotherapy but has not yet been shown with behavioral and cognitive-behavioral psychotherapy" (p. 1200).

Bieling and Kuyken (2003) concluded that for case formulation to be useful, the following questions need to be addressed:

1. Does case formulation have predictive validity?
2. Does case formulation lead to improved outcomes?
3. Does case formulation improve therapeutic alliance?
4. Do clinicians adhere to their case formulation once it is developed?

Essentially, the answers to these questions are unknown at present.

What can you, as a cognitive-behavioral clinician, take away from this discussion? It appears that outcome trials including case formulation as one of the components of treatment have good results, so despite the lack of research, there is good reason to suspect that a case formulation is a useful part of good clinical care. Most clinicians place great value on using an individualized approach, and taking many different variables into account to understand their clients and how they interact with their environment. Some practical suggestions that derive from the ongoing work in this area may help you think about it:

- Use the most reliable and valid assessment tools possible (see Chapter 2, this volume).
- Emphasize the use of descriptive and objective data where possible.
- Limit the range and number of inferences you draw from the available information.
- Use a consistent and structured approach to case formulation.
- Revisit and refine your case conceptualization as new data become available.
- Be open to alternative hypotheses.
- Test your hypotheses against what you observe over time in therapy; be especially open to new information that is inconsistent with your case conceptualization.
- Obtain feedback on your case formulation from the client and others who know him or her.
- Consider using a manual-based approach to treatment if the presenting problems are straightforward. Otherwise, you may be tempted to "overcomplicate" the underlying basis of a client's problems, leading to a more idiographic, but no more effective, treatment.

Mark was a practicing psychotherapist, with a background in psychodynamic and humanistic therapies. He came for supervision, though, to learn about cognitive-behavioral therapy. The supervisor found Mark to have very well-developed interpersonal skills, and a passion for helping distressed clients. At the same time, Mark could not seem to break away from case conceptualizations that were inconsistent with the evidence gathered in the therapy room, and that often made reference to hypothesized early developmental experiences. During sessions, he often would hear about a current issue or problem and strive to understand its genesis rather than work to find effective solutions with the client. In supervision, he more quickly asked the "why" questions about behavior than the "how" questions about strategies to help. He was drawn to the schema hypothesis, which, he recognized, had some similarities to psychodynamic ideas of unconscious processes.

The supervisor worked with Mark over a period of months and across several cases. He discovered that Mark was able to develop complex case conceptualizations quickly, and that he tended to focus on the core belief level of analysis with cases, but that Mark struggled more with the pragmatic and behavioral aspects of treatment. He especially struggled with the design and implementation of homework assignments.

The "breakthrough" in Mark's training came from a client who struggled with perfectionism. In session 4, just as Mark was beginning to offer a tentative case formulation to the client, she said: "I know all that. I just want to get over this problem." For some reason, this client at this point in training resonated with Mark. He stepped back from a schema focus with this client was able to use the methods he had learned, and was pragmatic and effective in his work. The client responded very favorably to the treatment and was grateful for the help she received.

STEPS IN CASE FORMULATION

We now turn to a description of a cognitive-behavioral case formulation process that compromises several steps. These steps include developing the problem list, developing the initial case formulation, and communicating the case formulation and assessment results.

Step 1: Developing the Problem List

Clients usually come to the initial assessment eager to talk about their problems. These problems often include items as diverse as general distress, symptoms indicative of a disorder, current stressors, relationships with other people, feelings about themselves, destructive behaviors in which they engage, outside events, and uncontrollable situations. Clients do not naturally describe their concerns in a way that makes it easy to develop a cohesive Problem List. Some clients have difficulties expressing their concerns clearly and succinctly. It can be challenging to create a Problem List to guide intervention planning on the basis of an initial assessment that is comprehensive and concise. Organization of the Problem List is one of the many reasons to conduct a good assessment.

Persons (1989) suggested that the Problem List should be inclusive and specific. When developing a Problem List in the assessment interview, attempt to have clients list all of the major problems related to their presentation to therapy. As the interview proceeds, however, it is important for the clinician to organize and categorize the problems. If a cognitive-behavioral assessment occurs as described in Chapter 2, this volume, this categorization will likely already be done by the time the assessment has been completed. Clients may also not be aware of all problems, or may not articulate all of the problems that they are experiencing, at the time of the assessment. It is important to observe carefully and ask the client about possible problems that they may not have expressed. For example, a client may appear to have poor social skills or be very anxious in the interview, but may not explicitly state either problem. Observing client reactions in the assessment and asking specific questions may elucidate problems not immediately apparent. Using a cognitive case formulation, it may also be possible for you to infer certain problems that the client has not directly expressed. For example, clients may present with a pattern of relationships that implies that they believe themselves to be unlovable, but they may not be aware of this belief. Noting this possible belief in the assessment results helps to shape future assessment and interventions.

After the comprehensive Problem List has been completed, the priority and importance of the problems to address in therapy must be selected. There can be several disadvantages to developing a very comprehensive and lengthy, treatment-oriented Problem List to include on the case formulation. Both client and therapist can become overwhelmed and have difficulty sorting out the primary from the more secondary problems. Rather than help the therapeutic focus, too many problems can detract from it. If asked simply, "What are your problems?", clients may include as many as they can think of, some of which may be relatively unchangeable or require considerable "massaging" to become a reasonable therapeutic goal. For example, a client may include the statement "I am too shy" as a problem, which may need to be translated into a workable problem that can become a focus of therapy, such as "lack of friends," "poor social support," or a belief about expecting rejection from others. From the first time a problem is named, you should be considering how amenable to change the problem is, and possible interventions to work with this problem.

A very helpful strategy is to consider the inclusion of one or two problems that lead directly to a quick and effective intervention. Early success in therapy helps to engage the client in the therapy process. For example, if a client presents with the problem of muscle tension related to anxiety, teaching the client progressive muscle relaxation may be a relatively quick intervention that leads to initial relief. Be careful, though, not to offer "quick fixes" that get the client to believe that he or she is better, and to flee from therapy before dealing with more central and difficult problems.

Should the client's diagnosis, if there is one, be on the problem list? We argue that it should not. It can be very useful to differentiate between *problems* and *diagnosis*; therefore, we recommend not including diagnosis or primary symptoms on the Problem List (see Figure 3.1 for a sample case formulation worksheet). In some settings, a formal diagnosis may not be necessary or appropriate, so only a Problem List may be required.

Name: _____ Date: _____

Identifying Information: _____

Problem List:

1. _____

2. _____

3. _____

4. _____

5. _____

Diagnoses:

Axis I: _____

Axis II: _____

Axis III: _____

Axis IV: _____

Axis V: Global Assessment of Functioning (GAF) _____

Medications: _____

Hypothesized Core Beliefs:

I am _____

Others are _____

The world is _____

The future is _____

Precipitants/Activating Situations: _____

_____

Working Hypothesis: _____

_____

_____

Developmental Origins: _____

_____

Treatment Plan/Goals: 1. _____ 2. _____

                         3. _____ 4. _____

                         5. _____ 6. _____

Potential Obstacles to Goal Attainment: _____

_____

_____

Potential Aids to Goal Attainment: _____

_____

_____

FIGURE 3.1. Cognitive-behavioral case formulation worksheet. Adapted from Persons (1989). Copyright 1989 by W. W. Norton. Used by permission of W. W. Norton & Company, Inc. Note that readers are not granted the right to reproduce this figure.

For example, clients who present in a private practice setting may not meet criteria for any diagnosis but still experience treatable problems.

Clients often come to the first session with a diagnosis as their main problem. Indeed, a number of materials about cognitive-behavioral therapy are oriented toward specific DSM-IV diagnostic categories. A client may have read some of these materials, or been diagnosed by another practitioner. In a cognitive-behavioral model, though, a diagnosis is the *result* of certain underlying beliefs, thoughts, and behaviors. The diagnostic problems may also have certain consequences, such as the exacerbation of avoidant behavior or changes in beliefs about self-efficacy.

We typically include the current factors related to the diagnosis on the Problem List, but not the diagnosis itself. For example, if a 36-year-old female client presents with symptoms that meet criteria for a generalized anxiety disorder plus additional symptoms that almost meet criteria for major depressive disorder, she may be experiencing many current problems that both lead to and result in anxiety symptoms. These symptoms may include difficulty managing daily activities, including work, child care, and family obligations. She may also experience low self-efficacy, negative thoughts about herself, and poor sleep patterns. A useful strategy in the initial stages of case formulation may simply be to complete two lists, one related to symptoms of a diagnosis or diagnoses, and another related to problems of living. The Symptom List helps to formulate the diagnosis, and the Problem List helps to guide the formulation. With appropriate interventions that help the client solve the problems, there should be a commensurate reduction of symptoms. The hope is that if the problems are resolved to satisfaction, the client will no longer meet diagnostic criteria. Conceptually, the main point here is that intervening at the problem level, rather than at the diagnostic level, is the major purpose of cognitive-behavioral therapy.

Step 2: Developing the Initial Case Formulation

The case formulation worksheet in Figure 3.1 is used to work through the steps of the formulation. In our experience, it is very difficult to have all of the necessary information to work through these steps after the initial interview. It can take several sessions before the case formulation has been completed to a satisfactory point.

During the assessment, and the development of the Problem List and diagnosis (if appropriate for your setting), you will have obtained considerable information about the client. You also will have had an opportunity to interact with the client during the interview(s). When developing the formulation, you need to consider the precipitants, activating situations, or current triggers that have led to the problem(s) that brought the client to therapy. It may be useful at this assessment stage to complete a chart that describes the interactions among life events, core beliefs and current thoughts, emotions, and behaviors (see Figure 3.2).

The core beliefs included in the case formulation are a result of what the client has told you in the interview, questionnaire data that you have gathered, as well as your hypotheses about beliefs that are likely to exist, based upon the problems reported. The working hypothesis seeks to explain the reasons why this person developed these problems at this point in time, based on the complex interaction among beliefs, precipitants, behavioral repertoires, and changes among factors over time. The working hypothesis must be viewed as preliminary and responsive to incoming data, just as any experimental hypothesis would be.

It is important to consider what obstacles are likely to stand in the way of treatment, and what factors may be used to assist treatment. For example, obstacles may include practical difficulties, such as financial limitations that preclude certain types of homework, lack of easy access to transportation or child care, or more individual characteristics (e.g., lack of psychological mindedness or difficulty with verbal expression). Some clients have a great deal of difficulty following through with therapeutic assignments. The information is taken from not only the questionnaire results but also client behaviors during the task (e.g., a client taking an unusually long time to complete tests may be perfectionistic or have difficulty reading). Obstacles need to be identified both to minimize their negative impact on therapy and to develop possible solutions to them. Put another way, treatment obstacles can, and probably should be, put on the Problem List. Factors that assist treatment may range from a great deal of distress, which tends to lead to a greater desire for personal change, interest in a cognitive-behavioral approach, high levels of motivation, or a supportive family.

The developmental origins of problems are the more distant factors and are likely to be more speculative in nature. Remember that the information you have received regarding the developmental origins of the problem relies on both the client's memory and his or her interpretation of events, often involving family, social relationships and other experiences over the course of time. Our general approach to such information, especially early in the course of therapy, is to take it "under advisement." Thus, you can perceive this information as the way the client has come to conceptualize the genesis of his or her problems but reserve judgment about the adequacy or completeness of the this model, until you learn more about the client and have the opportunity to see how his or her problems play out over the course of therapy. Generally, though, we encourage the use of a vulnerability model (also called the biopsychosocial or diathesis–stress model) as you consider developmental origins

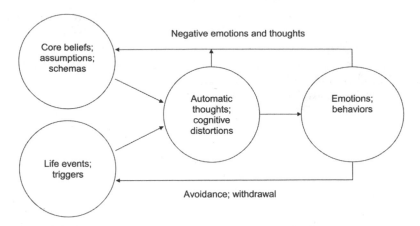

FIGURE 3.2. The cognitive-behavioral model of emotional distress.

of problems (Zubin & Spring, 1977); this model forces you to consider the broad range of biological, psychological, and social factors that may have been related to the problem genesis in the client's past. Our general view is that there are many pathways to developing problems, and many possible pathways to backing out.

> Tricia was a 21-year-old woman with problem eating patterns and ongoing depression. These symptom patterns caused her distress, as well as interpersonal problems, in the form of family tension and reduced involvement with her small circle of friends. After assessment, the therapist developed the following potential list of problems for work in therapy:
> - Problems that might underlie current issues, and might be addressed in treatment
>   - Past family relationships; family rules
>   - Dysfunctional self-schema
>   - Developmental issues in self-definition
> - Problems that likely underlie current issues and likely need to be addressed in treatment
>   - Perfectionism
>   - Family dysfunction
>   - Avoidance
>   - Limited social skills
> - Presenting problems
>   - Eating problems (bulimia nervosa)
>   - Depression
>   - Stress and anxiety
>   - Social isolation

Step 3: Communicating the Case Formulation
and Assessment Results

Communicating with the Client

Discussion of your case formulation with the client is a critical step in engaging him or her in the therapeutic process. Even though there has been minimal research on whether the therapeutic alliance is enhanced by this step, clinical experience would certainly suggest that it is. The collaborative nature of cognitive-behavioral therapy makes this communication process necessary.

It is generally helpful to be fairly transparent about the way you have begun to conceptualize the client's problems. The specific way you make this communication, however, should vary from client to client. Suggestions for communication include the following:

- Do not convey more information than is necessary, so that you do not overwhelm or confuse clients. Clients are often anxious as they receive assessment feedback, and they may not remember the details of questionnaire results or complicated conceptualizations. Pause frequently and ask questions to check on their understanding.
- Use everyday language or the typical language of the client, such as *thoughts* rather than *cognitions*, *feelings* rather than *affect*. Use frequent examples from the client's own experience, when possible.
- Consider using quotes from what the client has already told you during the assessment, particularly in relation to the client's core beliefs.
- Use the feedback process as an opportunity to check out the accuracy of factual parts of the formulation. Even though you may be confident about your facts, ask the client to verify occasionally. Doing so further engages the client in the process, increases his or her confidence in your respectfulness, and will likely augment his or her desire for participation.
- After you discuss the more factual components, raise the hypotheses as "informed possibilities." Convey an attitude of curiosity rather than certainty.
- If possible, use the feedback session to lead into a description of the cognitive-behavioral model of therapy. Remember that there are many ways to present an initial case formulation, and the "best" way is the one that works for your client. J. S. Beck (1995) presents a relatively complete cognitive conceptualization framework that can be shared with clients who are particularly bright or have past experience in cognitive-behavioral therapy. Consider other ways to present this information. For example, one of us (K. S. D.) often presents an initial case conceptualiza-

tion using a pictorial rather than written model, such as that described in Figure 3.2.

• Consider giving the client a written summary or graphic depiction of the initial case formulation, to take home and think about for homework.

• Therapeutic alliance may be enhanced, and client distress reduced, by "normalizing" a client's reactions; for example, by providing a statement such as "Your reactions appear to be a normal reaction to abnormal circumstances." Such statements may be particularly appropriate if the client experiences great stress in his or her life, or lives under difficult circumstances including poverty or family conflict. The client may have suffered through recent losses. Inclusion of these contextual factors in the formulation can "normalize" these reactions, offer relief to the client, and easily be included in the cognitive-behavioral formulation. Do not state this, however, if you do not believe it, or if it is obviously untrue; false statements of reassurance or normalization may have the unintended effect of being seen as patronizing, and undermine the therapeutic relationship.

• Ask for feedback and input about the formulation. Be collaborative and encourage a joint ownership of the case formulation. A statement such as "Even though I may know a lot about cognitive-behavioral therapy, you are the expert on yourself" can be useful.

• Ask the client to explain his or her understanding of the case formulation in his or her own words. This step allows you to assess the client's understanding of what you have said, and it can provide the client an opportunity to elaborate on certain components and seek clarification of points you have made, or allow him or her even to disagree with your ideas.

Communicating with Other Professionals

After you have completed your assessment and shared the results with the client, it is important also to communicate the necessary aspects of the assessment to other, involved professionals. If you work in an interdisciplinary team, these other professionals include colleagues within the same treatment setting. If you work in an HMO, these professionals may include an insurance company or organization administrator. If you work in a private practice setting, these professionals may include a referral source outside of your setting, such as the family physician or another third party. The needs regarding communication are different for each client, but you should develop a mental checklist of who needs to know what about your assessment.

Communication may be either verbal or written, depending on the nature of the relationship with the other professional. Communication may also be lengthy or be more succinct, depending on the other professional's need to know more or less. Of course, communication to others only occurs with the written permission of the client (unless circumstances, such as risk of harm to self or others, dictate otherwise). Here are some points to consider when communicating assessment results:

• Communication with other professionals who practice from a similar model is straightforward. This communication is only on a need-to-know basis, such as when consulting or obtaining peer supervision. Generally, such communication does not include any identifying information about the client. This type of communication can be stimulating and very helpful for obtaining new ideas and ways of viewing the problems. Colleagues can also provide opportunities to obtain second opinions.

• Communication with other professionals within a treatment team or setting, such as a day treatment program or inpatient unit, and in particular those who practice from a different model or who have different areas of expertise, can be both challenging and stimulating. Many practitioners work with other professionals who may play a role in the treatment of the client, including medical practitioners, social workers, psychiatric nurses, and occupational therapists. Diverse practitioners rarely agree on all interventions used and often negotiate components of the overall treatment "package" in some settings. Attempt to be both respectful of others and confident regarding your proposed plans when you communicate in case conferences or treatment planning meetings. See these meetings as an opportunity to highlight empirically supported cognitive-behavioral interventions.

• Expect other professionals to disagree with your case formulation and aspects of the treatment plan (but be pleasantly surprised if they do not!), and be prepared to explain and provide a solid rationale for what you plan. See Chapter 12 for a discussion of common myths that occur in some settings related to cognitive-behavioral therapy. Develop confidence in what you do and communicate accordingly. Develop resources that include the evidence base or practice guidelines that support your work. It is difficult for others to argue against a treatment that is in the best interests of the client. In treatment teams with a diversity of backgrounds and opinions, healthy debate can be stimulating and lead to improved treatments for clients if all members of the team listen respectfully to each other and follow through with plans that serve the client. For example, we have seen cognitive-behavioral therapists overemphasize the intrapsychic aspects of a client's problems, neglecting other aspects of client functioning, such as environmental or social factors.

• Consider the involvement of other team members in the treatment plan. A recreational therapist or dietician can not only provide balance for the overall treatment but also can dovetail with client self-care, behavioral activation or exposure (e.g., making telephone calls or going to a public place, in the case of an anxious client). For example, one of us (D. D.) frequently arranged exposure activities for anxious clients when she worked in a day treatment program. One such activity involved a whole social anxiety group collaboratively arranging to be "servers" at a celebratory luncheon activity for other clients and staff. Be aware, though, that such activities require planning and collaboration of other members of a treatment team. If you enlist other team members, be sure they understand the purpose of their involvement, and that they do not unwittingly undermine the treatment plan. An example of undermining would be doing the task for the client to reduce his or her anxiety.

• Formal assessment or intake reports may be required in some settings. These documents provide an opportunity to communicate the results of your assessment and formulation to family physician or mental health professional referral source, and to inform other professionals about cognitive-behavioral therapy. Figure 3.3 provides a sample initial assessment for cognitive-behavioral therapy report for a client struggling with anxiety and depression. This format is comprehensive and closely follows the case formulation worksheet provided in Figure 3.1.

• You can also routinely include a section entitled "Relevant Clinical Outcome Research" in your reports. Such a format was developed with colleagues in a cognitive therapy service in an outpatient mental health program. This section is helpful to the recipient of the report and also forces the writer to be aware of recent outcome literature in different problem areas. For samples of brief summaries of outcome research for different diagnoses, see Figure 3.4. Of course, it is necessary to update these summaries on a regular basis as new research becomes available and is published. It is also important to point out the differences between your client and the study sample.

The worksheet and sample report provided here need to be "customized" for your practice. It can be tempting to skip the completion of a formal case formulation, if you are busy and see many clients, or if you are involved in other activities. It may be tempting to omit the case conceptualization with more straightforward client presentations, and rely only on the case formulation with more complex clients. To fight against this tendency, it is prudent to attach a completed formulation sheet in an accessible and consistent place in each client's file. Return to it periodically for reexamination and revisions.

Bo, a seasoned cognitive-behavioral therapist, worked in a publicly funded mental health program. He had just completed the initial assessment and case formulation for new client Roger. Consistent with the usual practice in this setting, Bo wrote out the assessment and put a copy of it, including a paragraph about the evidence base for cognitive-behavioral therapy, into the case file. He also asked for Roger's written consent, and, with that consent, he mailed a copy of the assessment report to the family physician who had referred Roger to the program. Bo also made a drawing of the preliminary case formulation and put it on the inside front cover of the case file, so that it would be readily available to him for reference and editing over time.

Because the relationship with Roger's wife figured so strongly in the case, Bo pointed this out to Roger and used the pictorial case formulation to help explain his thinking at this stage of therapy. Bo suggested that, at some point in the future, it might be helpful to share the case formulation with Roger's wife, or maybe even to bring his wife into an information session or two. Roger agreed that this issue could be revisited at some future session.

FIGURE 3.3. Initial assessment for cognitive-behavioral therapy report. Adapted from Cognitive Therapy Subgroup, Outpatient Mental Health Program, Calgary Health Region. This report format may not be practical in all settings and will require adaptation.

Client Name: Anna C
Referral Source: Dr. X
Date of First Session: July 12
Date Assessment Completed: July 12

Referral Source and Presenting Concerns

Anna C requested a referral from her family physician for cognitive-behavioral therapy for depression and anxiety. She presented with a number of concerns, which included sadness, low motivation and energy, a negative sense of self-worth, and worries about her own and her family's health. She also reported some conflict and unhappiness in her marriage.

Identifying Information

Anna C is a 31-year-old married woman. She has a college certificate in office administration, and is a full time administrative assistant in a legal firm. Her husband Luka works full time as the manager of the men's wear department in a local department store. They have two children, Nate, who is 7 years old, and Alicia, who is 5 years old. Anna has been married for 10 years.

Current Situation

Anna was very cooperative and polite during the interview. She appeared to be motivated and interested in treatment. There were no indications of difficulties with her concentration or memory. She appeared sad, apologetic, and deferential, and frequently made self-deprecatory comments. She appeared somewhat anxious but had good eye contact, and the interviewer was able to develop rapport with her easily.

(continued)

FIGURE 3.3. (*continued*)

Anna reported numerous signs of both anxiety and depression. She worried "all the time" about her son's and her mother's health. She was not able to stop this rumination even though she realized that it was counterproductive. She was convinced that her mother would die within the next few years, and that her son's health was also in jeopardy. She reported insomnia at least five nights of each week. Anna's thoughts and feelings of agitation kept her awake for several hours when she went to bed. Even though she was often fatigued during the day, Anna tended to be very "jumpy" and was easily startled. A semistructured diagnostic interview revealed that she met diagnostic criteria for generalized anxiety disorder.

Although Anna reported some symptoms of depression, she did not meet criteria for a current mood disorder. She experienced self-blame and guilt over not being able to provide what she considered to be enough help to her family members. She did not believe that she was a good parent or an attractive partner to her husband. She had occasional suicidal ideation but no intention or plan for self-harm. Her appetite and libido were normal, but her energy, motivation, and interest in everyday activities were all somewhat reduced. She felt hopeful about the future in general; however, she doubted her own ability to make significant changes for herself.

Anna C's interpersonal style was passive and unassertive in the interview, and she acknowledged this pattern in all of her relationships. She described herself as a "nice" person who was loyal and hardworking, with high standards for her own performance. Anna stated that she was a good employee and tended to prioritize work above her own needs. She struggled with conflict and hoped that others would like her.

Anna C reported that she was generally in good physical health, but she had gained 20 pounds in the past year. She tended to eat "comfort foods" when she felt overwhelmed, or when she was alone. Anna reported that she seldom had time for exercise or other self-care activities. She had a migraine headache roughly once a month. She had been taking antidepressant medication for the past 6 months. She also took an anxiolytic medication approximately once a week. She admitted that she drank one or two glasses of wine each evening to relax.

Current Problem List

1. Uncontrolled worry
2. Decreased intimacy with husband
3. Lack of social support
4. Insomnia and fatigue
5. Lack of assertion and avoidance of conflict
6. Poor self-care
7. High standards and sense of responsibility to other people

Relevant History

Current Episode
Anna C's current symptoms date back to her return to full-time work 1 year prior to the assessment. Shortly after she started her job, her mother had a recurrence of breast cancer. Consequently, her responsibilities and her perceived need to support other people increased significantly. Anna has been more and more anxious, with worries about her mother's health, her father's coping abilities, and her son's health. Her daughter has been misbehaving since she began kindergarten and was placed in a child care facility. Anna feels guilty about her time away from her family and wonders whether she has been able to meet the demands of her job. She doubts her parenting skills. In addition, Luka has been working long hours at his job and frequently works

during the evenings and weekends. Because Anna spends most evenings alone after her children are asleep, she has been drinking alcohol and snacking more than usual, and has recently gained weight.

Treatment History

Anna C went to see her family physician 6 months ago due to her sleep problems. He completed a screening interview, noted her depressed mood, and placed her on antidepressant medication. He provided some information about depression and anxiety, and referred her for outpatient therapy. Anna reported that she has had some improvement, although she was concerned about possible side effects of weight gain and sexual difficulties. In terms of past treatment, she and her husband had six sessions of couple counseling 1 year after the birth of their daughter. She reported some benefit from the focus on their communication skills. They also came to appreciate the effect of their different cultural backgrounds on their marriage. There have been no inpatient admissions to psychiatric facilities and no previous individual psychotherapy. Anna has never attempted suicide.

Relevant Background

Anna C was born in Toronto, Canada. She is the eldest of three children and has two younger brothers. Her parents are retired and live within the community where she grew up. They have been married for 40 years. Her father worked as a city transit driver, and her mother was a homemaker. She grew up in a religious, Christian family that was involved in their church community. Value was placed on family and community contributions rather than on personal achievement or financial gain.

Anna stated that she was shy and nervous as a child and adolescent. She described being very close to her mother. When Anna was 14 years old, her mother was diagnosed with breast cancer and subsequently had a mastectomy with follow-up chemotherapy. As the eldest child, Anna assumed many responsibilities for household management and for her brothers' care. Her brothers were 10 and 13 when their mother was diagnosed with cancer. Anna's father was very distraught during the 18 months that her mother was ill and undergoing treatment. Several years later, her next-youngest brother began using drugs and alcohol. He dropped out of school when he was 16 years old and was charged with theft. These incidents were very stressful for the whole family. Anna wondered whether she was depressed during high school. She remembered feeling sad for lengthy periods of time, spending a lot of time at home cooking meals and taking care of the house. She does not remember joy in the home during those years or the pleasure of going out with friends. She worried a great deal about her family, particularly about her mother's health, her father's emotional well-being, and her brother's acting out. She tended to gain approval by working hard in school, taking care of other people, and being capable and conscientious. She lost faith in her religion during her late adolescence but retained many of the values inherent in the church, such as placing high importance upon self-sacrifice and family relationships.

Anna began dating in her last year of high school. Her first serious boyfriend broke off the relationship suddenly and without explanation. Because she did not understand the reasons, she blamed herself. She struggled with low mood and negative self-image for the 2 years that she attended college. When Anna was 22 years old, she met Luka, and they dated for several years prior to marriage. His parents had immigrated to Toronto from Croatia when he was 19 years old. His family was not at all religious. The war in Croatia had a strong influence on Luka during his adolescence. When Anna first met her future husband, she found him interesting and somewhat exotic. Gradually, they found that they had many values in common.

(continued)

FIGURE 3.3. (*continued*)

She bonded readily with his mother, who was warm and inviting, but found his father somewhat intimidating and aggressive. In general, Anna has found her husband and his family to be emotionally expressive and somewhat volatile, especially in contrast to her family. Her parents disapproved of the marriage and never formed a close bond with her in-laws. This situation improved considerably, however, following the births of the two children.

Anna worked full time as an administrative assistant at a law firm following her marriage until the birth of her son 7 years ago. He was diagnosed with asthma and a number of serious allergies when he was 2 years old. He has been seen in the emergency room on a number of occasions due to breathing problems. Anna remained at home, looking after the children, until her son started elementary school.

Cognitive-Behavioral Formulation

Anna C grew up in a family in which she obtained reinforcement for selflessness and nurturance toward other people. When her mother developed a life-threatening illness, Anna was placed in a role of sacrificing her own developmental needs to help the family continue to function. Over time, she internalized these beliefs, and she now has a very strong value system involving self-sacrifice in service to others. She developed core schemas of self-sacrifice, high standards, and vulnerability to harm. This vulner-ability schema includes physical harm from illness, as well as rejection by others. Her beliefs about men are mixed. Whereas her father modeled emotional vulnerability, her first boyfriend rejected her. Anna's husband is generally supportive. She has feared conflict and aggression most of her life. Suppression of anger was modeled in her family, whereas outward expression and high emotionality have been modeled in her husband's family. She tends to avoid bringing problems up for fear of reprisal.

Anna has recently been placed in a situation in which she has not had the time, energy, or resources to deal with the many demands placed upon her. Adjustment to all of these changes in her life has been difficult and has led to her heightened anxiety and a sense of being overwhelmed by the demands placed on her.

Diagnostic Evaluation

Axis I: Generalized anxiety disorder, major depressive disorder, in partial remission
Axis II: Deferred
Axis III: Migraine headaches
Axis IV: Problems with primary support group
Axis V: Current GAF = 65

Relevant Clinical Outcome Research

Many studies have demonstrated the benefit of cognitive-behavioral therapy for the treatment of depression and anxiety. This treatment focuses on behavioral assign-ments that increase behaviors associated with feelings of mastery and pleasure, the identification and restructuring of negative automatic thoughts and emotions, and the assessment and potential change of the client's beliefs. Meta-analyses demonstrate that cognitive-behavioral therapy is highly effective for depression (Feldman, 2007; Hollon, Thase, & Markowitz, 2005) and generalized anxiety (Hunot, Churchill, Teixeira, & Silva de Lima, 2007; Mitte, 2005a), with outcomes that surpass the effectiveness of other therapies and create longer-term change relative to drug therapies.

Recommendations and Treatment Goals

Cognitive-behavioral therapy sessions have been initiated with Anna. We have agreed to meet once per week, and the initial treatment goals have been set. Anna wishes to learn strategies to reduce her worry and increase her self-efficacy. She stated that she would prefer to stop taking medications if possible. She was advised to discuss this possibility with her family physician during the course of therapy. Treatment goals include the following:

1. Orientation to the cognitive behavioral model.
2. Provision of psychoeducation.
3. Monitoring of daily activities, including mastery and pleasure.
4. Assessing and working to decrease avoidance (particularly conflict).
5. Communication skills training, possible referral for skills group on assertion.
6. Monitoring of thoughts and restructure dysfunctional beliefs.
7. Worry exposure.
8. Monitoring of suicidal ideation and substance use.
9. Possible referral for parenting skills training.
10. Schema therapy near the later stages of treatment, if appropriate.

Anticipated Factors Affecting Outcome

Anna C is an intelligent, conscientious, and motivated individual. She made her own decision to seek out treatment, when she realized that she was worrying much more than necessary and that her coping skills could be improved. These factors made her an excellent candidate for therapy. On the other hand, she is eager to please and prefers to avoid rather than address negative emotions and difficult situations. These tendencies are likely to appear in the therapeutic relationship and may interfere with progress. If she is able to work on these issues within therapy and transfer this change to other aspects of her life, she may be able to change her core schemas. On a practical level, the many demands of her life may make regular sessions a challenge to maintain.

Keith S. Dobson, PhD, RPsych
Cc: Dr. X

FIGURE 3.4. Treatment efficacy summaries.

Major depressive disorder

Cognitive-behavioral therapy is an effective psychosocial treatment for depression, as well as for preventing relapse (Hollon et al., 2005). The National Institute of Mental Health (NIMH) study (Elkin et al., 1989) provides empirical support for the use of cognitive-behavioral therapy as a first-line treatment for acute episodes of depression. Other research using randomized control trials has determined that the efficacy of cognitive-behavioral therapy is equal to that of pharmacological medications in the short term (Hollon et al., 2005), and with even better long-term results than continued medication (Paykel, 2007).

Panic disorder

Cognitive-behavioral therapy is an empirically supported treatment with good outcome results for panic disorder. For example, research conducted with the Mastery of Your Anxiety and Panic (MAP-3) treatment program indicates that approximately 70–90% of people are panic free at its completion (Barlow & Craske, 2000). Reviews of the literature confirm that the results of cognitive-behavioral therapy for panic disorder are strong and generally long-lasting (Landon & Barlow, 2004; Mitte, 2005b).

Social anxiety disorder

Studies have demonstrated the effectiveness of cognitive-behavioral group therapy (CBGT) compared to supportive group psychotherapy for social anxiety disorder (e.g.,

(continued)

FIGURE 3.4. (*continued*)

Heimberg et al., 1990). Meta-analyses of outcome studies confirm that a combination of exposure and cognitive-behavioral therapy are highly effective in the treatment of social anxiety (Federoff & Taylor, 2001; Rodebaugh, Holaway, & Heimberg, 2004).

Posttraumatic stress disorder

Cognitive-behavioral therapy is an effective treatment for ameliorating symptoms of both acute and chronic posttraumatic stress disorder (PTSD). Exposure therapy and stress inoculation therapy are two main components of cognitive-behavioral therapy, and both are empirically supported methods for the treatment of PTSD. Cognitive-behavioral therapy has been shown to be very effective treatment for female survivors of sexual assaults (e.g., Foa et al., 1999). Reviews confirm that cognitive-behavioral therapy for PTSD is as effective as other methods and has good long-term results (Bisson & Andrew, 2007; Seidler & Wagner, 2006).

Obsessive–compulsive disorder

Cognitive-behavioral psychotherapy, particularly exposure and response prevention, is the psychological treatment of choice for adults with obsessive–compulsive disorder according to the Expert Consensus Treatment Guidelines (March et al., 1997). Clients who complete cognitive-behavioral therapy report a 50–80% reduction in symptoms after 12–20 sessions. Using cognitive-behavioral therapy in conjunction with medication may help prevent relapse once medication has been discontinued (Abramowitz, Taylor, & McKay, 2005).

Generalized anxiety disorder

In a meta-analysis, Borkovec and Whisman (1996) found that cognitive-behavioral therapy for generalized anxiety disorder produces significant improvement that is maintained following the end of treatment. Cognitive-behavioral therapy has also been found to achieve greater improvement than analytic psychotherapy, pill placebo, nondirective therapy, and placebo therapy (Mitte, 2005a).

Specific phobias

Exposure to the feared object or situation is considered to be an essential component of effective treatment for specific phobias. *In vivo* exposure sessions that are structured so that the anxiety drops significantly in sessions have been shown to result in clinically significant improvement in up to 90% of patients (Ost, 1989). Meta-analyses have confirmed the clinical value of cognitive-behavioral therapy for specific phobias (Choy, Fyer, & Lipsitz, 2007).

Anxiety and depression

Many studies have demonstrated the benefit of cognitive-behavioral therapy in treating depression and anxiety (Bandelow, Seidler-Brandler, Becker, Wedekind, & Rüther, 2007; Butler, Chapman, Forman, & Beck, 2006; Hofmann & Smit, 2008). Meta-analyses demonstrate that cognitive-behavioral therapy is highly effective for depression (Feldman, 2007; Hollon et al., 2005) and generalized anxiety (Hunot et al., 2007; Mitte, 2005a), with outcomes that surpass the effectiveness of other therapies and create longer term change relative to drug therapies.

Individualized statements

It is also important to add the following individualized statements for your clients, as appropriate:

• Individuals with comorbid concerns, such as depression or other anxiety disorders, are likely to require either longer treatment or adjunctive therapies.
• Postpartum depression is similar to a clinical depressive episode and is not necessarily treated differently (Bledsoe & Grote, 2006).

Chapter 4

Beginning Treatment

Planning for Therapy and Building Alliance

The assessment and the clinical case formulation have been completed, and you are just beginning to discuss therapy goals with your client. You have considered whether a diagnosis is appropriate, and have provided this information to the client during the assessment feedback. A positive therapeutic alliance is just beginning. If you are fortunate, you have had time to research the most current, empirically supported therapies for the client's presenting problem. Now what? How do you translate the client's hopes into reachable goals? This chapter reviews the steps in treatment planning and goal setting: establishing a contract and enhancing client motivation. We also make suggestions for establishing a positive therapeutic alliance with your client.

Many textbooks, training programs, and workshops focus much of their time and energy on the assessment and formulation components of therapy, and spend much less time on what actually occurs in therapy after the first few sessions. Many students and interns ask the "Now what?" question, and are uncertain how to proceed after completing the most structured and clearly delineated parts of the process. In some respects, this focus on assessment makes sense. Clients referred for treatment typically receive an interview assessment, and many will receive a diagnosis. Not all clients, however, receive all other aspects of treatment. The first step after the assessment and formulation involves treatment planning, goal setting, and developing a therapeutic contract.

Although initial goals are set during the case formulation, they must be developed further during the first few treatment sessions.

We believe that relationship factors are vitally important in psychotherapy. In the most extreme case, a client who is uncomfortable with his or her therapist, or who feels disrespected, may stop attending sessions. A client with a good therapeutic alliance is more likely to engage in the difficult work of change. In the second part of this chapter, we briefly review the relationship factors that affect psychotherapy, particularly cognitive-behavioral interventions. During the early phases of treatment, the therapeutic relationship is new, and the client may not yet feel comfortable or fully trust the therapist. We review some of the "common factors" that affect cognitive-behavioral interventions, in particular, the development of a therapeutic alliance to facilitate change, as well as some of the ways these factors differ with this approach.

TREATMENT PLANNING, GOAL SETTING, AND THE THERAPEUTIC CONTRACT

The case formulation you have developed helps you understand the relationships among the various problems that the client is experiencing. It also assists you with treatment planning and goal setting. The choice of interventions depends only on the client's particular problems, client (and therapist) preferences, availability of different interventions (e.g., virtual reality or some types of *in vivo* exposure may not be readily available), the training and skills level of the therapist, the evidence base for the intended interventions, and other variables (e.g., the urgency of certain problems). Goal setting is a critical part of therapy that may appear to be deceptively simple but is surprisingly difficult for many clients. Indeed, in some ways, you can imagine that the reason the client has come to you is because he or she was unable to master this step on his or her own in the past. Treatment planning is an ongoing process that provides the bridge between the assessment and intervention. Certainly, communication and agreement with the client on formulating and planning the treatment of his or her problems is an intervention in and of itself, and leads directly to goal setting.

Researchers have a number of suggestions about goal setting. For example, it is crucial for the client be involved in, and committed to, both goal setting and the process of working toward his or her goals. Agreeing on goals is a component of the working alliance in therapy, which has been measured with the Working Alliance Inventory (Reddin Long, 2001; Horvath & Greenberg, 1986). The working alliance has been found to be related to outcomes across different types of therapy. Safran and Wallner (1991), for example, found that the perceptions of goal consensus obtained early in therapy (after the third session) are associated with clinical improvements after 20 sessions of cognitive-behavioral therapy for depression. Commitment to goals prior to treatment has been positively related to remission in a 12-session cognitive-behavioral group treatment for bulimia (Mussell et al., 2000). Tryon and Winograd (2002) report a positive relationship between goal consensus and outcome on at least one of the measures used in 68% of the studies they reviewed.

It is difficult to measure goal consensus in most clinical settings. Tryon and Winograd (2001) state that "to maximize the possibility of achieving a positive treatment outcome, therapist and patient should be involved throughout therapy in a process of shared decision making, where goals are frequently discussed and agreed upon" (p. 387). They further state that "patients who achieve better outcomes are those that are actively involved in the patient role, discussing concerns, feelings and goals rather than resisting or passively receiving therapists' suggestions. When patients resist collaborating with therapists, poor outcomes ensue" (p. 388).

Berking, Grosse Holtforth, Jacobi, and Kroner-Herwig (2005) have argued that although goal attainment is an essential measure of the success of psychotherapy and strongly associated with other measures of success, the goals that clients propose are often vague, unrealistic, or not necessarily appropriate or feasible. They used the Bern Inventory of Treatment Goals in their study to formulate cognitive-behavioral therapy goals and to categorized goals that were more or less likely to be attained. They proposed that success with comparatively easy goals early in the course of treatment helps clients build confidence and a sense of self-efficacy, and strengthens the therapeutic alliance. (It is noteworthy that they reported the lowest levels of goal attainment when dealing with sleep problems and resolution of physical pain.)

Explicit agreement on goals may lead to early improvement, whereas the lack of an explicit treatment contract may be related to negative outcomes. For an example of a treatment contract, see Figure 4.1. The development of a treatment contract is an intervention in and of itself (Reddin Long, 2001). Otto, Reilly-Harrington, Kogan, and Winett (2003) discuss the benefits of formal and informal treatment contracts in cognitive-behavioral therapy. *Formal contracts* are defined as explicit agreements between all involved parties that outline the responsibilities for everyone. Agreement is formalized through signatures on a contract. Otto et al. suggest that the benefits of formalized treatment contracts may include improved adherence and motivation. The contract also may help the client provide a clear statement of his or her intentions and goals for change. Otto et al. also suggest that outcomes may be improved with *less* therapist input and *more* input on the part of the client.

This is an agreement for cognitive-behavioral therapy, between _____ , client, and _____ , therapist. This treatment will address the following problem(s):

1. _____   2. _____

3. _____   4. _____

5. _____   6. _____

    I understand that cognitive-behavioral therapy is a type of psychological treatment that focuses on solving current problems. There is no guarantee that this treatment will solve all of my problems, but signing this form reflects my commitment to work towards this goal. I understand that cognitive-behavioral therapy is a treatment that involves a relationship in which the client and therapist work together to solve these goals. It is also a treatment that typically involves assignments between one treatment session and the next. I am aware of these facts, and enter into this treatment of my own free choice.

    I have been advised that this treatment will likely take about _____ sessions. We will review progress towards goals at regular intervals. I am free to ask questions about progress, and to re-set the treatment goals or to stop therapy at any time.

    The information gathered during the assessment and treatment will be held as confidential, within the limits of the law. I understand that the therapist may be forced to release information about me if there is a perception of potential harm to myself or others, if there is a report of child abuse, if there is an investigation by a professional licensing body, or if there is a legal requirement to release information. Otherwise, no information will be released about myself or the treatment without my expressed and informed consent.

    I understand that the therapist deserves to be fairly compensated for providing this treatment. I agree to pay a fee of $_____ per treatment session. I also agree to provide 24 hours notice of any need to revise or cancel an appointment, or pay the agreed to fee for a missed appointment. I agree to discuss with my therapist any significant changes to my financial status, which might affect my ability to continue in treatment.

    This agreement is signed with my free and informed consent. All of my questions have been answered to my satisfaction.

Signed today, _____ , at _____ .

_____   _____
Client   Therapist

FIGURE 4.1. Sample treatment contract.

Just as therapists may recommend but not necessarily adhere to formal case formulations for all clients, the same is true for formal treatment contracts. Informal contracts are much more common in most clinical settings. These contracts are developed between therapist and client through a collaborative process, and may change from session to session as part of regular agenda setting. Generally, the onus is on the therapist to adhere to the overall treatment goals. Unfortunately, therapists tend to become sidetracked more easily without a formal contract. Formal contracts tend to be more common in settings where client "acting-out" behavior is a problem. For example, contingency contracts may be used to enforce consequences for poor attendance or self-harm behavior. The goals of these types of contracts generally are to control client behavior, and are the not the same as the goals in a treatment contract.

Steps in Treatment Planning and Goal Setting

1. Be collaborative, and listen carefully to the client's goals for change. Work with him or her to formulate goals that can lead to possible interventions. Even if you do not necessarily think that some of the goals are critical to the Problem List, it will to help the therapeutic alliance to establish early goals related to the client's wishes. However, if a client's goals are unrelated to the Problem List, then point that out to him or her. Let the client know that he or she is free to work on other goals outside of therapy and that he or she may learn transferable skills that help in doing so. For example, if a client needs financial management skills, or has a legal problem, then it would be appropriate to acknowledge the importance of the goal and help the client to obtain that service elsewhere.

2. If possible, set an early goal that is likely to lead to quick success or a reduction in distress. The act of establishing clear goals often reduces distress, because it provides a therapeutic direction and gives clients a sense that they are doing something about their problems rather than "just talking" about them. For example, when seeing a depressed client, an early goal might include increasing daily activities, such as leaving the house once a day. These goals can lead to early therapeutic activities, such as adding increased structure to the day and obtaining information about possible community activities. These preliminary goals not only help reduce distress but they also enhance motivation for change, increase self-efficacy, and help to establish the therapeutic alliance. They also increase the "buy in" to the cognitive-behavioral model for not only the client but also other individuals who may be involved in the process, including both family members and members of a treatment team who initially may be skeptical about cognitive-behavioral therapy.

3. When setting goals, it is important to establish ways to assess outcome, so that the client knows when outcomes are successful. A helpful method to keep you and your client on topic is to name and set a series of goals, and to assess your client's goal attainment periodically. *Goal attainment scaling* is a fairly simple process, in which you initially name certain goals that are antithetical to the problems developed in the Problem List. For example, if social isolation is a noted problem, developing an active social life might be a goal. You need to establish some benchmarks or concrete criteria for knowing that this goal is being met.

Indeed, goal attainment scaling is most useful when you set some achievable behavioral goals that are obvious when reached by the client (e.g., leaving the house once per day). From time to time, you can revisit the list of goals and see how well you and the client are working toward them. In this respect, goal attainment scaling serves to develop a collaborative set and to keep the treatment focused on both solving problems and developing positive areas of functioning.

4. It can be surprisingly difficult for some clients to set goals that are conducive to cognitive-behavioral interventions. Many clients initially list goals that are vague, ambiguous, or that frequently change or are seemingly unrelated to their problems. Examples include "I want to be happier" or "I need to get a different job ... partner ... life." Some goals may be completely unreachable or beyond the control of the client. Some goals may be reasonable in theory but completely impossible to assess in any reliable or valid way. Frustrated clients often mention changing other people, such as partners, parents, or supervisors! In addition, although cognitive-behavioral therapists are accustomed to working in a future- and goal-oriented manner, some clients are not. Their lives may move primarily from day to day, with little future orientation. Clear and specific goals may be a foreign notion. All of these styles require flexibility and ingenuity on the part of the therapist to aid the therapist–client collaboration to set goals for change. For clients who struggle with goal setting, it is helpful to set very short-term, easily reachable goals. Also bear in mind that learning how to set goals is itself a skill that some people need to learn, so problems in goal setting itself might become a problem to name and work to overcome.

5. Goals can be divided roughly into those that involve the reduction of something negative (e.g., decreased tension and anxiety) or the increase of something positive (e.g., increased skills, pleasure, mastery, and self-efficacy). At least part of your plan should be to increase the positive, with the eventual outcome of decreasing the negative. For example, when working with an angry client, think about interventions that reduce anger, as well as those that increase the amount and quality of positive interpersonal interactions.

6. Goals can also be divided into affective, behavioral, cognitive, interpersonal, and environmental realms. A client may also have other goals (e.g., spiritual or existential ones) that generally are beyond the scope or practice of most cognitive-behavioral clinicians. An affective goal might be to learn emotion regulation skills, so that the client does not react impulsively or become uncontrollably upset. An interpersonal goal might be increased awareness of other people's reactions in certain types of work or social settings. An environmental goal might be something as simple as requesting a change in one's work space to be closer

to other people. Imagine a client who feels left out at work, but whose work space is not in the "line of traffic." A simple request for a change of desk placement can make a significant different in the client's feelings of being left out, particularly if the client sees that reduced contact is not intentional on the part of his or her coworkers.

7. For some goals it is helpful to use an acronym, such as SMART, that provides guidance relative to suitable goals and can be easily recalled. SMART goals are Specific, Measurable, Achievable, Realistic and Relevant, and Time limited (*time limited* refers to the idea that outcomes will be assessed in the near future to reduce procrastination). Any goals can be subjected to a SMART evaluation; however, the SMART model tends to be most suitable for behavioral goals.

8. Goals may also be divided into immediate, short-term, medium-term, or long-term. *Immediate goals* are those that can be set and achieved within a therapy session. For example, if a client is reluctant to practice a new skill outside of session or doubts his or her capacity to do so, then the goal may be set to practice, monitor, and assess outcomes within a single therapy session. *Immediate goals* may include many types of communication, affective or cognitive awareness, interpersonal feedback, and so on. Immediate and short-term goal setting tend to be in the "service" of long-term outcomes. For example, learning improved communication might be a medium-term goal that is an interim step serving the long-term goal to improve relationships with other people.

What If Your Client Does Not "Buy In" to the Model?

Some clients may not agree with setting specific goals or be interested in a cognitive-behavioral model of change. It is important to consider hypothesized reasons behind this lack of "buy in." Possible reasons include the following:

• *Lack of understanding of the model.* The solution for this problem may be as simple as more explanation of the model, particularly as it relates to the client's concerns.

• *Lack of credibility of the model.* Some clients state that the cognitive-behavioral model is "simplistic" or "common sense." Other clients may be convinced that although this therapy may work for others, a straightforward approach cannot help their problems. The best solutions to this problem are likely to combine providing evidence about the success of the model and some early treatment success, personalizing the model to clients' concerns, and listening carefully to clients' feedback.

• *Disagreement about the case formulation.* If your client does not accept the case formulation, stop and understand their perspective. Have you been unclear in expressing the case formulation to the client? Is there some important information you missed or misunderstood? Do you need to do more assessment? Maybe you and the client need to respectfully agree to disagree, even while you begin therapy and try to solve some initial problems. Generally, though, if you and the client do not concur about the major problems or their bases, you need to spend more time at this phase, before plunging into treatment. In the extreme, if you and the client do not agree on the problems to be addressed, or their bases, it may be more appropriate to refer the client to another form of therapy that is more consistent with his or her worldview. For example, if a client believes that his or her anxiety disorder is the result of an unconscious conflict, as a result of having been in some form of psychodynamic therapy in the past, then referring that client to such a therapist may be preferable to battling about the "right" case formulation and optimal treatment.

• *Lack of suitability of the model.* Sometimes the standard model for a given set of problems may not particularly fit the client. At such times, you need to be honest with the client about this issue, and ask him or her to suspend judgment and instead adopt a "Let's see what happens" attitude to therapy. At other times, it is important to be humble and realize that neither you nor cognitive-behavioral therapy can help all clients. Despite good effort, some clients do not benefit. If a client does not experience early success, struggles over time with goal setting, has problems with follow through on homework (see more on this topic below), or continues to be distressed by his or her concerns, then consider a referral to another therapist who uses a different approach.

• *Persistence in asking "why?" questions.* Despite the therapist's best efforts, clients may persist continue to ask questions such as "Why am I having these problems?" or pursue discussion of their early childhood development. The reasons for these discussions might be a natural curiosity to understand their own functioning, previous therapy experience that encouraged such discussion, or avoidance of problem solving and concrete action. Many clients come to therapy expecting to review early childhood experiences, even though the therapist may try to dissuade them from lengthy explorations. Sometimes it is possible to negotiate with the client; for example, you might agree to spend part of the session on a historical topic of interest to the client, and the remainder on present concerns. If you do so, make sure that you cover the current issues first, so that the session is not "hijacked" by what could be a lengthy discussion of a fascinating personal story! Again, if you are able to obtain some early treatment success, you can use this evidence, suggesting to the client that understanding the past is less likely than concrete and specific goal setting and follow through to lead to changes in the present. It is particularly important to identify whether discussion of past issues is a form of avoidant client behavior. Sometimes, talking about issues is easier than confronting problems. In such cases, you need to listen skillfully to the story of the past but reorient the client to current displays of the problem and strategies for change that can be implemented in the short-term future.

> Jenna did a careful and comprehensive assessment of Miriam, a new client who was referred to her cognitive-behavioral practice. Miriam was found to have some fairly apparent core beliefs about the need to please others and to sacrifice her own needs in the service or relationships. These beliefs were related to various interpersonal problems, stressful interactions, and symptoms of anxiety and anger. When Jenna shared this case formulation, Miriam expressed a strong opinion that her beliefs reflected unconscious conflicts that required exploration of her early history. When questioned, Miriam said that this idea had been stated by a previous therapist, and it made sense to her.
>
> Jenna briefly explained the idea of cognitive schemas, and how they are addressed in cognitive-behavioral therapy. She also noted that treatment typically begins with a focus on current issues rather than on the past or on unconscious problems. She acknowledged that other models of therapy focus on these concerns, and offered referral to another therapist. Jenna was careful not to challenge Miriam's beliefs about her own psychological functioning or the existence of unconscious conflicts.
>
> After asking some questions about the cognitive-behavioral model, which Jenna answered in a pragmatic and nondefensive manner, Miriam agreed to begin this type of treatment. Jenna encouraged Miriam to keep her skeptical attitude toward cognitive-behavioral therapy, and to report any serious reservations she might harbor about their work together. They also agreed to reevaluate the credibility of the treatment for Miriam at the end of five sessions, to ensure that Miriam thought the treatment was on the right track.

What If the Client Is Not Motivated to Change?

Our experience is that the typical client who comes for cognitive-behavioral therapy is motivated to solve his or her problems. Problems such as anxiety and depression, which together comprise the most typical problems seen in outpatient mental health settings, are most often distressing to the client and intrinsically unpleasant. It is difficult to imagine someone who is motivated to be anxious or depressed. Even with other problems in which motivation may be more complicated, such as substance use disorders or eating disorders, clients do not present for help unless they want to change some aspect of their functioning.

Our belief is that when most people face problems in their lives, they naturally try to solve these problems. Many people do not need the assistance of a mental health professional to undertake this work, because they have the needed skills or social support to overcome life's obstacles. Humans are a remarkably adept species. That said, sometimes problems are truly overwhelming, or the individual does not have the skills, mental ability, emotional toughness, cognitive flexibility, social support, or motivation to make the desired changes. These individuals have likely failed in past efforts to change, and motivation may be an issue for them.

Motivational interviewing methods have been widely used, researched, and written about in the field of addictions (Miller & Rollnick, 2002; Sobell & Sobell, 2003). These strategies have moved beyond the addictions field, however, and can easily be adapted to a cognitive-behavioral approach. Rather than being viewed as a basic instinct or trait, motivation is viewed as a state that can be influenced by a clinician. *Motivational interviewing* is defined by Sobell and Sobell (2003) as a way of talking and interacting with clients that either avoids or minimizes resistance to change. Miller and Rollnick (2002) point out that it is normal to experience ambivalence about change, and that most people have an "approach–avoidance conflict" with respect to changing. Initially, change may seem like a great idea, but when a client realizes not only the work involved but also all of the consequences of change, his or her desire to follow through with a change plan may wane!

Miller and Rollnick (2002) describe *motivational interviewing* as a method of communication that focuses on the resolution of ambivalence. It is fundamentally collaborative in nature and generally uses basic therapeutic skills, such as therapist provision of support, empathy, and acceptance. Sobell and Sobell (2003) provide a list of "dos" and "don'ts." These ideas include open-ended questions, reflective listening, elicitation of self-motivational statements, and helping clients to provide their own arguments for change. Some of these methods are similar to Socratic questioning (A. T. Beck et al., 1979), in which the therapist asks questions that lead the client to a certain conclusion. In the case of motivational interviewing, these reflective statements and Socratic questions are used to help the client reaffirm his or her reasons for change.

Miller and Rollnick (2002) provide four general principles of motivational interviewing:

1. Express empathy by using acceptance and reflective listening. Let the client know that ambivalence about change is normal.
2. Develop discrepancy. Help the client perceive the discrepancies

between their present state and his or her goals or values. If a client engages in behavior that is highly discrepant with his or her own values, then the situation will very likely lead to discomfort, particularly once the client's awareness of that discrepancy increases.

3. Roll with resistance. Never argue with the client, because the client is then pressed into defending his or her actions. Also, do not impose different perspectives on the client. Rather, help the client become engaged as the primary resource to find his or her own solutions to the problem(s).

4. Support self-efficacy. Therapist confidence in the client's ability to change can help to build the client's confidence. Use cognitive tools to increase the client's belief in his or her abilities. Build on early successes to increase self-efficacy.

Motivational interviewing typically includes using change talk to support and enhance client self-efficacy. *Change talk* includes discussion of the disadvantages of the status quo, the advantages of change, reinforcement of the intention to change, and the therapist's expression of optimism for the client's capacity for change. To this list we would add the importance of reinforcing small changes made early in therapy and the client's intention to change by coming for therapy, and exploring other changes that the client has made in the past. Discussion of past changes might focus on how these changes came about, and highlight evidence that supports the client's capacity to change.

RELATIONSHIP FACTORS WITHIN COGNITIVE-BEHAVIORAL THERAPY

The therapeutic relationship as a major change component of psychotherapy has been extensively studied, written about, and discussed for many years. A comprehensive text and a task force of the American Psychological Association have reviewed the vast literature in this area (Norcross, 2002). The relative importance of the therapeutic relationship has been energetically debated. Some proponents suggest that it accounts for the majority of change, whereas others believe that a positive working alliance between therapist and client is "necessary but insufficient" for change (A. T. Beck et al., 1979).

Throughout the history of cognitive-behavioral therapy, therapist characteristics and relationship qualities that lead to a working alliance have been emphasized. These factors, similar to those in other types of psychotherapy, include warmth, empathy, unconditional positive regard, and respect for the client (cf. Castonguay & Beutler, 2006). To provide effective cognitive-behavioral therapy, it is necessary to have a good therapeutic relationship. A number of items on the Cognitive Therapy Scale (see Appendix A), the most commonly used measure of cognitive-behavioral therapy competence, assess "common factors" rather than the "specific factors" related to cognitive therapy. Understanding the client's internal reality, demonstrating warmth and concern for the client's welfare, and developing a collaborative working alliance are all required for cognitive-behavioral therapies. The *working alliance* has been defined as therapist–client agreement on therapeutic goals and the tasks through which the goals will be achieved, and the formation of a bond between the therapist and the client (Borden, 1979).

For a brief review of the research support in this area, please see Chapter 11, this volume. We now turn to some of the ways these principles can be applied in cognitive-behavioral therapy relationships. We assume that you have had training, supervision, and practice with the development of therapeutic alliances with your clients. In this section, we do not review the common factors or how to develop them in general, but we do discuss how some of them may be used in cognitive-behavioral treatment.

The Role of the Therapist

Clients look to their therapists to be experts in the provision of treatment, as well as to behave in a professional manner, which includes having good professional boundaries and excellent interpersonal skills. Cognitive-behavioral therapists must balance a number of interpersonal demands in their role, remaining sensitive to the needs of their clients.

"Expertise" versus "Equality"

You are an expert on certain matters, which include cognitive-behavioral treatment, normal and abnormal psychological functioning, and specific disorders and problems. When treatment begins, acknowledge your expertise graciously, describing your areas of competence and experience. If a client asks you a question about a treatment matter, answer it to the best of your abilities. If you do not know the answer and it is something that relates to the client's treatment or disorder, it is fine to say so and, if possible, access the information and bring it to the next session. At the same time, having an area of expertise does not mean that you are an expert regarding the client. The client is the expert on his or her own history, psychological functioning, and current concerns. He or she also may have areas of expertise unrelated to treatment, which, if acknowledged, can lead to a relationship of two experts with different skills sets working to solve a set of problems.

The relationship between cognitive-behavioral therapist and client is never one of complete equality, however, because the client is consulting the therapist as an expert and professional. You need to be aware that many clients will view you as powerful and, indeed, your role tends to be more powerful than theirs, particularly when they feel vulnerable and distressed. This role is played out in a number of ways, including the way the client addresses you (e.g., Dr. vs. first name), the setting of the sessions (e.g., formal office vs. community), and the payment arrangements for your work.

As an expert, you are also an educator. When you provide information to your clients, the qualities of a good teacher are important. These include being clear and frequently assessing your clients' understanding of the materials or exercises being discussed. Gear what you say to their language—neither talk down to clients nor use language that they are not likely to understand. Some clients see the provision of scientific articles as a sign of respect; others are overwhelmed by such material. Always remain sensitive to your clients' levels of understanding, education, needs, and interests when teaching concepts or providing information.

"Coping" versus "Mastery"

As a therapist, you often are a model for your clients, either implicitly or explicitly. For example, it is common to utilize role plays and other types of modeling exercises during sessions. When practicing communication or other skills, you are not expected to be an expert in all areas. In fact, it can be unhelpful for you to appear to be "perfect" to your clients. It can be intimidating to clients to make their own attempts at change in the presence of a highly skilled and knowledgeable person. Consequently, clients often learn more from a coping model than from a mastery model. It can be reassuring for clients to see their therapists make mistakes, acknowledge them, and work to improve their own behavior. It can be useful at times to make mistakes deliberately during practice exercises, so that clients have a chance to offer suggestions. If a client gives you feedback on your own performance in the session, it is a sign that he or she feels comfortable doing so, and it is important for you not to become defensive. The ability to learn from mistakes, attempt changes, and take alternative perspectives are all important characteristics to model for your client. Similarly, when you provide feedback or suggestions, frame them as "just an opinion" rather than as definitive answers. Also, encourage your clients to obtain opinions from other people they trust and respect.

Use of Self-Disclosure

Self-disclosure can be an effective tool in cognitive-behavioral therapy. It includes a number of different types of communication that can be roughly broken down into the disclosure of content versus process. Content disclosure includes your response to questions asked by the client (e.g., "How old are you?"; "Do you have any children?"). One useful guideline for self-disclosure is not to answer questions with which you do not feel comfortable, by simply stating that fact ("I'm not comfortable answering that question"). We recommend that you not follow such a statement with another that implies that the client was wrong to ask, or that turns the question back to the client ("Why do you ask?"). Consider the intention of the client, however, who may be attempting to establish your credibility or experience, or simply to make conversation and be polite. It is your responsibility to answer questions regarding your training, background, and experience. Clients are naturally curious about their therapists, and sharing some information can help them see you as a normal human being. In fact, it is virtually impossible not to share information. Clients may view your family photographs in the office, look at the books on your shelves, or form opinions on your clothing or hairstyle!

You also may choose occasionally to disclose problems you have encountered in your life and how you dealt with them. A useful guideline for this type of self-disclosure is that it should always be in the service of treatment and have the interests of the client at its center. If you disclose a personal problem, then it should be one that you have solved and certainly not something that leads a client to be concerned about you or your well-being. Consider the purpose of the disclosure carefully. Will it help to "normalize" the client's concerns? Will it help him or her see you as a person who may struggle with problems at times and use cognitive-behavioral strategies to resolve them? Are the strategies that you used similar to what you are proposing in treatment? For example, one of us (D. D.) sometimes notes that she has had difficulty in the past with public speaking but overcame it through repeated teaching (exposure).

Process-oriented self-disclosure in cognitive-behavioral therapy includes sharing your automatic thoughts or emotional responses, particularly with clients who may have interpersonal problems. This type of disclosure can be invaluable to your clients, because many people seldom receive honest feedback from the people in their lives. For example, a client who appears angry or aggressive may experience interpersonal rejection from others without explanation. It can be extremely helpful to provide feedback, including your own responses during the session. Similarly, the disclosure that you have become sad or worried in response to your client can be very useful information to him or her. Sharing your own automatic thoughts can lead to increased interpersonal understanding for your client. It also models a skill that you are likely to encourage a client to use in his or her life outside of treatment. If you share your reactions, then it is important to frame them as one example of a reaction, rather than as the definitive or the only response the client is likely to receive. Be sure to take personal responsibility for your own reactions; you cannot speak on behalf of how people in general might react to your client.

Use of Metacognition

To use self-disclosure regarding the therapeutic relationship, you must be aware at a *metacognitive* level and use that information during the session. This process means being aware of not only the immediate needs of the client, in terms of the content of what he or she is saying, emotional reactions to the situation, and attention to the strategies used in the session, but also your own reactions. It involves being aware of the nuances of the client's reactions, such as not only what the client says, but also what he or she does not say. Your observation can then be posed as hypotheses to the client, so that he or she can agree, disagree, or simply reflect on the comments. This skill requires the ability to sit back, listen, and observe both the client and yourself (e.g., "Listen with your third ear; watch with your third eye"[1]). It takes time and practice to develop this skill, because the perspective required may be diminished by therapist anxiety, frustration, or merely focusing on the matters at hand.

Use of Affect

One of the "myths" about cognitive-behavioral treatment is that it is dry, technical, and without emotion. Clients, virtually without exception, are distressed and express negative emotions when they begin treatment. Although expression of emotion for its' own sake is not encouraged as an intervention, many emotions are expressed by clients during the course of treatment. Affect is typically triggered by many of the interventions (e.g., exposure) and is required for them to be effective. Therapists may also express their own emotions, including sadness at a client's plight, enthusiasm and excitement at a client's efforts toward change, frustration at lack of progress or effort, and poignant pleasure when the treatment has been successfully completed. Humor

---

[1]With apologies to Theodor Reik (1948).

and irreverence can at times be very helpful, partly to ease tension and partly because levity can provide a different perspective for the client. At times, the activities you may ask a client to engage in may have a genuinely humorous side to them (e.g., touching dirty objects for exposure in obsessive–compulsive disorder; teaching a client to tell jokes in social anxiety disorder). Similarly, if you are genuinely touched by your client's story, it can be very helpful to let him or her know. You may be brought to tears by some clients' situations, such as a history of traumatic abuse. Although it is obviously not helpful for your clients if you begin to sob in therapy, if they see a tear or two on your face, then they are likely to feel more understood.

Encouraging Courage

As therapists, we may lose sight of the difficulty of the tasks that we set for our clients. Clients may have spent much of their lives avoiding situations, people, or certain emotions. In treatment, we ask them not only to become more aware of their problems but also to face them head on. It is natural for clients to hesitate, avoid, and procrastinate. It is crucial to encourage clients to be courageous in their quest for change; without these efforts, change will not occur. As a therapist, you can support change through encouragement, support, and reinforcement of any small change that you see. Remind your client that their efforts will pay off, and regularly point out ways in which they have done so already.

In addition to the role of the therapist, a number of other issues that arise in cognitive-behavioral treatments have an effect on the therapeutic relationship. These include the use of structure, the provision of hope and positive expectations for change, and collaborative empiricism.

Balance between Structure and Flexibility

One of the major differences between cognitive-behavioral treatments and other psychotherapies is the use of structured sessions. We review the typical structure of sessions in the next chapter. Although the structure makes sense, it can be very difficult for therapists to provide focus in sessions, particularly with very distressed, talkative or effusive clients. You may feel that you are being rude and interrupting your clients, particularly when they are upset. Indeed, it is often necessary to interrupt clients gently to refocus the session. Some clients may require clear rather than subtle redirection, such as "we have 10 minutes remaining" or "In order to complete our agenda, we must move on." One of us (D. D.) had a client who tended to respond negatively to ending sessions, commenting that she felt rushed. After discussing several ways to address this concern, we agreed on a "10-minute warning," so that she had a sense of when the session was drawing to a close. Many clients talk freely if they feel comfortable; however, they seldom respond negatively to redirection. Certainly, setting the initial agenda and summarizing at intervals during the session, then again near the end, go a long way in structuring your time together. A practical suggestion is simply to have a clock visible to both therapist and client. The structure of sessions is typically reassuring rather than problematic to clients.

At the same time, it is important to be flexible and responsive to the needs of clients, so that they have opportunities to contribute to the session, provide feedback, and offer their own suggestions. There may be times where it is important not to follow the typical structure, such as during a client's crisis or if there is a problem with the therapeutic alliance. Clients may respond negatively to structure if they feel that you are not attending to their interests or needs. Be attentive to your responses to clients. At times if therapy is not going well or with overly dependent clients, you may be tempted to provide *more* rather than *less* structure, particularly if you are becoming anxious about the outcomes. Resist this urge and discuss clients' reactions to treatment instead. To be flexible also may involve "rolling" with the situation and doing things that you did not expect. If a client suddenly asks to bring a partner to a session for support, or a child, if he or she could not find child care, then certainly consider the request. If it seems reasonable, or if it might be useful, be flexible. One of us (D. D.) once had a client bring her cat with her during a thunderstorm, which led to a different type of session!

Provision of Hope and Positive Expectations for Change

Many clients have doubts about their own ability to change and occasionally have a profound hopelessness about themselves and their own futures. Clients who begin treatment, however, are likely to have at least a small degree of hope for change; otherwise, they would not have initiated the process of therapy. When clients report that they are not at all hopeful, it can be helpful to point this fact out to them as a discrepancy. Building on any hopes a client has, without promoting false or unrealistic hope, can be crucial, particularly in the early stages of treatment. Saying to the client, "I am hopeful for you, because.... Others, similar to you, have made big changes in treatment" or "Feeling hopeless can be a sign of depression rather than a sign that you cannot change" may also begin to instill hope. It may be useful to discuss the client's automatic thoughts about coming for treatment as a further step. Use of these thoughts for cognitive restructuring can lead clients to feel less negativity about the future. Once the client experiences an increase in hope, it is possible to promote a positive expectation for change.

Other cognitive-behavioral strategies may also instill hope and build on positive expectations. These include keeping track of small steps toward change, providing feedback to the clients, and looking at other times in clients' lives when they have shown themselves capable of change or of carefully monitoring their own progress. When clients express discouragement about lack of change, you might go back in their progress notes and read aloud some of their earlier comments or review their initial symptoms or concerns at the time of assessment. Comparing their current status with earlier problems can reassure clients that they are indeed making changes. Obviously, this strategy is only useful if you believe that change has actually occurred.

Promotion of Collaborative Empiricism

Collaborative empiricism (A. T. Beck et al., 1979) means that you and your client work as a team to solve his or her problems and reduce distress. The stage is set for this teamwork when you review the assessment results and clinical case conceptualization, and engage in treatment planning. To promote this approach, it is helpful to be actively curious and question clients' experience and worldview. This curiosity is an expression of interest in the client as a person, and typically helps him or her feel a bond with you. The stance of empiricism involves developing hypotheses, asking questions, and engaging in experimentation—all in service of helping the client. This position forces both of you to be objective and take a perspective that the client typically is likely not to take. Many people do not normally "stand back" and review their thoughts, feelings, and reactions to situations or people. It tends to be "proactive" rather than "reactive," and encourages perspective taking on one's problems, which in and of itself is helpful. It is similar to the metacognitive stance of the therapist that we described earlier.

Collaborative empiricism also involves transparency about the therapy and the therapeutic process. A rationale is typically provided for all interventions, which may include expected outcomes or problems that could arise. The purpose of strategies is discussed at each step of treatment. Clients are actively involved in planning the interventions, and they do all of the work involved outside of the session. The client participates as a "researcher," gathering data from behavioral experiments, thought records, or interpersonal practice assignments. The results are "analyzed" when the client comes back for the next session to discuss outcomes and plan the next strategy. The eventual goal is for the client to learn how to engage in this process independently, but the therapist actively teaches, supports, and guides it during treatment.

Use of the Relationship as a Measure for Change

The sessions in the early phases of cognitive-behavioral therapy are quite structured, and the therapist may tend to be somewhat didactic and use more "formal" methods compared to those in the latter phases of treatment. As the treatment proceeds, the client typically becomes more comfortable with both the therapist and the treatment. The client is familiar with the process and takes a very active role in setting the agenda. It is a sign of comfort and trust if he or she is able to raise concerns, express opinions, and disagree with the therapist. If a therapist comes across as authoritative or defensive, clients are not likely to speak up, but they may "vote with their feet" by not returning or may not speak up again. We have seen therapists who urge their clients to use assertive communication outside the sessions, but who become very uncomfortable when clients are assertive with them. Reinforce clients verbally when they voice their opinions, disagree, or are assertive with you. As therapy nears completion, it is common for the relationship to become more and more egalitarian, and for clients sometimes to converse more with you, rather than raise any problems. If you recognize this pattern of communication, then you might reassess the initial problems, and consider whether more treatment is necessary, or whether the client is ready to "strike out" on his or her own.

At this point early in treatment, you likely have established many of the factors for success, including a flexible case formulation, concrete and specific goals, client motivation, and a positive therapeutic alliance. We review in the next chapter some of the basic skills in cognitive-behavioral therapy.

Chapter 5

Beginning Treatment

Basic Skills

Now what? What do you actually do once treatment begins?
Most cognitive-behavioral treatments include common components, such as structured sessions, assignment of tasks outside
of sessions, psychoeducation, and problem solving. This chapter
reviews the basic skills for beginning treatment once you have
established goals and developed a positive therapeutic alliance
with your client.

In this chapter, we cover the components of treatment included
in most cognitive-behavioral interventions. These components include
orientation to cognitive-behavioral treatment and its session structure,
psychoeducation, and problem solving. All of these processes occur near
the beginning of treatment, although they may recur over the course of
therapy. Another basic intervention of all cognitive-behavioral treatments is the assignment of homework, which tends to occur at the beginning and continue throughout treatment. All of these strategies in and
of themselves may lead to change, as well as ease the transition toward
more formal behavioral and cognitive interventions, which we cover in
Chapters 6–8, this volume.

Prior to discussion of the structure of individual sessions, we briefly
review the typical sequence of overall treatment in cognitive-behavioral
treatment. This sequence is approximate and must be tailored to the individual needs of the client.

SEQUENCING AND LENGTH OF TREATMENT

Treatment manuals are inconsistent with respect to the relative ordering of behavioral and cognitive interventions. Some begin with behavioral interventions (e.g., A. T. Beck et al., 1979), whereas others begin with psychoeducation regarding cognitive distortions and cognitive restructuring (e.g., Antony & Swinson, 2000). Our recommended practice is generally to start with behavioral strategies, then "interweave" cognitive interventions into therapy fairly quickly thereafter. In this way, we obtain objective change in functioning, even as we continue to understand better the client's patterns of thinking, and the optimal ways to intervene with negative thinking. The sequencing of cognitive-behavioral therapy usually proceeds in the following manner, although movement back and forth across the various phases may occur, if necessary:

1. Assessment.
2. Clinical case formulation.
3. Feedback to the client and reformulation, as needed.
4. Goal setting.
5. Psychoeducation.
6. Client monitoring of behaviors and emotions.
7. Behavioral interventions.
8. Client monitoring of cognitions.
9. Cognitive restructuring.
10. Reassessment and discussion of schemas.
11. Schema monitoring (if needed).
12. Schema change therapy (if needed).
13. Relapse prevention, maintenance, and ending therapy.

As noted in Chapters 2 and 3, this volume, assessment and formulation are ongoing processes. Although the preceding order is common, the sequence must be flexible and adapted to each client, according to the clinical case formulation. For example, some clients require minimal psychoeducation but a greater focus on their cognitions. Other clients may respond very well to behavioral interventions and promptly state that they do not require any more help. Still other clients may require the full treatment "package." In some cases, it is necessary to move back and forth among these treatment stages, because the client may initially improve, then suffer a setback that requires more basic interventions. Also, for some problems, a behavioral strategy is necessary and sufficient for change, but for other issues, cognitive interventions are needed. Obviously, behavioral interventions affect cognitions, and cognitive interventions affect behavior. It is extremely difficult to tease apart the effect of the many components of treatment. Your initial formulation may suggest that the client requires schema change treatment; however, these underlying beliefs may gradually start to shift during the early phases of therapy, making this type of treatment shorter or at times even unnecessary.

The average duration of interventions in treatment studies varies but averages between 12 and 16 sessions. The average duration of therapy in clinical practice is much more variable, and ranges from one session to many sessions. Consequently, the interweaving of behavioral and cognitive interventions is crucial, because each reinforces the other. For example, behavioral experiments may be conducted during early, middle, or late phases of therapy. These experiments may not only help the client practice behavior change but also challenge his or her underlying thoughts and beliefs. Consequently, an astute cognitive-behavioral therapist constantly assesses the client's in-session reactions to behavior change experiments and points out discrepancies with the client's identified and expressed beliefs. One of us (D. D.) sees clients with social anxiety and fears regarding public speaking. Early in therapy, she has them plan an experiment in which they talk for 2 minutes about a topic of interest to them. This exposure exercise typically generates anxiety, but most clients are able to rise to the occasion. Following the activity, their predictions about not being able to engage in public speaking are challenged, because obviously they were able to do so! The discrepancy with their typical thoughts is pointed out and alternative predictions for future exercises are proposed.

ORIENTATION AND SESSION STRUCTURE

Although orientation to a theoretical model is not specifically an intervention, it is crucial to the success of treatment. Successful therapy orientation increases the client's "buy in" to the therapeutic model, in the process enhancing his or her motivation, compliance, and willingness to take some of the risks required in therapy. Orientation begins during the initial interview or even before the therapist meets the client. Some clients who come to therapy are already aware of cognitive-behavioral therapy; consequently, they may already have accepted the model to some extent.

Therapy orientation occurs in a number of different ways and varies depending on the needs of the client and the goals of therapy. One of the ways that orientation occurs is through the structure of cognitive-behavioral sessions. The typical format for a cognitive-behavioral therapy session includes the following:

1. A general check-in, including a mood or distress rating and a comment about, or "bridge," from the previous session.
2. A brief review of homework that was assigned, attempted, and completed.
3. A discussion of any pressing issues for the current session.
4. Agenda setting, including the setting of priorities and approximate time allocated for each topic.
5. Discussion and work on each agenda item.
6. Summary of the session's main points.
7. Feedback about the session.
8. Discussion of the overall homework, including anticipation of problems, practice regarding any concerns, and final homework assignment.

It is very common for new therapists to overestimate the amount of work that can possibly be completed in a session, and to find that they have only a few minutes remaining at the end of the session to summarize and plan homework. If homework assignments are rushed, then they are less likely to be collaborative, flexible, and successful. Mentally dividing each session into three "chunks" is helpful—*beginning* the session (items 1 to 3), the *work* of the session (items 4 to 6), and *ending* the session (items 7 to 8). In this way, neither the beginning nor the end of the session receive short shrift, and therapist expectations for the work that can be completed are reduced. In general, a 10–30–10 rule for the minutes allocated for each chunk can also be utilized, assuming a 50-minute session. Thus, in a typical session, you should begin winding down, or moving to the conclusion, about 10 minutes before you actually plan to end the session.

Although the 50-minute therapy hour is a tradition and is often a convenient way to organize our schedules, there may be good reasons to vary the length of sessions at times. Exceptions to the usual length of session can include planned exposure exercises or group interventions. Exposure sessions are frequently longer than 50 minutes, particularly for clients with obsessive–compulsive disorder, posttraumatic stress disorder, or for clients whose anxiety takes longer than 30 minutes to reduce in intensity. When planning an exposure session (see Chapter 6, this volume), it is wise to schedule longer sessions, if possible. Although cognitive-behavioral group sessions typically last 90–120 minutes, the rough division of the sessions into thirds can still be followed. Occasionally, 30-minute sessions may be scheduled for clients nearing the end of therapy, who require only a maintenance session. It also is helpful to consider briefer sessions for clients with concentration or other cognitive problems, particularly near the beginning of therapy. For example, clients with severe depression or psychotic disorders may require shorter but more frequent sessions to promote therapeutic change.

PSYCHOEDUCATION

Psychoeducation is defined as teaching relevant psychological principles and knowledge to the client. This aspect of therapy takes place in a variety of ways, using a variety of formats. The types and extent of methods to impart this information depend on the learning needs of the client. Some types of information are routinely used, whereas others are only used occasionally. Table 5.1 provides a number of considerations, and further suggestions regarding psychoeducation.

Given the veritable explosion of available client information, can be very difficult to separate the "wheat" from the "chaff." We suggest that you not recommend a pamphlet, book, video, or website you have not reviewed, to ensure that the quality and types of information to which you want your client exposed are embodied within that source. Also, we suggest that rather than routinely making the same recommendations to all clients, you should tailor recommendations to each client. In some cases, it may be better simply to give verbal information and not assign any reading.

Norcross et al. (2000) have conveniently provided ratings of the self-help books, autobiographies, movies and Internet resources, and self-help/support groups that are widely available in the United States. This text can help to guide your choices of available materials up to the date of its publication. Remember that many clients are not as interested in reading as most therapists are, and that brief, concise materials are often suitable and sufficient for the purposes of basic psychoeducation. Some clients, however, appreciate direct access to research studies and see the provision of these references as a sign of respect for their intellect. In such cases, discussion of these materials can enhance the therapeutic relationship and provide opportunities for applications to clients' particular situations. It may also be helpful for some clients to conduct their own research and find their own educational materials.

Here are some of the major considerations we recommend when choosing materials:

- How the education, language, and literacy levels of the client match the materials.
- The skills of the client (e.g., computer or library research skills).

- The interests of the client, and his or her desire for more or less information.
- The resources available to the client (e.g., computer or Web access).
- Privacy issues (e.g., if family members are not aware of the problem, then the client may be reluctant to take written materials home).
- The distress level and concentration ability of the client (e.g., high distress and poor concentration impede the client's ability to engage in psychoeducation, so adjust the materials accordingly).
- The quality of the materials (e.g., timeliness of the information, its accuracy, its technical quality, and the consistency of the material's message with the treatment you are trying to develop with the client).

What do we know about the efficacy and benefits of psychoeducation? Although few studies have directly evaluated psychoeducation as a separate component of cognitive-behavioral therapy, many studies have reviewed the efficacy of brief educational interventions and clinical practice guidelines, often recommending information or "bibliotherapy" as a first step in treatment or as a first-line treatment for individuals with mild problems. Numerous self-help manuals, websites, and workbooks that have been developed are included in "stepped" care models for mental health clinical practice guidelines. These models work to match service delivery to client needs and have been used by some health care organizations, such as the National Health Service (NHS) in the United Kingdom.

Most practitioners believe that psychoeducation is helpful above and beyond increasing compliance with interventions. In our experience, the benefits are multifold. Knowledge typically leads to a sense of control over problems, and it begins to shift beliefs. Some clients who come for psychotherapy are convinced that a "biochemical imbalance" has caused their symptoms. Such a belief typically leads to thoughts regarding lack of control and feelings of helplessness. A client who begins to understand some of the precursors and triggers for depressive symptoms *in general*, typically also considers how the information applies to his or her own situations. Benefits of psychoeducation also include clients' sense of relief that their problems have been written about, researched and discussed, leading to feelings of validation, support, and hope. Clients who are exposed to such materials may offer statements such as "I know that I'm not alone," "My problems are more common than I thought," and "Many people improve with this treatment, so I am likely to feel better after this therapy."

Other types of psychoeducation have the benefits of increased knowledge and skills. For example, some of these materials teach the client about the principles of reinforcement, or the potential effect of cognitive change on behavioral outcomes. The onus is on the therapist to determine what type of information might be helpful to the client above and beyond diagnostic, treatment rationale, and research findings. Information on disorders and cognitive-behavioral interventions can be found online and easily printed off for your clients. See Table 5.1 for a list of downloadable resources.

> Kerry was finishing the first session with his new client Natasha. He was describing the cognitive-behavioral model of depression, which was Natasha's major presenting problem. Somewhat surprisingly, Natasha seemed uninterested in this information, and when he asked if she had questions, she declined to ask any. When Kerry offered her some reading materials, she said she was not that interested. Kerry asked whether she ever liked to learn by reading rather than by doing. Natasha clearly expressed an interest in "getting going" and finding out what would work by experience.
>
> Rather than try to force the issue of education, Kerry took note of Natasha's learning style. He tried to ensure that active homework was integrated into every session. He carefully explained the rationale for each assignment to ensure that Natasha could explain why each assignment was important, but he did not emphasize reading materials. He hypothesized that Natasha might also be reluctant to do written homework. This prediction turned out to be largely true; Natasha did not like writing things down on homework forms to bring in to therapy. They did discover, however, that she was fine with the use of a whiteboard during the session and to demonstrate how the homework might be done. In fact, she found the use of diagrams on the whiteboard particularly effective. Over time, she also was able to use written reminders in the form of notes or cue cards. Together, Kerry and Natasha always discussed how to remember and implement each assignment, always respecting Natasha's particular learning style.

HOMEWORK ASSIGNMENT

Homework is an essential component of cognitive-behavioral interventions. The many goals for homework include learning and generalizing change beyond the therapy sessions. The numerous types of homework assignments include reading educational materials, completing Activity Schedules and Dysfunctional Thought Records, conducting behavioral experiments, or practicing communication skills. Clients are generally taught that homework is a necessary component of cognitive-behavioral treatment, without which significant change is unlikely to occur. See Table 5.2 for some suggestions for homework assignment. Generally, successful homework must be developed collaboratively with the client (see Figure 5.1). Further discussion regarding homework for behavioral and cognitive interventions can also be found in Chapters 6–8. Difficulties with homework adherence are discussed in Chapter 10 (see Tables 10.1 and 10.2, this volume).

Contrary to what most cognitive-behavioral therapists say to their clients, homework compliance has not been positively associated with outcome in all studies. Keijsers, Schaap, and Hoogduin (2000) reported a positive outcome in four studies but not in seven other studies. However,

TABLE 5.1. Psychoeducation Considerations

Consider the use of psychoeducational information for this type of material:
- Relative to diagnostic criteria, many clients are quite interested in seeing and discussing the symptoms that constitute a disorder. Only consider using this information if you are confident that the client's symptoms actually meet the criteria.
- Cognitive-behavioral explanations and models for symptom development and maintenance.
- Cognitive-behavioral interventions and their efficacy.
- Principles of behavior change, such as reinforcement, punishment, shaping, and extinction.
- Information regarding clinical practice guidelines for clients' problems. For example the NHS in the United Kingdom publishes evidence-based practice guidelines for a wide variety of mental health problems: *www.nice.org.uk*.
- Related problems that clients may be experiencing, such as sleep disorders, general "stress" and anxiety, and parenting or communication difficulties.

A number of available modalities for psychoeducation include the following:
- Didactic information presented by the therapist in the session.
- Professionally produced pamphlets or brochures. Books, movies, or Internet materials (see Norcross et al., 2000, for examples and ratings).
- Local resources and public presentations.

Useful websites for downloadable brochures for clients:
- *www.cpa.ca/public/yourhealthpsychologyworksfactsheets*: Canadian Psychological Association; fact sheets on many different topics, including evidence-based treatments.
- *www.apa.org*: American Psychological Association; see Psychology Topics.
- *www.adaa.org*: Anxiety Disorders Association of America.
- *www.anxietycanada.ca*: Anxiety Disorders Association of Canada.
- *www.abct.org/mentalhealth/factsheets/?fa=factsheets*: Association for Behavioral and Cognitive Therapies; explore symptoms of disorders and highlight the ways cognitive-behavioral therapists treat them.
- *academyofct.org*: Academy of Cognitive Therapy; see Consumers section.

TABLE 5.2. Tips for Successful Homework

1. Ensure that decisions regarding homework are collaborative rather than decided on by the therapist or the client alone.
2. Leave sufficient time at the end of each session to discuss and develop homework assignments.
3. Ensure that there is a mutual understanding regarding the assignment. It can be helpful to have clients paraphrase their understanding of what the homework is.
4. Provide a good rationale for the homework, so that it is clear how this particular assignment is related to the overall treatment goals.
5. Obtain a commitment on the client's part to complete the homework.
6. The assignment should be specific and clear rather than general (e.g., "Practice eye contact with three different people per day" rather than "Practice nonverbal social skills").
7. Evaluate success by client efforts and homework process rather than outcomes, which is consistent with collaborative empiricism (e.g., if the client practiced eye contact as in item #6, it was successful, independent of whether other people responded positively).
8. Ensure that the client has both the resources (e.g., financial, emotional, motivational) and skills (e.g., literacy, social, knowledge) to complete the homework.
9. Use memory aids, such as homework sheets or the Prescription for Change (see Figure 5.1). Clients may be anxious in session and have good intentions to complete their homework, but they may genuinely forget exactly what they were to do.
10. Have clients predict the likelihood that they will complete the homework. If it is less than approximately 70%, consider changing or simplifying it, or finding a strategy that will increase the chances of completion.
11. Ensure that you ask about the homework during the following session and verbally reinforce homework efforts and completion.
12. Consider assigning yourself homework, so that you can model homework completion. Your homework might include accessing psychoeducational material or finding out information relevant to a client's problems.

Kazantzis and Dattilio (2007) suggest that there are compelling theoretical and empirical grounds to use homework in treatment. A recent, published text is on the use of homework in psychotherapy (Kazantzis & L'Abate, 2007). There is also a recent finding that learning and successful incorporation of cognitive therapy interventions did lead to lower rates of relapse for moderate to severely depressed clients followed up for 1 year after successful treatment (Strunk, DeRubeis, Chiu, & Alvarez, 2007).

PROBLEM-SOLVING INTERVENTIONS

In a sense, all of cognitive-behavioral therapy is solving problems. We help clients who come for treatment to name and define their problem(s) as accurately as possible. We then join with them in a collaborative relationship to determine the methods and order in which to tackle their

Prescription for Change

Homework agreed on:

_____

_____

_____

_____

_____

_____
Dr. Deborah Dobson
_____
Client
Next Appointment (date and time): _____
Phone: (403) xxx-xxxx

FIGURE 5.1. Prescription for Change form.

problems. On the way to solving these problems, we assess for concerns about or deficits in their behaviors, cognitions, and beliefs. If we see these concerns, or if clients appear to have any skills deficits, we provide education and training to help them develop more adaptive skills to employ for both current and future problems. The techniques we use vary, depending on the case formulation for each client, but involve some of the typical interventions we discuss in succeeding chapters (see Chapters 6, 7, and 8) of this volume.

Although cognitive-behavioral therapy uses a general problem-solving format, it is important to recognize that *problem solving* has been defined as a stand-alone treatment format (Chang, D'Zurilla, & Sanna, 2004; D'Zurilla & Nezu, 2006). There is evidence that problem-solving therapy alone can produce significant treatment effects for clients who struggle with depression or chronic health problems, such as cancer. Problem-solving therapy involves a flexible strategy for problem solution that can be adapted to suit different cases. It can also be incorporated into case-formulated cognitive-behavioral therapy in either a more general way or as a specific methodology taught to help clients approach and resolve problems.

In the general problem-solving model, which can be seen in Figure 5.2, the process begins with identification and naming of a specific problem. The problem might be a sign or symptom of a psychological disorder (e.g., avoidance; sleep dysfunction); it might be the occurrence of a psychosocial stressor (e.g., a critical parent or partner, job stress) or an ongoing issue in the client's life (e.g., a child's asthma). When the process begins, therapist and client determine the parameters of the problem (e.g., how often it occurs, how long it lasts, the triggers or onset factors

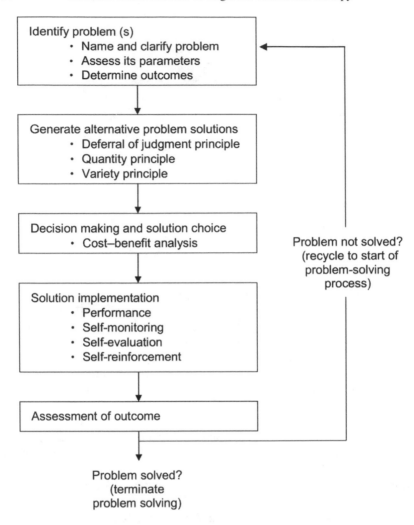

FIGURE 5.2. The general problem-solving model.

for the problem, and how it usually resolves), and develop an assessment strategy for the problem. It is important to understand fully and measure the problem before intervention, so that the outcomes can be assessed.

The second step encourages a problem-solving orientation in which the client is asked to entertain the idea of change and begin to consider how to promote change. The concept of behavioral experimentation is provided, and the client is urged to forgo any past thoughts or feelings about the problem, especially those related to helplessness or passivity. Instead, some possible ways to approach or solve the problem are discussed. In doing so, the client is strongly encouraged not to jump to conclusions about the usefulness of any given strategy, but to defer judgment until as many alternatives as possible are identified. This process of solution generation is often called *brainstorming*. During this step, the therapist encourages the client to use both the quantity (as many as possible) and quality (as many types as possible) principles to generate alternative strategies, and to open up a range of options for discussion. Because some clients struggle with the generation of new ideas, it can be helpful to propose some creative, impractical, or even humorous suggestions as a way to open the client's eyes to possible solutions.

In the third step, a process of cost–benefit analyses is conducted, in which each problem-solving option is evaluated in turn. The key criterion for judging each option is how likely it is, if implemented well, to solve the original problem. Issues such as cost, time, effort, or other considerations need to be taken into account, of course, but even difficult solutions should be considered, if they will more fully resolve the problem. This process is done collaboratively and explicitly with the client, and discussion about how different options might be implemented is often part of this problem-solving step.

A "best" strategy is chosen for the fourth step in this process. This is the optimal strategy that considers current facts, information, and resources of the client, and that is a best guess about the likely outcome of the different options considered in the third step. The precise way to implement the strategy is discussed, including when it will begin, how it will be conducted, for how long, and so forth. If necessary, the client may receive instruction or be taught how to implement the strategy, if he or she is at all uncertain. At times, it may be helpful to practice these strategies during the session. It may also be important to break the overall strategy into a series of smaller subgoals, which can be done in a planned order. Following the choice, the client implements the strategy as homework. In doing so, he or she tries to ensure that the performance matches the expectation and that he or she self-monitors his or her use of the strategy, provides ongoing evaluation of him- or herself as a change agent, and gives him- or herself credit for the efforts made. It should be recognized that even though the client may be doing a wonderful job, the strategy may not change the problem, so the reinforcement here is for effort, not for outcomes. Clients can be encouraged to include their own efforts and problem-solving attempts as a very important part of the outcome.

In the fifth step, client and therapist evaluate the outcome of the problem-solving effort. If the problem was solved, then they can work on the next issue and build on the current success. If the problem was not solved, or was partially solved, or maybe changed somehow during the problem-solving exercise, then therapist and client cycle back to the start of the process, and reevaluate the problem and the strategies that might now be attempted. This step is often easier, because the other solutions generated in the "brainstorming" phase can be re-introduced as possible strategies to consider. The client has also learned from his or her efforts and may have generated new ideas. In our experience, it is not uncommon for a somewhat easier but suboptimal strategy to be chosen the first time through, so it may be appropriate in such cases to discuss the need to try a more difficult but potentially more effective alternative with the client.

As noted earlier, the problem-solving model is a metaphor for cognitive-behavioral therapy in general, and therapists are encouraged to also approach their clients' problems from a generic problem-solving orientation. When working with an individual client, though, we might or might not be explicit about the model itself. Our sense is that the process of going through the steps is the key to solving problems for many clients, and that naming the principles for generating alternative problems, for example, is not necessary for them to use the method. For other clients, though, particularly if they are somewhat disorganized or tend to have relatively poorly developed coping strategies, it may well be worth the time and effort to outline a generic problem-solving model, then work through in a more explicit manner the way the model might be applied to their unique situations.

> Thomas's client Joshua came into a session with a clear issue to discuss. When it was addressed in the session, Joshua said that he had a major problem with his mother-in-law Penny that he did not know how to approach. His mother-in-law was providing some needed care of his young daughter Chloe, because both he and his wife Samantha were working outside of the home. They needed and appreciated the care, and really could not afford to pay for it.
>
> The problem was that Penny was not as careful as Joshua and Samantha would have liked. Just two days before the session, Joshua had come home to find the safety gate to the basement wide open and Chloe perched at the top of the stairs, almost ready to fall. He and Samantha had at other times found kitchen drawers open or objects with which Chloe could have hurt herself left on tables. As a consequence, Joshua came to the session concerned about his daughter, somewhat angry toward his mother-in-law, and unsure how to approach this issue with his wife.
>
> Thomas and Joshua generated the following possible solutions to this situation:
>
> 1. "Firing" the mother-in-law and paying for help.
> 2. Getting rid of anything unsafe and locking the safety gates.

3. Posting a list of rules for the household that everyone had to follow.
4. Having Samantha confront her mother, so that Joshua could "stay out of it."
5. Having a family meeting with the mother-in-law to express concern.
6. Trying to have the mother-in-law appreciate how dangerous her behavior was.

As much as possible, Thomas used questions to help Joshua generate the list of possible problem solutions. Thomas kept a mental note about Joshua's ability to do this task, and how his emotions seemed at times to cloud his judgment.

Having generated the list, they went back over each strategy and looked at its possible advantages or disadvantages and ease of implementation. In the end, they agreed that the best strategy to try was for Joshua first to have a discussion with Samantha, to ensure that they both agreed on the problem and proposed solution. Then, together, the two of them would speak to Penny to try to get her to appreciate the danger that Chloe might be facing, and to get Penny, if possible, to come up with ideas to change her apparent carelessness. They agreed that Joshua would discuss the idea first with Samantha. They could either implement right away, if there was agreement, or Joshua and Thomas could discuss it in the next week's session, if the discussion with Samantha proved problematical.

To conclude this discussion, Thomas took a few minutes to explain to Joshua the problem-solving process that they had just completed. He suggested that this general strategy could be used in a variety of situations, and that he would watch for other, potential situations in which Joshua could practice this idea. Joshua agreed also to watch for similar situations, and they moved on to the next item on the agenda.

Another important note is that the problem-solving model does not prescribe which strategies need to be used. Whatever strategy will ameliorate or solve a problem is acceptable from this framework. In general, the strategies tend to focus on external problems, such as relationships or real-life stressors, or internal problems, such as symptoms or emotional concerns, and some methods are more likely to be used for each class of external versus internal factors (see Table 5.3). At the end of the day, it is really up to you and your client to develop, select, and strategize the optimal method to solve the problems, so the method is highly individualized. Finally, note that not all of the selected strategies need necessarily to be monitored by you, as the therapist. For example, if the client's major problem is financial, then consulting a financial planner may be much more effective than ongoing sessions with a therapist.

Now that we have reviewed the basic cognitive-behavioral skills, as well as general problem-solving strategies, we turn in Chapters 6–8, this volume, to the behavioral and cognitive strategies of treatment. You are likely to find yourself cycling back to the basic skills in circumstances when your clients do not do their homework, when they require psychoeducation about a new problem, or when the therapeutic alliance feels strained. Although the sequencing in this text follows a logical model, it is intended to be flexible, and it is important always to keep the particular needs of clients in mind.

TABLE 5.3. Common Problem-Solving Strategies

Problem-focused coping skills	Emotion-focused coping skills
• Communication skills training	• Cognitive restructuring
• Job finding and interview skills	• Relaxation methods (progressive muscle relaxation, breathing, meditation)
• Parenting or child management	• Structured routine
• Financial education or training	• Positive mental imagery
• Educational upgrading	• Behavioral self-control strategies
• Conflict resolution skills	• Distraction from problems
• Developing social support	• Physical exercise
• Obtaining self-help	• Positive or coping self-statements
• Interpersonal relationship skills	• Sleep hygiene
	• Emotional distancing or perspective taking

THE CASE OF ANNA C, continued (from Chapter 3, this volume)

Following the assessment, Anna C was provided with verbal information regarding her diagnoses of generalized anxiety disorder and major depressive disorder, in partial remission. The rationale for making the diagnoses and criteria for them were discussed. Many clients are anxious when receiving feedback and may not recall the details of the discussion; consequently, written information was provided, using pamphlets from the Academy of Cognitive Therapy website, Consumers section. The clinical case formulation was also reviewed with Anna, along with the typical treatments for these problems. Anna was deferential during this discussion; however, she was encouraged to ask questions, and her opinions regarding the accuracy of the formulation were sought. The overall goals for treatment were reviewed, as well as the steps toward the creation of specific goals. For homework after the first treatment session, she was asked to read the pamphlets. Anna was asked to purchase a therapy binder and insert the handouts in it. Although the general goals for treatment had been discussed during the assessment, the guidelines for goal setting were discussed, including a handout on setting SMART goals (see Chapter 4, this volume). Anna noted that some of her major concerns were ongoing worry, fatigue, and lack of communication with her husband.

During this session and the subsequent one, Anna received orientation regarding the cognitive-behavioral model, which was one of the first treatment goals. It was described as an active therapy to help her solve the problems in her life, and a treatment that the therapist and she would work on together. Anna reacted positively to this information and asked several questions. The therapist set the agenda for the first session, which included the provision of feedback on the assessment, discussion of the formulation, and goals for treatment. Cognitive-behavioral treatment was described, and Anna was given a handout on this approach from the Academy of Cognitive Therapy website. As Anna commented about her fatigue, she was provided with basic information regarding sleep hygiene to review for homework.

Anna reported that she had read all the materials the following week and had tried out some of the recommendations regarding sleep. Anna was surprised that she felt somewhat better, and she noted that she felt slightly hopeful.

Chapter 6

ℬℐ

Behavior Change Elements
in Cognitive-Behavioral Therapy

In this chapter we cover the common behavior change elements included in cognitive-behavioral therapies. In doing so, we recognize that some manual-based cognitive-behavioral approaches offer a session-by-session description of treatment but, by definition, idiographic treatments do not. The strength of clinical case formulation is its flexibility, which can be daunting for new therapists who are accustomed to manuals and structure in their practices. A goal of this chapter is to help you learn to adapt behavior change elements for clients rather than necessarily use manuals applicable to specific diagnoses. For example, a client who presents with anxiety and avoidance is likely to require strategies similar to those for a client with a diagnosable anxiety disorder.

T he behavioral elements of treatment that are relevant to most clients in cognitive behavioral interventions can be divided roughly into two broad categories: (1) behavior change strategies that increase knowledge, skills, and change-enhancing behaviors, and (2) those that decrease avoidance and self-defeating or problematic behaviors. Because there are some areas of overlap between behavioral and cognitive elements of change, the division in this text is by necessity approximate and somewhat artificial. There is an interaction among all components of therapy, which, we hope, results in a therapeutic outcome that is more than the sum of its parts. Researchers attempt to "tease apart" the effective components of therapy to determine the relative efficacy of each one. Clinicians cannot typically predict which strategies will be most effective or useful for an individual client. What works for the average subject in a randomized clinical trial may be ineffective for your own client. Thus, the evidence from randomized trials suggests likely intervention strategies, but the clinical case formulation guides treatment, and helps you to plan the interventions that are likely to be most useful for your client.

BEHAVIORAL INTERVENTIONS TO INCREASE SKILLS AND TO PLAN ACTION

Behavioral interventions to increase skills and to plan action have been mainstays of cognitive-behavioral therapy since its inception. In this chapter, we chose to separate traditional behavioral methods, whose major purposes are to increase reinforcers and decrease aversive consequences, from behavioral activation, whose major purpose is to decrease avoidant patterns of coping. Although there is overlap between these two approaches, they are distinct in the literature, and considerable confusion between them has arisen (Farmer & Chapman, 2008; Lewinsohn, Sullivan, & Grosscup, 1980; Martell et al., 2001).

Traditional Behavioral Methods and Activity Scheduling

Consider traditional behavioral methods for the following:

- Clients with low activity levels.
- Clients who struggle with low motivation and energy, regardless of diagnosis.
- Clients who complain of loss of pleasure, low productivity, and low self-esteem.
- Clients who are depressed (either as a primary or secondary diagnosis).
- Clients who are on disability benefits, with low activity level and decreased self-efficacy.
- Clients with emotional distress resulting from chronic medical conditions or pain (assuming they are medically able to increase their activity).

Behavioral activation methods were primarily developed for the treatment of depression, because most clients who struggle with depressed mood also have decreased reinforcement from their environment. Decreased activity leads to further loss of reinforcement, including loss of pleasure, social support, and social reinforcement. We have seen countless clients who become less active due to depression, anxiety, chronic medical conditions, or pain. Reduced activity usually provides short-term relief from these problems, but usually this behavioral reduction creates many more problems than it solves. These problems include further reduction of mood, loss of self-worth, increased avoidant behavior, increased anxiety about avoided situations, feelings of isolation, and loss of productivity.

Negative coping behaviors can result from reduced behavior, such as increased eating, lack of exercise, or substance abuse. A depressed individual who is home alone during the day typically has an increase, rather than a decrease, in negative, self-derogatory thoughts. An anxious person usually develops increased levels of avoidance. A person with chronic pain often becomes more out of shape, sedentary, and physically disabled. Even though these individuals may be admonished for these patterns by people in their lives, and may be advised to increase their activity levels, they are usually unable to do so without the structure of everyday life activities. They often feel overwhelmed and unable to do the things that previously gave meaning to their lives, which leads to shame and further negative affect. Family burden may also exist, due to other people "picking up the slack" for the person who is at home. Interpersonal and family conflict can be an unfortunate result of this sequence of events.

Since its development by Ferster (1973) and Lewinsohn et al. (1980) as a behavioral treatment of depression, behavioral activation has been used in many ways. The goal of the original treatment was to help people to increase the quantity and quality of positively reinforced behavior, as well as improve coping behaviors to deal more adaptively with negative life situations. This type of approach can be used with clients who have decreased activity and reduced reinforcement, even if they are not clinically depressed. Behavioral strategies may be considered early in therapy, because typical results include improved mood and higher levels of energy. If clients become more engaged in their lives, then it becomes much easier to identify and to work with any skills deficits or negative thinking patterns that become apparent.

It is important in this stage of treatment to differentiate between reduced activity due to low mood, disinterest, and low motivation, and reduced activity due to anxiety and avoidance. The first step to make this distinction, if it has not been done during the assessment, is to assess client activity patterns through self-monitoring. Different forms exist for activity recording, but a straightforward sheet listing the days of the week across the top of the page and the times of day (broken down into morning, afternoon, and evening) down the left side will suffice (see Figure 6.1).

If the client does not like the formality of such a record (which is useful information in its own right), the same information can be collected

Time	Day						
	Monday	Tuesday	Wednesday	Thursday	Friday	Saturday	Sunday
7:00							
8:00							
9:00							
10:00							
11:00							
12:00							
1:00							
2:00							
3:00							
4:00							
5:00							
6:00							
7:00							
8:00							
9:00							
10:00							
11:00							

Note: List your major activity for each hour. If the activity provided a sense of mastery or accomplishment, write **M** beside the description in that box. If the activity provided a sense of pleasure, write **P** beside the description in that box.

FIGURE 6.1. Example of a self-monitoring schedule.

on a piece of paper in a free-form list of major activities. If your client keeps an electronic calendar, this can be printed to examine behavioral patterns. As a final strategy, you can rely on the client's verbal report of behavior, but remember that such reports can be biased by the client's clinical state, or by issues such as social desirability (i.e., the client might tell you what he or she thinks you want to hear).

Guidelines for Behavioral Activation

When beginning behavioral activation, make sure that you start where the client is, not where the client thinks he or she should be. Be very careful to avoid any judgment about the client's level of (in)activity. If the client spends much of the day in bed, in his or her pajamas, it is important that the client feels able to admit to this to you. Some clients are reluctant to talk about their daily activities for fear of disapproval. They often receive "just get over it" messages from other people in their lives, which can lead them to feel inadequate and to have self-derogatory thoughts. Replicating this problematical interpersonal process in therapy is unlikely to lead to positive behavior change.

Differentiate between activities that are simply pleasurable, and those that provide a sense of mastery or success. Some clients struggle to understand this distinction, so use examples from their lives. Examples of primarily pleasurable activities include massage, eating chocolate, watching a television show or reading an escapist novel or magazine (what might be called "mind candy"). Lists of pleasant activities exist, such as the Pleasant Events Schedule (MacPhillamy & Lewinsohn, 1982). Some of these activities may have purposes other than pleasure, such as relaxation or improving concentration. Examples of primarily mastery activities include exercising for 10 minutes, preparing a nutritious lunch, doing a single load of laundry, paying a bill, or completing a therapy assignment. Many activities combine components of both pleasure and mastery, such as phoning a friend, playing with young children, watching an educational television show, or organizing an outing.

Although pleasure and mastery activities are commonly considered and used in behavioral aspects of treatment, bear in mind that other categories of behaviors may also be monitored and scheduled (Farmer & Chapman, 2008). For example, if your case conceptualization makes it clear that social behaviors are important determinants of your client's mood, then you can monitor the frequency of social events in the client's life, and schedule such events to examine the impact of this change on client mood and overall functioning. Indeed, we suspect that behavioral monitoring and scheduling can be used with any class of behaviors.

Create a list of simple, concrete activities with clients. If clients are unable to think of any possible activity they might do, ask them what they have enjoyed in the past. Some clients are able to imagine what might be helpful for someone else, so this question can perhaps lead to ideas about things to try. It can be helpful to organize a list of 10-minute activities that are readily available in the client's home. Be sensitive to possible barriers to the client, such as cost and inconvenience. For example, registration for a discounted gymnasium program located across the city has a very low chance of success. Have the client make small, incremental steps, and record his or her activities until they become more habitual. Build on each prior step. Each step should be slightly more difficult than the client thinks he or she can accomplish, but not so taxing that the client is likely to fail; in this way, completion of any given step is seen by the client as a success. Verbally reinforce the client's efforts and, if possible, have the client make positive statements about his or her efforts. Try to encourage the client to make an internal attribution for the completion of behavioral assignments. Ask the client to assess success by efforts, not outcomes. This guideline applies to all behavior change strategies.

Before you agree to any behavioral assignment, try to ensure that the client has the skills and resources needed to complete the activity. One of us (D. D.) had a client who had avoided completing her tax return since the death of her husband, several years prior to the beginning of therapy. She was unable even to bring out and start to sort materials related to her taxes. When she tried to do so, she became overwhelmed and made predictions about financial ruin. Her grief had not been resolved by prior grief counseling. Another approach clearly was required to resolve her tax problem, which included asking her daughter for assistance and obtaining the services of a tax consultant who offered pro bono services. Once this client was able to start the process and obtain some practical assistance with it, her sense of mastery blossomed and she eventually was able to complete the returns.

For clients with extreme inactivity and symptoms that affect their motivation and energy levels, consider the use of activities that likely help clients increase their chances of success. Clients sometimes state that they will become more active when their motivation and energy increase. They can be advised that motivation and energy are a consequence of behavioral activation rather than a requirement for it. Rather than debate this point, however, use clients' ideas as a chance to engage in a behavioral experiment. Have them design an assignment to see whether they feel more or less energized afterwards.

One option for an early behavioral assignment is to have the client commit to a scheduled activity with a family member or friend, outside of the house. In general, people are more likely to show up for activities if someone else is waiting for them. Collaborate with the client to schedule the therapy appointment in the morning if he or she has trouble at the start of the day. Begin the homework within the session, or have the client plan to do one of the homework activities immediately after the session. Use community resources when they are available, such as self-help groups or leisure programs. In some cases, a day program or clubhouse for people with mental health disorders may be an option. The International Center for Clubhouse Development website (*www.iccd.org/clubhousedirectory.aspx*) provides a list of centers in many countries around the world. These centers can be very helpful to increase daily structure, as well as provide other social benefits, but they are most appropriate for clients with severe or persistent mental disorders. Volunteer work a few hours per week can be very useful for many clients, because it can lead to greater structure, productivity, and self-efficacy.

Contingency contracting can be helpful a client who struggles with inactivity or the completion of a specific task. In this procedure, the client agrees to complete the assignment in exchange for a particular contingency or outcome. The contract may be verbal or written, between you and the client, or between a trusted friend and the client. Self-reward may be a component within the contract, following the completion of prescribed tasks. Use these strategies only when you think the client will be able to exert sufficient control to make them effective. Many inactive people are prone to reward themselves indiscriminately (e.g., with unhealthy foods or large amounts of television), then feel guilty later. Ensure that the reinforcement matches the intensity of the homework assignment itself.

Mastery activities are often more important and useful than pleasurable activities. Although pleasurable activities may temporarily elevate mood, mastery creates not only elevated mood but also improved self-efficacy. The client is more likely to make personal attributions for success and feel a greater sense of control after the completion of a mastery activity. In addition, he or she is likely to have completed a small task that needed to be done, such as paying a bill or making a phone call. Completion of several of these tasks gradually reduces the client's feeling of being overwhelmed.

Reassess progress every week, adding steps and other strategies indicated by the client's case formulation. Few clients require more than 2–3 weeks of behavioral activation to get started, unless they are severely depressed or have a pattern of chronic inactivity. Once you have moved on to other strategies in therapy, ensure that your client continues to be active.

Skills Training and Practice

Many types of skills can be taught within cognitive-behavioral sessions over and above the provision of information during the psychoeducational portion of therapy. Consider skills training for the following:

- Clients who appear to have a skills deficit in an area in which you are able to provide training (e.g., relaxation or communication skills). Communication skills training is one of the most important behavioral elements in a therapist's repertoire of tools (see below).
- Clients who are anxious about their skills and might benefit from added practice, feedback, and generalization to fine-tune skills and improve their confidence.
- Clients who have a skills deficit in an important area related to their referral problem, but for whom you cannot provide training (e.g., client has a driving phobia, with doubts about his or her

skills). Refer for appropriate services, preferably to an instructor who may be sensitive to your client's problems.

- Other commonly taught skills, including relaxation, mindfulness meditation (typically included during relapse prevention, see Chapter 9, this volume), and problem solving (see Chapter 5, this volume).

Communication Skills Training

The terms *communication skill training*, *social skills training*, and *assertiveness training* have been used somewhat interchangeably in treatment manuals and textbooks. These interventions have long histories of research and applications in behavior therapy and are commonly used by most cognitive-behavioral therapists when needed.

Apparent social skills deficits can arise for a number of reasons, and it is important to assess and understand them when they appear. Some clients do lack skills and may not previously have been socialized for the interpersonal situations in which they find themselves. Very commonly, though, clients are able to use good skills in some settings or with some people, but become tongue-tied with certain people, such as authority figures or potential romantic interests, or in public speaking or conflict-ridden situations. Consequently, their major barrier is anxiety or certain types of negative predictions (e.g., "Other people won't like me or will become angry") rather than lack of skill. It is difficult to differentiate between a true skills or interpersonal deficit and anxiety that affects social expression, particularly because clients may present with a combination of these problems.

There is likely little risk (except for the loss of time), and there may be considerable benefit in offering some social skills training and opportunity for practice during sessions. The practice may be used to assess skills further, as well as boost your client's social confidence and experience. Some clients may lack basic skills due to disadvantaged or chaotic backgrounds, severe illness (either mental or physical) during childhood or adolescence, lengthy periods of avoidance, or a lack of "social intelligence" that leads them to be insensitive to some social cues or indirect feedback. In the extreme, some clients may present with clinical problems, such as schizophrenia or Asperger syndrome, that directly affect their ability to process social cues and be socially appropriate. These clients may benefit from basic skills training and practice.

Communication skills training includes the teaching and practice of basic verbal skills, such as how to start conversations, engage in chit-chat or superficial conversations, make topic transitions, and make and respond to requests. This training also includes nonverbal communication skills, such as pacing, rate of speech, modulation of loudness of voice, and the identification and reduction of extraneous or habitual vocal patterns, such as "ums" or "ahs." In addition, nonverbal communication includes tone of voice, which can portray the speaker's affect and intention (e.g., a questioning or blaming tone). Communication skills training may include the use of appropriate body language, such as physical proximity, facial expressiveness, and hand gestures. Many people are relatively unaware of the subtleties of their communication patterns, which often are very habitual and automatic. Table 6.1 lists areas for social skills practice that can be used in either individual or group sessions.

Clients commonly have adequate basic skills but struggle with "more advanced" skills, such as assertive communication and dealing with conflict. Communication with intimate partners may also be a difficult area that may be associated with frightening feelings of vulnerability. These feelings can result in clients' difficulties addressing issues in their relationships.

TABLE 6.1. Social Skills Exercises Inventory

 1. Listening skills—attending and remembering.
 2. Listening skills—topic transitions (keeping the conversation going).
 3. Listening skills—what is paraphrasing?
 4. Selfdisclosure skills—what is appropriate disclosure? What is not?
 5. Flexibility exercises—thinking of different ways to introduce someone, ask someone out for coffee, make a request, and so forth.
 6. Introductions to a group of people—practice remembering names.
 7. Coping with having one's mind going blank in a social setting.
 8. Coping with social silences—practice and time silences.
 9. Talking in front of several people.
10. Awareness of body language.
11. Awareness of tone of voice.
12. Awareness of vocal mannerisms.
13. Making requests of other people.
14. Saying no.
15. Giving and receiving compliments.
16. Giving and receiving criticism.
17. Asking questions in different settings.
18. Dealing with difficult people (e.g., critical, angry, rejecting, blaming).
19. Making telephone calls and leaving messages.
20. Extending invitations, asking someone out on a date.
21. Job interview skills.
22. Doing an activity in front of other people (e.g., writing, eating, dancing).
23. Dealing with conflict.
24. Dealing with passive–aggressive people.
25. Taking emotional risks.
26. Making mistakes on purpose.
27. Accepting imperfection in self and others.
28. Being gracious—practicing tolerance of other people's mistakes.
29. Empathy skills—putting oneself in another person's shoes.

There are relatively few absolute "rights" and "wrongs" regarding good, effective communication. There is considerable variability in social expression across cultures, age groups, and work settings, and no single pattern is inherently better than any other. We have met people who are charming and engaging but have "quirky" social habits. What we may believe as therapists (e.g., "It is important to communicate honestly and directly, and always treat others with respect") may not always be effective in reality.

Similarly, we have known other people who have relatively limited ranges of social skills, or what we might consider poor social skills, but seem to get by just fine in their environment. Unfortunately, in some social situations, it may be aggression rather than assertion that leads the person to obtain attention or to get certain needs met. For example, a customer who complains loudly in a shop may be more likely to be served compared to a respectful, assertive person. We are typically open with our clients, and state that we have certain opinions and values about what constitutes good social skills. We also think that it is wise to get a range of opinions and feedback from others about this topic. One of us (D. D.) has had male clients working in blue-collar settings, such as construction sites, find her suggestions ("I would prefer it if ... ," "I feel hurt when ... ") quite humorous! These men have said that they would be teased mercilessly if they attempted such communication strategies. Therapist and client together are often able to formulate a compromise. At the least, this discussion prompts some reflection and speculation about optimal ways to communicate clients' desires and needs in their environment.

Group settings are extremely helpful for any type of social skills training. If your client lacks basic skills, or clearly might benefit from social practice, consider referral to a social skills or assertiveness training group as an adjunct to individual therapy. Although a therapist can provide feedback, suggestions, and opportunities for practice, other clients in a group context provide multiple sources for all of these aspects of treatment. A number of other benefits to a group include all of the common therapeutic group factors, such as the chance to provide feedback to others, and a sense of not being alone or different from other people. Different types of practice opportunities also may be created in a group, such as role playing in social settings or speaking in front of a number of people. Table 6.2 lists some of the methods for training social skills.

Other skills deficits identified during therapy may relate to problem solving (see Chapter 5, this volume), time management, sleep hygiene, knowledge of nutritious foods, exercise habits, or healthy lifestyle. Most therapists are not experts in all of these areas. If you are confronted with such problems, we generally recommend that you obtain professional

TABLE 6.2. Methods and Strategies for Social Skills Training

1. Use psychoeducational materials (e.g., McKay, Davis, & Fanning, 1995, for general communication skills; Paterson, 2000, for assertive communication).
2. Identify problematic skills through therapist assessment and observation.
3. Offer *specific* verbal feedback to the client, providing concrete examples, preferably those gleaned through direct observation in session.
4. Point out the consequences of the problematic skills (e.g., "I find myself tuning out of the conversation when you avoid eye contact with me"; "I notice that when you are fidgeting with your hands, I become distracted and don't always hear what you are saying").
5. Discuss other options, providing specific suggestions (e.g., "Could you try starting three sentences with the words *I feel* … or *I think* … ?"; "Try pausing and waiting for me to answer following one question").
6. Use video feedback if at all possible. Tape a short sequence in which a problematic behavior is identified and have clients observe themselves. Many clients become quite anxious observing themselves, but very direct, moment-by-moment feedback becomes possible. They are then able to see exactly what you mean and are more likely to be able to change it. Use video feedback for attempted changes as well, to fine-tune and reinforce client efforts. With digital cameras and monitors, it has become relatively easy to access the equipment needed for taping. Assure clients that the information will be deleted after the session, unless they give permission for later research, training, or other use.
7. Use modeling. Differentiate between a mastery and coping model. Clients are likely to react more positively to a therapist who has imperfect skills and is willing to make a mistake or look foolish compared to one who has expert skills. Clients are also more likely to make an effort themselves after observing an inexpert but somewhat competent model. Clients appreciate therapists who take risks in the session; such actions make it easier for them to take risks also.
8. Provide ample but honest positive feedback, as well as specific suggestions for change. It is usually possible to provide some positive and specific feedback, even for clients who are quite offputting socially.
9. Use role-play exercises in different ways, such as having the client take on an "expert" role or the role of someone with social skills very different from his or her own. For example, a very shy, anxious client might feel somewhat liberated when role playing an aggressive, loud person. It is unlikely that the client's behavior will be inappropriate, and it can be interesting to attempt this type of exercise. Switch roles, so that you play the role of the client. Try out different types of responses so that the client can see what the change looks like. Be flexible and approach these exercises with a sense of fun. Create an atmosphere in which your client feels supported and encouraged to take risks.
10. Encourage risk taking and effort rather than perfection. Demonstrate to the client that most people warm up to someone who makes an effort but feel intimidated by experts. A useful exercise may be to identify celebrities whose social skills the client admires, then help him or her determine the reasons for this admiration. Often, it turns out that the admiration is not due to perfect skills, which can lead to a discussion of other positive features that people may have and a broader perspective on the issue of social desirability.
11. Encourage small steps for homework practice. Attempt one skill at a time, and observe and monitor the results. For example: "Practice increased eye contact and smiles to your coworkers on three occasions each day at work this week. Count the number of people who return the smile").
12. Social skills practice provides many opportunities for behavioral experiments, such as the example just described. These experiments not only provide practice in social skills but also the chance to challenge some of the client's thoughts (see Chapter 7, this volume).

materials on the topic, consult with other professionals who may have such expertise, and consider the use of other resources in your community. The world wide web has a veritable cornucopia of ideas about how to manage various behavioral problems. If you use this source, ensure that the authors of the web-based materials are credible.

It did not take Sebastian long to realize that his client Lauren had some organizational skills deficits in her life. Lauren seemed to be unable to set up and to keep a tidy apartment, and she fairly often misplaced materials related to therapy. As a result, progress was slower and more difficult than Sebastian thought it "should" be, and he was somewhat frustrated in the treatment.

At the ninth session, and after Lauren again said she was not able to organize some aspects of the homework assignment, Sebastian took the tack of stepping back from the content of treatment to focus instead on the process of getting homework accomplished. In a nonpunitive way, he pointed out the pattern he had observed, and asked for Lauren's assessment. Lauren agreed that she was chronically disorganized, but she did not know how to deal with this issue. Together, Sebastian and Lauren agreed that this issue was itself a problem, and agreed to devote the session to develop ideas to help Lauren get more organized, so that the other ideas could be put into practice. They developed a series of ideas that Lauren began to implement with at first limited but then growing success over the next few weeks.

By putting this issue on the agenda for discussion, Sebastian found that his frustration decreased. Lauren was somewhat embarrassed at first, but over time she came to appreciate new ways to organize her activities. Most importantly, as these skills became more regular features of her lifestyle, they allowed Lauren to get on and deal with the other pressing issues that had brought her into therapy.

Relaxation Training

Relaxation skills are taught in many different places and settings, ranging from aerobics and yoga classes to stress management programs. Given their ubiquity, we do not discuss these methods in detail. For a good overall source of information on relaxation training, see Davis, Eshelman, and McKay (2000).

Most therapists find it useful to have several different types of relaxation scripts available, such as progressive muscle relaxation, breathing retraining, autogenic relaxation, or visualization exercises. It can be helpful to create for your clients a personalized audiotape that uses strategies planned collaboratively with them, such as combining different types of relaxation strategies. These tapes can be made in session, simply by tapping the script as the client practices the exercise (have the client bring his or her own tape to keep after the session is completed).

Building relaxation into one's lifestyle is helpful and recommended for everyone. Relaxation may be beneficial in the following ways:

- As a personal self-care activity.
- For clients who are easily agitated and have trouble calming themselves.
- As a way to decrease physical tension through progressive muscle relaxation.
- As a way for clients who are always "on the go" to relax and learn to pay attention to internal sensations.
- For clients who are prone to hyperventilation, or those with panic attacks and/or panic disorder who may benefit from breathing retraining.

Although there is limited evidence that relaxation benefits to exposure treatments for anxiety disorders (Antony & Swinson, 2000), most clients appreciate its effects when they are tense or agitated. Our experience is that clients usually report immediate benefits from relaxation; however, they often state that they forget or are unable to use the skills when they are highly anxious. Use of these methods can be increased by visual reminders, frequent practice, and the pairing of relaxation with a regular daily activity, such as practicing immediately before or after taking a shower in the morning. Once relaxation becomes a new habit, its use is more likely to continue, and clients are able to call upon the skills when needed.

You might be surprised if your client has a panic attack during a relaxation session, but people occasionally have counterintuitive responses to relaxation and letting go of control, instead becoming agitated and having a panic attack or a dissociative episode. Anxiety and panic can be triggered by relaxation or meditation in vulnerable clients (Antony & Swinson, 2000; Barlow, 2002). These responses may be due to feelings of loss of control or increased awareness of physical sensations, which a client may perceive as frightening. It is best to treat this experience in a matter-of-fact way and attempt other types of relaxation to help the client in the session. Be sure, though, to use the client's experience as an opportunity to assess the process that led to this reaction. In particular, be sure to identify the triggers (e.g., certain physiological sensations or cognitions) associated with increased anxiety, because these will help you to understand your client better. Also, ensure that relaxation is not used as a safety behavior (see below) to minimize the effects of anxiety during exposure exercises.

BEHAVIORAL INTERVENTIONS
TO DECREASE AVOIDANCE

Effective cognitive-behavioral therapists know how to manage avoidance, both in therapy and in their client's lives. Regardless of the specific problems, it is a natural tendency to avoid distressing emotions, thoughts, memories, sensations or situations. Avoidance is a feature of all the anxiety disorders and avoidant personality disorder, but it also occurs in many other disorders and problems. Clients may procrastinate when they have to deal with a difficult problem at work, ask an attractive person out on a date, apply for a new job, or otherwise make changes in their lives, even if these actions might lead to long-term improvement and positive change. Avoidance not only increases anxiety but it also leads to lower self-esteem and other emotions, such as depressed mood or frustration with oneself. Cognitive-behavioral therapy is a change-oriented approach; consequently, the reduction of avoidance is a central component of virtually all interventions. Two types of behavioral interventions that specifically target avoidant behavior are exposure treatments and behavioral activation.

Exposure Treatments

Exposure-based interventions are among the most studied and effective components of cognitive-behavioral therapy (Barlow, 2002; Farmer & Chapman, 2008; Richard & Lauterbach, 2007). This treatment can be defined simply as exposure to a feared stimulus, with the goals of habituation of physiological anxiety, extinction of fears, and provision of opportunities for new learning to occur. Gradual and systematic exposure over lengthy periods of time can facilitate new learning as the client's avoidance patterns gradually start to dissipate within the exposure session.

Consider exposure treatment for the following:

- Clients who are anxious, regardless of whether they meet diagnostic criteria for an anxiety disorder.
- Clients who are avoiding something that has a negative impact on their lives or functioning (e.g., an activity, situation, person, emotion, or event) due to anxiety or fears.

Although skills training and traditional behavioral activation components of treatment increase exposure in a natural way for most clients, they are not typically planned exposure sessions. It is sometimes possible, however, to combine activation and exposure within a treatment plan. The following excerpt is from a client handout on exposure drafted by one of us (D. D.):

> Exposure treatment means gradually and systematically exposing yourself to situations that create some anxiety. You can then prove to yourself that you can handle these feared situations, as your body learns to become more comfortable. Exposure treatment is extremely important in your recovery and involves taking controlled risks. For exposure treatment to work, you should experience some anxiety— too little won't be enough to put you in your discomfort zone so you can prove your fears wrong. Too much anxiety means that you may not pay attention to what is going on in the situation. If you are too uncomfortable, it may be hard to try the same thing again. Generally, effective exposure involves experiencing anxiety that is around 70 out of 100 on your Subjective Units of Distress Scale. Expect to feel some anxiety. As you become more comfortable with the situation, you can then move on to the next step. Exposure should be structured, planned, and predictable. It must be within your control, not anyone else's.

In the early days of behavior therapy, systematic desensitization combined progressive muscle relaxation with imaginal exposure to a phobic stimulus. Research has demonstrated that the relaxation component is not necessarily beneficial, and that *in vivo* exposure leads to greater benefits than does imaginal exposure (Emmelkamp & Wessels, 1975). *In vivo* exposure, however, is not necessarily practical for some fears or situations; imaginal exposure may be better in some sessions. Possible targets for exposure can include many different stimuli (see Table 6.3).

Planning Effective Exposure Sessions

A crucial element of effective exposure is the provision of a solid rationale to encourage your client to take the risks involved in this strategy. A good therapeutic alliance is absolutely essential for exposure to occur. The completion of the behavioral assessment (see Chapter 2) is required to determine the specific elements of the feared stimulus, which can range from certain thoughts, emotional responses, consequences, or situations. Once the alliance and the targets have both been established, try to find some exposure practices that have a high probability of working, so that the client's "buy in" is increased.

TABLE 6.3. Possible Targets for Exposure Therapy

1. The feared situation(s) in specific phobias.
2. Obsessive thoughts in obsessive–compulsive disorder.
3. Ruminations and worries in generalized anxiety disorder (or for a person who worries a lot).
4. Social "gaffes" or mistakes in social anxiety disorder.
5. Being the center of attention or public speaking in persons with social anxiety and public speaking fears.
6. Imperfection in self or others for clients with perfectionistic traits.
7. Ambiguity or uncertainty for clients with a high need for control.
8. Increased affect for clients who fear loss of emotional control.
9. Angry affect for clients who fear loss of control over anger, or who have anger problems.
10. Physiological sensations (e.g., dizziness, increased heart rate) for clients with panic symptoms.
11. Being far away from sources of help for clients with panic disorder with/without agoraphobia.
12. Being in situations from which escape is difficult for clients with panic disorder with/without agoraphobia or claustrophobia.
13. Feared memories or images for clients with posttraumatic stress disorder.
14. Spending time alone for anxious, dependent clients.

Exposure is most effective when it is performed frequently and continues until the client's anxiety is reduced. The client's focus should be on the feared stimulus, rather than on his or her own reactions, distractions, or other aspects of the environment. Lengthy periods of exposure are generally more effective than briefer ones, and, based upon the results of some studies, "massed practice" has been recommended, particularly for obsessive–compulsive disorder (Foa, Jameson, Turner, & Payne, 1980). Massed practice sessions are those longer (e.g., 90–120 minutes) sessions that occur several times per week.

Most therapists are familiar with the development of *hierarchies*, which are structured, gradually paced steps from stimuli or situations expected to lead to low levels of anxiety, through those that are likely to engender strong anxiety. Exposures to easier stimuli are practiced until the client becomes more comfortable, then the next item on the hierarchy is introduced. It can be difficult for a client accurately to predict his or her anxiety levels for exposure practices. Some clients underestimate the degree of anxiety they will feel as they plan the sessions, and find that they are overwhelmed when exposed to the triggers. They may have a strong urge to flee or to escape the situation. These reactions indicate that the intensity of the situation needs to be reduced somewhat. For exposure to be effective, the anxiety should be moderately intense but not extreme or overwhelming. Clients should expect to feel some discomfort. If anxiety is nonexistent or very low, the exercise will not be helpful. For some fears, modulating the intensity of the stimuli can be very difficult. This problem tends to be particularly true for social fears, because other people's responses are not within a client's control. Early on, plan practices that are as controlled and predictable as possible, then build into the practice, uncertainty or negative reactions on the part of other people.

Although imaginal exposure is more convenient for therapists and can be helpful for some fears or the early stages of some exposure hierarchies, exposure that is performed in the actual situation or its closest approximation is more realistic and credible for most clients. Encourage your clients to practice with a variety of situations, settings, or people to promote generalization. In addition to practice of within-session exposure, clients should be instructed to practice regularly outside of the session as part of their homework. It is helpful for clients to repeat the in-session practice on their own using imaginal or *in vivo* exposure. Most clients feel more comfortable when they practice in the therapist's office, so independent homework practice can boost their confidence in themselves. Suggest to clients that they practice either the same or a slightly easier situation on their own to avoid heightened anxiety. Have clients record their practices and progress, so that they can review them regularly. Positive coping thoughts help to counter anxious automatic thoughts.

A critical feature of exposure therapy is the client's interpretation of that exposure. Ideally, you will be able to have clients recognize that they can learn through exposure that the situations they have avoided are not as scary, unpredictable, or out of control as they might have imagined. Also, we hope clients learn that they can cope with situations they previously avoided and, consequently, increase their sense of self-efficacy. If you have clients articulate these thoughts in therapy, then practice them by themselves as they engage in assigned exposure, their self-talk will likely become more consistent, with a generally more effective approach to difficult situations and stimuli.

Therapists use exposure therapy far less than the empirical literature suggests it should be used. Freiheit, Vye, Swan, and Cady (2004) surveyed doctoral-level psychologists who regularly treated clients with anxiety disorders about their approaches. Most of the respondents (71%) identified themselves as having a cognitive-behavioral orientation. For treatment of panic disorder, 71% of cognitive-behavioral therapists reported the use of cognitive restructuring and relaxation, whereas only 12% used interoceptive exposure. For social anxiety disorder, 69% used cognitive restructuring and 59% used relaxation training, whereas only 31% used self-directed *in vivo* exposure, and 7% and 1% used therapist-directed and group exposure, respectively. Fully 26% of sample participants reported that they never used exposure and response prevention for obsessive–compulsive disorder. These results suggest that although therapists may be aware of the empirical support and treatment recommendations for anxiety disorders, they choose to use strategies other than exposure. Hembree and Cahill (2007) have reviewed the problems with the dissemination of exposure treatments, as well as other obstacles to their use.

Therapists do not regularly employ exposure methods for a number of reasons. These include therapist anxiety, particularly with highly anxious clients or those with posttraumatic stress disorder. This anxiety typically includes a negative prediction that exposure might retraumatize the client or make the symptoms worse. It can be easy for therapists to avoid this treatment, especially if the client is reluctant to face his or her fears. Be aware of your own cognitions as you begin to do exposure treatment, and counter negative predictions with a "wait and see" attitude. You can model a good evidence-based approach to exposure with your client as you begin this work. Having had some successes with this approach, you will likely find yourself using it with more confidence and less reticence as time goes by.

Exposure often takes more time and creativity than other components of treatment, because stimuli have to be gathered or situations must be re-created. We have both scoured the shoreline, collecting insects of different sizes; have been on the lookout for movies involving copious amounts of vomit or blood, or have gone shopping for life-like renditions of rodents! *In vivo* exposure can involve anything from having your client observe you receiving a needle in a blood donor clinic (done by K. S. D.) prior to his or her own injection (for blood–illness–injection phobia) to repeatedly riding in elevators (specific phobia), to spinning in chairs (interoceptive exposure). Exposure sessions can take therapists beyond their offices and their own "comfort zones."

Practical problems can arise in exposure therapy. Therapist-guided exposure can be time-consuming and inconvenient, because it may involve activities such as traveling to an airport, riding on public transportation systems, or going to a shopping center. If you work in a private practice and charge your client for the service, costs can be high for the client or whoever funds treatment. Consequently, the use of additional resources can be very helpful and cost-effective. A trusted partner or friend of the client can be incorporated into the practices. This person can be invited to attend a psychoeducational and planning session with the client. Other professionals may be used in some circumstances, although, again, it is critical that they understand the principles of effective exposure. We have sometimes used the services of other staff if a client was admitted to a hospital or seen by other members of an interdisciplinary team. Students and other trainees can easily be incorporated into the treatment, and they also gain excellent training experiences through *in vivo* exposure practice.

It is important to be clear with clients about the purpose of any exposure sessions that take place outside your office, and to discuss appropriate therapeutic boundaries with them. Some clients confuse the therapeutic purpose of an exposure session, for example, going to a coffee shop, with a social purpose. Talk with your client before you go to such settings about appropriate topics for discussion in public places, so that clients do not disclose personal information that others may overhear, or ask you about personal issues you do not want to share. You might role-play what you and the client should say if you encounter someone whom either of you know. Decide how you will handle paying for amenities, such as bus tickets or coffee.

Be cautious in some aspects of preparing for out-of-office exposure sessions. We generally recommend that you do not drive together to the exposure site. Plan to meet there, or use public transit, if that is more convenient. Take a cellular phone with you in case of any unexpected concerns, and leave contact information with your office receptionist or other staff person. Nowhere are these concerns more relevant than if you plan a visit to your client's home. It is wise to be cautious regarding unaccompanied house visits, even if you know the client quite well. Again, ensure that the client understands that this is not a social visit, but a treatment session being conducted in his or her home. Anticipate any problems that might arise, so that any discomfort or problems can be avoided.

Minimizing Factors That Inhibit Successful Exposure Therapy

When you introduce the concept of exposure, clients may comment that they have already attempted exposure on their own, and that it has not been helpful. Ask some questions about what clients have attempted to see whether you can determine why they were unsuccessful. There are many ways in which clients inadvertently reduce the efficacy of exposure, without awareness that what they are doing actually obstructs their recovery. Even as you support their initiative and effort, you can provide some education about how you conduct exposure, and how it differs from their past efforts.

Most cognitive-behavioral therapists are aware of the anxiety reduction function of mental rituals and/or compulsive behaviors in obsessive–compulsive disorder. Exposure and response prevention are the most commonly recommended psychological treatments for this disorder. Clients are instructed to avoid mental or behavioral compulsions that serve to reduce anxiety while they expose themselves to obsessive thoughts. The concept of response prevention has not been promoted for other anxiety problems, yet most anxious clients typically have mental or behavioral habits that are functionally similar to compulsions, and serve to decrease their anxiety and minimize the effectiveness of exposure. For example, if exposure to social situations were all that is needed to treat social anxiety, then it would not exist in the first place, because virtually all people have ample opportunities for social exposure during their school years!

Salkovskis, Clark, and Gelder (1996) coined the term *neurotic paradox* to describe the fact that people with anxiety disorders do not necessarily benefit from repeated experiences of being unharmed in the situations they face. Many clients have developed numerous actions, inactions, attentional processes, or attributional styles that inadvertently neutralize the effects of exposure or even incorporate in-session experiences into their dysfunctional belief systems.

Anxiety neutralization and maintenance, even with exposure, can take place in a variety of ways, including subtle avoidance, safety behaviors, and self- or anxiety-focused attention. Gelder (1997) categorized these behaviors as avoidance, escape, and subtle avoidance (usually within the situation). People may perform these types of behaviors before, during, or following an exposure practice. Conceptually, these "maintenance" behaviors have the same function and are the behavioral equivalent of *defense mechanisms* in psychodynamic theory, which are defined as unconscious processes used to escape anxiety. The purpose of any maintenance factors is temporarily to reduce anxiety, generally inadvertently making treatment less effective. However, just as "stripping away" defenses would likely lead to overwhelming anxiety for the client, it is not typically feasible or advisable to eliminate neutralization responses completely without planning.

Of the various maintenance factors, safety behaviors have received the most research attention (e.g., Wells et al., 1995). *Safety behaviors* are either mental or physical activities performed to reduce anxiety in an anxiety-provoking situation. For example, a socially anxious client might wear sunglasses to avoid eye contact. A person who is afraid of a panic disorder might carry anxiolytic medications, even if he or she has no real intention to use them. Such actions typically have negative consequences, including increased focus on anxiety, prevention of new learning, and prevention of true involvement in the exposure practice. Consequently, *anxiety neutralization* or *maintenance factors* can be defined broadly as any factors that minimize the effects of exposure. They are usually performed automatically and habitually, and may include affective, cognitive, and behavioral factors. For a conceptual model of the interaction between exposure and anxiety maintenance factors, see Figure 6.2.

Examples of these maintenance factors vary from client to client and

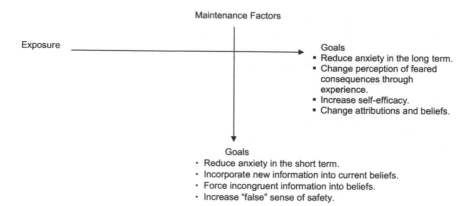

FIGURE 6.2. Exposure and anxiety maintenance factors.

disorder to disorder. They may include anticipatory behaviors (e.g., drinking alcohol prior to attending a social function, taking Ativan before an exposure session), in-session safety behaviors or actions following a session (e.g., checking to ensure that one did not make a mistake or washing one's hands following exposure). Because these actions typically are quite automatic and the client thinks of them as helpful rather than harmful, they can be difficult to identify and to reduce. They are probably crucial to change, however; the likelihood of improvement is reduced if they are not identified, reduced, and eventually eliminated.

Examples of subtle avoidance strategies that should not be used during the exposure include the following:

- Use of alcohol or drugs to reduce affective arousal (prescribed or unprescribed).
- Distraction.
- Internal avoidance (e.g., daydreaming, "tuning out").
- Sitting near exits, knowing the location of all exits or bathrooms.
- Avoiding eye contact or conversation.
- Wearing plain clothes to avoid calling attention to oneself.
- Going only to "safe" places, or at "safe" times of the day.
- Telling oneself that decontamination can take place after the exposure session.
- Reassuring oneself that exposure is OK, because the therapist said so, and the therapist would not put the client in a "dangerous" situation.
- Telling oneself that the therapist's materials for exposure are "safer" or "cleaner than average," so risk is minimized.

It is important that clients grasp the effects of these subtle patterns, so that they can identify them on their own. It is often helpful to reduce these behaviors systematically in a gradual fashion, building their reduction into the exposure. Many clients are overwhelmed with the immediate reduction of all avoidance patterns.

> Alishia had been working with Carl regarding his depression and social anxiety over a period of weeks. Carl was beginning to be more active, but he had placed a number of restrictions on his behavior, due to the perception of risk, danger, and potential embarrassment. Alishia was able to help Carl identify some of his thoughts about social situations, and the role of safety behaviors in maintaining this anxiety. Together they agreed that eliminating safety behaviors would be a way to test out these predictions. They developed a list of these behaviors, which included shopping on certain days, avoiding busy shopping malls, wearing darker and loose-fitting clothes, being quiet at work and in group situations, not asking that errors be corrected, pretending not to be home if the phone rings or if someone comes to the door, and avoiding public washrooms. Over time, and at a pace that Carl was willing to accept, they began to test out Carl's ideas, and to eliminate these safety behaviors. Alishia and Carl both knew they were making progress when Carl went home to another city for a holiday, wore new, well-fitting clothes the whole weekend, and openly disagreed with his mother over a difference of opinion on a political topic.

The choice to use deliberate avoidant strategies with your clients in the short term may be called reliance on "crutches," which are described as methods to be used only if absolutely necessary to help clients feel more in control in the short term. A planned, temporary "time-out" is an example of such a crutch. Calling a confidante when one feels overwhelmed is another crutch. For example, a client with agoraphobia may go to a shopping center and experience panic symptoms that do not abate. Rather than leave the situation completely, the client could take a brief "time-out" and sit on a couch in the mall. Or the client might call his or her confidante and talk about the situation. Once the anxiety reduces slightly, the client potentially can then reenter the situation, or at least reevaluate the commitment to this exposure task while not in an anxious state. It is better to use a "crutch" than to leave the situation. Just as crutches are used only temporarily for broken and healing limbs, psychological crutches are meant to be used while the client is building resolve and confidence. The permanent use of crutches obviously is not recommended. For more suggestions on reducing avoidance and helping clients maintain gains from exposure therapy, see Table 6.4.

TABLE 6.4. Methods to Minimize Avoidance and Maintain Gains from Exposure Therapy

1. Identification of major maintenance factors through functional analysis.
2. Therapist vigilance and close observation. Maintenance factors may be subtle and automatic for your client.
3. Client education and assistance with identification. Help your client to become aware of avoidance and understand its function.
4. Partner/family assistance in identification. Help your client's significant others to develop awareness and understanding about how they can help to minimize avoidance (with your client's consent and collaboration).
5. Differentiate between *coping* with anxiety and *avoidance* of anxiety.
6. Identify outs versus crutches. *Outs* lead to increased avoidance and are harmful in the long run, whereas *crutches* gradually help the client to decrease avoidance, with some assistance along the way. One way to differentiate between outs and crutches is that the former help the client to avoid a situation and the latter help to get him or her into the situation.
7. Gradually and systematically reduce maintenance factors in collaboration with the client, as he or she is able to tolerate this reduction.
8. Gradually help the client learn to tolerate anxiety. Anxiety tolerance is often an important part of exposure.
9. Use the therapeutic relationship. Enhance both trust in you and in the approach itself.
10. Ensure that the client attributes success to his or her efforts rather than to outside factors or to your efforts or presence.
11. Assess and modify the client's beliefs about personal efficacy and his or her ability to cope.
12. Assess and modify the client's beliefs about specific danger. Restructure these beliefs through typical techniques, such as systematic data gathering with regard to feared outcomes.
13. Repeat exposure, and have the client practice more than you think is necessary.
14. Encourage perspective taking and use humor where possible and appropriate.
15. Use relapse prevention near the end of therapy. For example, set future goals, predict setbacks, predict and overcome avoidant strategies, and space follow-up or "tune-up" sessions over longer and longer intervals.

BEHAVIORAL ACTIVATION

"Third-Wave" Behavioral Activation

"Third-wave" behavioral activation (Martell et al., 2001) takes a contextual approach to depression and suggests that avoidance works to maintain depressed mood. This explanation is similar to the approach of Lewinsohn (1980), discussed earlier, and there is overlap between these two approaches. The third-wave approach, however, primarily concerns the function or process of depressive behavior rather than its form or content. Martell et al. clearly state that an increase in pleasurable activities is *not* a goal for this approach. Just as avoidance maintains anxiety, avoidant coping patterns maintain depressed mood and some of the other symptoms and consequences of depression. Third-wave behavioral activation targets avoidant coping as a primary problem in depression. Martell et al. work to understand contingencies that maintain depression, then share this analysis with the client. Third-wave behavioral activation works from the "outside-in" rather than the "inside-out." It is completely contextual, and the client is encouraged to become more deliberately active in spite of how he or she is feeling. Just as the function of behaviors is addressed, the function rather than the content of thoughts is addressed as well (see Chapter 7, this volume).

Consider behavioral activation for the following:

- Clients struggling with depressed mood.
- Clients with avoidant behavior patterns.
- Clients who procrastinate or appear not to approach problems in their lives.

In our opinion, this simple but elegant approach can be applied to avoidance in general. The first step in behavioral activation is to conduct a functional analysis to determine the client's avoidance patterns. Some of the strategies used in this approach have already been covered. They include the client's use of a detailed activity chart, and completion of mastery and pleasure ratings; the encouragement of increased general activity levels; and minimization of avoidance. Specific interventions that are particularly useful are the identification and analysis of TRAP (trigger, response, avoidance pattern) and TRAC (trigger, response, alternative coping) model (Martell et al., 2001; see Figure 6.3). This strategy involves identification of the triggers for avoidance and delineation of its consequences, prior to naming and practicing behavioral alternatives to avoidance.

A FINAL COMMENT REGARDING SOCIAL CONTEXT

Many of our clients live in difficult circumstances and have had unfortunate, sometimes tragic events in their histories. It is important to be realistic about our interventions and remember that no amount of individual behavioral activation, exposure, or skills training can change their histories. Our hope is that these clients will become better equipped to change their present and future circumstances. If they are able to minimize their avoidance, reduce symptoms and problematic behaviors, as well as increase their skills level in different areas, we hope that they will be better able to improve their lives and have a positive influence on the people around them.

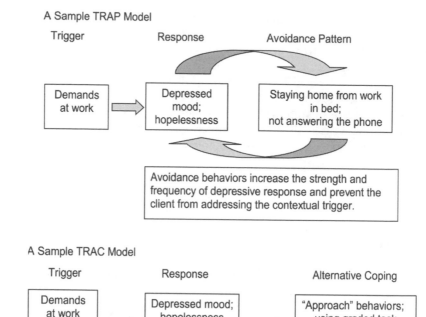

FIGURE 6.3. TRAPS and TRACS models.

The Case of Anna C, continued

Following the orientation and psychoeducation for Anna C, the therapist spent several sessions reviewing her daily activities and determining the relationship between her behavior, thoughts, and mood. Because the overall model had been discussed previously, the therapist took frequent opportunities to point out the connections between not only avoidance and negative mood, but also approach and positive mood, and increased self-efficacy. Anna noted that she was starting to look forward to coming to sessions. She was asked to monitor her activities and provide mastery and pleasure ratings, using the form in Figure 6.1. Her tendency to engage in activities for other people was noted, as was her difficulty with saying "no." She spontaneously reported some of her automatic thoughts in session, such as "Luka would become angry with me if I wasn't at home when he arrived" or "My mother might feel abandoned if I didn't take her for treatment." The therapist emphasized how these predictions might lead Anna to neglect her own needs and affect her behaviors but did not begin formal cognitive restructuring.

After activity scheduling, Anna was encouraged to consider her own needs for self-care in conjunction with others. The therapist discussed assertive communication, emphasizing the relationship between assertive beliefs and behavior. Problem-solving steps were used to "brainstorm" possible strategies, which were then practiced within the session as role plays. The therapist participated in the role play, first as Anna, demonstrating coping skills, then as Anna's partner. Several different versions of assertive skills were practiced, and the therapist noted that there is no single, "right" way to communicate with others. Reading materials on assertive communication skills (from Paterson, 2000) were provided as homework, and Anna was encouraged to practice three different types of specific skills during the week.

Later on in therapy, Anna began to be aware of how her worrying interfered with her ability to solve problems. She had been under the impression that worrying was a positive attribute that showed she cared about others and was a responsible mother. A hierarchy of worries was established, and worry exposure was begun. Initially, Anna was asked to develop a written script for a homework exercise regarding her fears about her son's asthma attacks. She read this script aloud four times during the next session, and the therapist audiotaped the reading. Anna listened to the tape daily over the next week and reported much lower anxiety levels regarding this specific worry in the next session. Anna spontaneously noted that she also had been more proactive in dealing with her son's asthma. She had made an appointment with a respirologist and had contacted the local branch of the Allergy and Asthma Association. She had previously avoided both of these activities, for fear of what she might find out.

Chapter 7

Cognitive Restructuring Interventions

Clients may come for treatment with the knowledge that their thinking is negative or pessimistic. These thoughts may be so "powerful" that they feel overwhelmed and unable to respond to them. Often these thoughts seem "true" to clients, so there does not seem to be any effective way to counter them. In this chapter we discuss some common strategies to help clients develop effective ways to recognize and respond to these problematical cognitions. First, we describe some of the ways you can help your clients to recognize negative thinking, and some methods for collecting this information. We provide a framework for differentiating among different types of thoughts, and we suggest some effective strategies for working with such thoughts, which we generally refer to as *cognitive restructuring*. We end the chapter with some of the common stumbling blocks that you may face in doing this work, to help you problem-solve your own possible difficulties.

Before describing how to identify and work with negative thoughts, we want to underscore the general point we introduced in Chapter 6, this volume, which is that the major goal of practical cognitive-behavioral therapy is to help clients resolve their problems. In some instances, behavioral interventions on their own lead to a significant reduction of the problems. At times, treatment may be complete, following the behavioral interventions alone. Cognitive change may occur without specific cognitive interventions. Adopt a practical attitude, particularly if your setting focuses on short-term interventions. For example, the provision of new information can significantly shift the way that clients conceptualize their own problems. At times, the fact that a conceptualization can be provided encourages a more active orientation to solving problems. We also know that behavior change techniques do not just change behavior. Clients are active observers of their own behavior, and they draw conclusions about what they see themselves doing. A male client who was afraid of social situations but now sees that he is approaching other people cannot help but recognize that his thoughts about these situations have changed. The previously depressed and hopeless client who is now reengaged in her life and trying to solve her problems cannot help but notice that she has changed her fundamental attitude toward her future self. In most cases, you need to track these cognitive changes and help clients note that these changes are occurring in support of the behavior change strategies they have initiated. In turn, awareness of the cognitive changes is likely to help maintain and enhance further behavior change.

In most cases, though, we recognize that your clients have negative thoughts that not only reflect but also actually perpetuate their problems. In these cases, we believe that you assist your clients by exposing the linkages between their thoughts, behaviors, and emotions. Such clients benefit from education about these linkages, and from strategies that directly modify these cognitions. These strategies are the focus of this chapter.

Consider cognitive restructuring for the following:

- For most clients.
- Clients with significant emotional distress or dysfunctional behavior.
- Clients with evidence of cognitive distortions.
- Clients who demonstrate resistance to more direct behavioral change methods.

IDENTIFICATION OF NEGATIVE THOUGHTS

Before you can help clients to change dysfunctional thoughts, you need to help them become aware of their thoughts and report these experiences to you. At a general level, you are encouraging them to step back from their immediate experience and to instead introspect or reflect on their experience. This act of metacognition (Wells, 2002) is itself a skill that needs training and practice. Some clients are quite "psychologically minded" and understand these ideas fairly quickly, whereas others struggle with some of these notions and exercises. Indeed, some clients come to therapy ready and able to engage in these interventions, whereas others need practice to become even moderately adept. We encourage you to anticipate individual differences and ready to respond to your clients' abilities and skills levels. The language you use to teach your clients may be modified to ensure that they understand or do not react negatively. Some clients may object to terms such as *dysfunctional* or *distorted thoughts*. The onus is on the therapist to find substitutions that have the same meaning but are more palatable to clients. For example, we may use the phrase "thoughts that make us feel bad" or "thoughts that lead to negative emotions."

A good way to assess your clients' abilities to engage in metacognition is to wait for a situation to emerge, early in therapy, in which you realize that clients' thoughts are affecting how they feel and react. You can use the example and describe a basic version of the cognitive-behavioral mediational model, by identifying the situation–thought–response chain. You can ask the client whether he or she understands how the thought led to the emotional or behavioral response. If the response is positive, you can ask the client to describe the sequence in his or her own terms, so that you can evaluate his or her understanding. Alternatively, you might ask the client to describe comparable situation that demonstrates the same principle. If the response is negative, you can rephrase the explanation, use another situation that has arisen in therapy, or use yet another hypothetical situation to teach the skill of metacognition.

Once you have established with the client that there is a linkage between his or her thoughts in different situations, and responses to that situation, you can encourage him or her to start to pay attention to similar response patterns. You may make an informal request early in treatment that the client become more aware of these thought patterns. If you do so, be sure to follow up with the client in the next session. Ask for a description of the situation–thought–response process, and ensure that the client understands this pattern. If possible, you might draw out this process, as in Figure 7.1. Writing out the process helps the client to see his or her response as more abstract than when he or she is in the middle of the situation. This exercise often leads to a helpful "distance" from the reactions. It also allows you to talk to the client about the process to determine his or her ability to think about these issues and use appropriate terms.

Some of problems that can arise in identifying thoughts include the following.

The Client Who Struggles with Identifying Events or Triggers

One reason that clients struggle with identifying triggers is that the situation is not clearly in mind when they are discussing it. When you col-

Situation	Thought	Response
At a party, trying to talk to an interesting person there and show her that I am also interesting.	"She thinks I'm boring." "I don't know what to say." "She thinks I'm making things up."	Feel anxious. Feel worried. Feel frustrated.

FIGURE 7.1. A sample situation–thought–response pattern.

lect the client's description of the situation, ensure that it is clear and detailed enough in your mind that you can imagine yourself in that situation. Remember that "situations" can involve interpersonal interactions, solitary events, or even imagined events. They might include memories, partial images of events, or mental pictures to which the client is responding. Events can also have multisensorial components and include sounds, smells, or tactile elements. They are often locked into a certain time of day, so asking about the contextual aspects of the situation can help to trigger the client's memories. Although it is unlikely that you need to attend to all of these aspects of situations in every instance, be mindful of these various possible elements as you collect the situation description.

In some cases, you may find it helpful to have the client close his or her eyes and mentally imagine the situation with you. Ask the client to describe it aloud in vivid detail. The client can visualize the space he or she occupied and identify sights, sounds, or other sensations, in an attempt to enhance visualization and memory of thoughts in the moment. If the situation involved an interpersonal process, then an alternative strategy is to have the client describe the other person's behavior. You can then role-play that person, to help the client reimmerse him- or herself in the situation and recall thoughts and reactions.

One issue that emerges fairly often is that the situation is not just a single, static moment, but it actually evolves over time. For example, an interpersonal dispute may begin with a fairly minor insult or perceived hurt, then quickly escalate into mutual insults. A final action might range from aggression to your client leaving the situation in an angry state. It is likely that the client's thoughts and emotions will evolve throughout this transaction, which also changes over time. In such cases, it is sometimes helpful to break the set of events down into discrete moments and chart the changes in thoughts associated with various reactions. Although this exercise may seem detailed and tedious, it typically yields for the client the fruit of enhanced understanding.

In some cases, the client who struggles with naming feelings may demonstrate a mood shift during the therapy session. Such occurrences represent wonderful opportunities to help the client focus on internal experiences, and to improve emotional self-expression. The skillful cognitive-behavioral therapist watches for such mood shifts, and, if it seems appropriate, usually gives the client a moment to react (e.g., to cry), then offers a supportive statement followed by a cognitive assessment. This assessment includes a debriefing about the client's emotional response(s), the thoughts that precipitated the responses, then the statement, image, or other trigger in the session that initiated the response. The use of in-session mood changes can provide effective ways to examine the situation–thought–response chain and also an opportunity to demonstrate your sensitivity to the client's emotional responses. Cognitive-behavioral therapists should be ready to discuss emotions in the present moment, and to be comfortable with a client who expresses strong emotions in their offices. That said, we discourage too much focus on in-session emotional experiences, because the general focus of this treatment is on solving problems in the client's real world. For example, imagine learning that your client is anxious about coming to a therapy session because he or she is afraid you will be angry or disappointed because he or she did not complete the homework. It is obviously important for you to understand that emotional reaction, and addressing it in the therapy session itself, can be helpful. However, we would encourage you to determine fairly quickly whether this type of reaction also occurs in client's other relationships rather than focus only on the client–therapist relationship.

The Client Who Has a Difficult Time Identifying Emotions

Generally speaking, most people can identify and name their emotions, but there is considerable variability in these skills. Clients who come from emotionally impoverished backgrounds, who perhaps were discouraged from talking about their feelings in the past, or who are simply not very psychologically minded, may struggle with this process. If so, you might help clients use different terms to describe these processes. Such terms include *feelings*, *gut reactions*, *reactions*, *heart*, *experiences*, or *emotions*. Some clients pay more attention to their internal physiological reactions, so helping them learn emotional terms they can tie to these responses may help them to label these feelings more accurately. In more extreme cases, you might actually need to spend some time presenting and defining different emotion-related terms to clients, so that they can use these terms in future situations.

In some cases, a client needs help to improve the range and quality of his or her emotional vocabulary. The client who uses the term *upset* or *bad* to communicate an emotional reaction, for example, is certainly telling you that he or she has experienced something negative but it is not clear what that negative experience is. Such a client should be discouraged from using vague terms, and instead substitute words that are more descriptive and specific. For many examples of words to label emotions, see *www.psychpage.com/learning/library/assess/feelings.html*. Some clients prefer visual images of emotions, such as *www4.informa-tik.uni-erlangen.de/~msrex/how-do-you-feel.html*. It is often helpful to have clients not only name the type of emotional reaction they have had but also describe its intensity. Intensity ratings might involve a variety of terms, such as *not at all, a little, some, moderately, a fair bit, quite a bit, strongly, a lot,* and *intensely*. Numerical ratings from 0 to 100% on a Subjective Units of Distress Scale can be used to describe the intensity of any emotion.

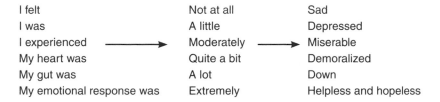

I felt	Not at all	Sad
I was	A little	Depressed
I experienced ———▶	Moderately ———▶	Miserable
My heart was	Quite a bit	Demoralized
My gut was	A lot	Down
My emotional response was	Extremely	Helpless and hopeless

As an example, imagine the different ways an experience of sadness might be expressed. If you can help your client to be more accurate and precise in the way he or she describes the experience to you, then you may better appreciate how much of a problem this is for your client, and how to optimally intervene.

The Client Who Is Confused about the Nature of Feelings

Some clients use terms that we associate with emotions or action impulses to describe their thoughts. A client might say, for example, "I thought how disappointed I was with my child" or "I thought sad thoughts" or "I felt that I should leave." In such cases, you need to spend some time to help the client to differentiate more accurately among feelings, thoughts, and behaviors. The definitions of these terms help, but it is also helpful to use the client's own experiences to help him or her understand these differentiated responses.

The Client Who Struggles to Identify Thoughts

Even though you have helped the client to clarify the nature of the event, situation, trigger, or stimulus, and you have spent some time discussing how to differentiate thoughts from feelings and behaviors, the client may still struggle to identify his or her thoughts. In such cases, you might use a series of questions to help the client pay attention to his or her thought processes and identify ideas (see Table 7.1).

TABLE 7.1. Questions to Help Elicit Thoughts from Clients

1. What were you thinking in that situation?
2. What might you have been thinking at that time?
3. Does this situation remind you of other, similar situations, in which you knew what you were thinking?
4. Could you have been thinking _____ (supply a likely thought)?
5. Could you have been thinking _____ (supply an unlikely thought, to contrast what the client was *not* thinking)?
6. Did you have any particular images in your mind?
7. Can you recall any memories related to this situation?
8. What did this situation mean to you?
9. What would someone else think in this type of situation?
10. If I had been there, what would I have thought?
11. How would you think, if this were the situation (provide a hypothetical variation of the situation, to see whether the client's thoughts are similar, or different)?

Note. Adapted from J. S. Beck (1995). Copyright 1993 by Judith S. Beck. Adapted with permission from Judith S. Beck and The Guilford Press.

The Client Who Poses Thoughts Stated as Questions

Some clients recognize that they ask themselves question in response to problematical situations: "Will I be accepted?", "What if I fail?", "Why does this always happen to me?", or "How can I get out of this situation?" These questions generally indicate the client's heightened levels of anxiety but belie the actual negative thought itself. Most clients do not just raise questions to themselves; they also typically answer the questions in a negative fashion. For example, the client who asks "Will I be accepted?" likely predicts that he or she will not be accepted. The client who worries about the consequences of failure probably believes that this outcome will occur. The client who worries about how to get out of a situation may be afraid that he or she cannot escape. When you hear a client raise these types of questions during the session, ask the client to answer the questions with his or her best guess. If the client does have evidence to answer the questions, then this information can be the focus of intervention (see below). The inability to answer the questions may also be instructive, and you and the client can then work together to gather the information.

THERAPIST: Do you think that you could take action on this problem this week?

CLIENT: I don't know if I can try. What if I can't do it? I'm going to be pretty busy this week.

THERAPIST: What do you mean? Could you answer that question— "What if I can't do it?"

CLIENT: I suppose I'm thinking that I won't be able to do it. That's pretty scary. I might fail and be back where I started. Even worse, I will have tried and failed. At least now I realize that I could have the option to try in the future.

THERAPIST: It sounds like you are anxious about making an attempt. I wonder if one of your predictions is that your efforts will lead to failure.

The Client Who Confuses Thoughts with Beliefs, Schemas, or Assumptions

In some cases, clients can provide not only their thoughts or appraisals of situations or events, but also their inferences about these thoughts. For example, a depressed client who is unable to accomplish assigned homework might react by saying, "I could not do my homework, because I felt unable to start, which once again proves what a failure I am." The first reaction in this statement reflects a situation-specific thought related to inaction (although the thought still needs to be clarified), but the latter part is the result of an inference, or conclusion, drawn from the inability to start. Early in therapy, it is helpful to note the inference the client has drawn and to incorporate it into the developing case conceptualization rather than comment on it. It is more helpful simply to focus on the first part of the response, which is the "automatic thought" (A. T. Beck et al., 1979) in the particular moment connected to the inability to start the homework assignment.

Even though we encourage the therapist in this situation to focus on the situation-specific thinking, particularly in the early sessions of therapy, we may note that the thought reflects a deeper concern related to a core belief or schema. In the previous example, the core belief is related to a theme of failure or incompetence. Given the strong negative reaction that this client has had to being unable to start the homework assignment, the therapist in this case may continue to assign homework around the theme of accomplishment and success, to see whether (1) perceived success is related to improved mood and (2) perceived failure or incompetence is related to increased depressed mood and/or feelings of helplessness. Both of these predictions would be consistent with the cognitive formulation of this case, and both reactions can help to confirm the developing case conceptualization.

The Client Who Responds to His or Her Negative Thoughts

Even though the focus of your work initially is the assessment of automatic thoughts, many clients may accurately perceive that your next step is to intervene with them. Some clients are familiar with cognitive-behavioral interventions prior to coming to treatment. Many Thought Record forms have columns in which clients write down their responses to negative automatic thoughts. Given these prompts, it is not surprising that some clients may start to respond to their negative thoughts in advance of your work with them. Although these responses are positive in some respects, because they demonstrate clients' eagerness to engage in this work, and allow you to assess clients' spontaneous ability to do so, we discourage them for several reasons. First, clients are likely to engage in unsuccessful strategies, as reflected in their ongoing problems and attendance in therapy. Such lack of success likely leads to disappointment with therapy and might even precipitate loss of confidence in treatment and early termination. Furthermore, these responses interrupt the flow of negative reactions to the situation, thus interfering with your ability to understand fully your client's thoughts and other responses to adverse situations.

METHODS FOR COLLECTING NEGATIVE THOUGHTS

Many cognitive-behavioral therapists use the daily Dysfunctional Thoughts Record (DTR; A. T. Beck et al., 1979; J. S. Beck, 1995). Indeed, the DTR has almost become the defining characteristic of cognitive assessment, and numerous versions of the DTR have been created over time. This method is no doubt an effective strategy for collecting thoughts, and we have used it extensively with clients. However, the classic version of the DTR does have the following potential limitations:

1. Placement of the emotions column before the thoughts column is not consistent with the cognitive model.
2. Whereas the rating of the intensity of emotions is helpful, because you can use the strongest emotional responses to orient your assessment, our experience is that rating the strength of belief in the thoughts is not very helpful. Most clients typically believe their own thoughts strongly.
3. The form fails to collect information about behaviors that follow automatic thoughts.
4. Inclusion of the cognitive distortions column suggests to clients that their thinking is distorted or "wrong." Although some distorted negative thoughts require particular interventions, many other thoughts are not particularly distorted, so this column can be problematical.
5. Inclusion of the rational responses column sometimes encourages

clients to begin responding to negative thoughts before they are ready.

We have generally chosen to use a modification of the traditional DTR. We may ask the client to purchase a notebook at the beginning of therapy to bring to sessions. The notebook is very useful for writing down homework assignments, keeping treatment notes, and collecting negative thoughts. When it comes to collecting thoughts on a Thought Record, the client writes a set of columns, as seen in Figure 7.2, into the notebook, to initiate the data collection process. This columnar format may also be reproduced in a computer, if the client wants to generate such a form, or printed out on an actual form sheet. Another option is to have the client purchase a three-ring binder to collect all thought records, as well as handouts and other therapy information. Other ways to collect this information also may be useful. For example, the client may use the point form as follows:

Situation (date, time, event)	
Automatic thoughts	
Emotions (list type and rate intensity from 0 to 100)	
Behaviors or action tendencies	

A diary format may also be utilized, as long as the requisite information is included. Although we have not had this experience, a client might even use a digital voice recorder, and have his or her computer transcribe the recording into a file that he or she could e-mail to you! Our point, of course, is that the information collected in the Thought Record is more important than its format. The client must be an active collaborator in decisions about how to record the information, so that it is useful and increases the likelihood of follow through with the homework assignments.

Sometimes the content of negative thinking is less important than other dimensions of these thoughts. For example, a client may have repetitive thoughts about the same problem rather than negative thoughts about different matters. In such cases, a Frequency Record may be the optimal form of Thought Record to create. Such a record could be a golf stroke counter, or any other frequency count system, as long as it is a reasonably accurate and reliably completed record. In another case, a single thought may be behind most of the client's distress (e.g., taking responsibility for a child's poor health). In such a case, having the client rate and rerate the strength of belief in the thought may be the best index of thera-

Situation (date, time, event)	Automatic Thoughts	Emotions (list type and rate intensity 0–100)	Behaviors or Action Tendencies

FIGURE 7.2. Dobson adapted Thought Record (for assessment only).

peutic success. Of course, any such single system loses other information, such as the settings in which such thoughts occur, and the outcomes of this pattern of thinking, but in some cases your judgment may be that this extra information is not as critical to track as other issues.

Some clients struggle to write the information into a Thought Record outside of therapy sessions. Before assigning a Thought Record for homework, ensure that the client feels comfortable writing down such information, that the system is one the client can remember, that it is something that will be available, and that the client can keep the system confidential (e.g., most clients would not want their Thought Records to be discovered at work!). If the client expresses reticence about this assignment, you may need to negotiate a different strategy.

Clients may tell you they prefer not to write the information down, that they will be able to remember it. We are generally skeptical about such a claim, but if the client is insistent, we let him or her try to collect this information without a written record as an experiment. Typically, the client acknowledges that his or her memory is more fallible than he or she originally believed, and agrees to try a written Thought Record. Clients often remember the general nature of their thoughts but not specific details. Sometimes clients are reluctant writers because of poor penmanship, worry about the quality of their writing, or concern that their efforts will be judged. Some people have low literacy levels that may not be apparent in the assessment. They may also make efforts to hide their difficulty with reading and writing because of shame. Be sure to reinforce any efforts that clients make to record their thoughts, even if the results are different than what you discussed in the session. Modifications can be easily made as treatment proceeds. If clients get the sense that they did not do the homework correctly, then they may be reticent to try again. You and your clients can reevaluate the process and utility of the information together.

INTERVENTIONS FOR NEGATIVE THINKING

Once you start to collect negative thoughts, you soon find yourself working with a wealth of information. Some beginning cognitive-behavioral therapists may actually be overwhelmed by the information and do not know where to start to intervene. Points about negative thoughts include the following:

- Look for the negative thoughts that are connected with strong emotional reactions. Generally, we recommend that you attend to and work with the most emotionally loaded thoughts, or "hot cognitions."
- Look for thoughts that are connected to a strong behavioral response pattern. Just as some hot cognitions have emotional valence, others have behavioral valence, and these patterns can help to identify these thoughts.
- Look for thoughts that have a strong degree of belief associated with them, because these are likely going to be the hardest ones to change.
- Look for repetitive thoughts, because these are more likely to help determine themes in thinking, and for core beliefs that cut across different situations.

When you begin cognitive interventions, it is possible that you may choose a thought that turns out not to be very fruitful or productive. At the least, this choice shows you how well the client can work with the method, and you can use this information to determine where not to intervene in the future. Generally, our belief is that if there is a dysfunctional thought pattern, then it is not going to go away without intervention. Give yourself another chance to refine your case conceptualization, and make another effort with the client. It is also helpful for clients to see that their therapists make mistakes!

Three Questions to Challenge Negative Thinking

If you have carefully worked through a Thought Record and identified the client's most distressing cognitions, you are ready to begin the more formal process of cognitive restructuring. Once you have identified a cognitive target for intervention, you can use three general questions to try to modify a negative thought:

1. What is the evidence for and against this thought?
2. What are the alternative ways to think in this situation?
3. What are the implications of thinking this way?

The questions that are most helpful depend on the nature of the thought itself, the phase of therapy, and the client's success with these methods.

Each of these general questions represents a series of interventions. The first question is most useful in situations where you think the negative thought likely represents distorted thinking, or thinking that is at least more negative than the situation warrants. The second question, which you can sometimes explore after examining the evidence-related question, asks the client to question whether his or her thinking is the only, or the most helpful, way to think about the situation. The third general question encourages the client to examine whether the situation has activated core beliefs, and whether maladaptive inferences are being made in the situation. The wording of each question may be modified to ensure maximal understanding for the client. We discuss each of these types of questions in turn below.

What Is the Evidence for and against This Thought?

Generally speaking, evidence-based interventions are most successful when the therapist is able to determine that the client is using a cognitive distortion. There was a strong emphasis on distorted thinking in the earliest descriptions of cognitive therapy (A. T. Beck, 1970; A. T. Beck et al., 1979), and a variety of descriptions of these distortions exist (e.g., see Table 7.2). These distortions all share the idea that clients have somehow misperceived or distorted their perceptions of what "really" happened. Put another way, the real events may have been modified to be more in line with clients' beliefs than with the facts of the situation.

A relevant, important philosophical note here is that cognitive-behavioral therapists generally subscribe to the idea that a "real world" exists independently of our perception of it. A tree that falls in the forest does make a sound, even if no one is there to hear it. This realist assumption (Dobson & Dozois, 2001; Held, 1995) is consistent with the idea that mental health is associated with a more accurate appraisal of the events in the real world, and that, by implication, problems in mental health are associated with misperceptions or distortions of the real world. As we discuss briefly in a later chapter, this epistemological

TABLE 7.2. Common Cognitive Distortions

Title	Description
All-or-nothing thinking	Also called black-and-white, or dichotomous, thinking. Viewing a situation as having only two possible outcomes.
Catastrophization	Predicting future calamity; ignoring a possible positive future.
Fortune telling	Predicting the future with limited evidence.
Mind reading	Predicting or believing you know what other people think.
Disqualifying the positive	Not attending to, or giving due weight to, positive information. Similar to a negative "tunnel vision."
Magnification/minimization	Magnifying negative information; minimizing positive information.
Selective abstraction	Also called *mental filter*. Focusing on one detail rather than on the large picture.
Overgeneralization	Drawing overstated conclusions based on one instance, or on a limited number of instances.
Misattribution	Making errors in the attribution of causes of various events.
Personalization	Thinking that you cause negative things, rather than examining other causes.
Emotional reasoning	Arguing that because something feels bad, it must be bad.
Labeling	Putting a general label on someone or something, rather than describing the behaviors or aspects of the thing.

Note. Adapted from J. S. Beck (1995). Copyright 1993 by Judith S. Beck. Adapted with permission from Judith S. Beck and The Guilford Press.

perspective is somewhat at odds with some of the more recent developments in cognitive-behavioral therapy.

Another relevant theoretical note is that the model holds that our perceptions are based on two sources: (1) the facts or circumstances of the situation in which a person finds him- or herself, and (2) the person's beliefs, assumptions, and schemas. It is the interaction between these two sources that conspires to lead to situation-specific thinking. By implication, this model holds that whereas accurate appraisals of the world are driven more by perceptual and specific elements observed in moment-to-moment experience, distorted thinking is driven more by core beliefs, assumptions, or schemas that are consistent with the situational automatic thoughts. In a very real way, then, *the identification of cognitive distortions represents the royal road to the schema* (Strachey, 1957; with our apologies to Sigmund Freud). For this reason, the cognitive-behavioral therapists are sensitive to, and work to understand, the important distortions they observe in their clients.

Predicated on the idea that our clients may distort reality, and that distortions are related to the core beliefs and schemas that clients hold, cognitive-behavioral therapists often begin their treatment programs by trying to modify these distortions. In the following section we describe some of the main methods to do this work. Other sources also exist, and we encourage you to examine them (J. S. Beck, 1995, 2005; Leahy & Holland, 2000; McMullin, 2000).

GENERAL PRINCIPLES

The goal of comparing automatic thoughts and their evidence base has several overarching principles. These principles may be demonstrated through various techniques, as discussed below. They include helping the client to realize that whereas thoughts *feel* correct, they can be evaluated in their own right. As such, cognitive-behavioral therapists hold that probabilities are not certainties, that feeling a certain way does not validate the thoughts that lead to the feelings, and that thoughts can be either accurate or distorted.

To plan interventions, cognitive-behavioral therapists need to know the range of possible distortions that clients may demonstrate, and become adept at recognizing them. A general strategy is to have a list of cognitive distortions available to yourself and the client. Clients who have accepted the principle that these distortions exist can help you to identify their tendencies to distort. Some clients like to carry the list with them, so that as they write down their thoughts in the Thought Record, they can identify whether any of the thoughts are potentially distorted. Indeed, one of us (K. S. D.) had a client who became so fluent in his ability to identify distortions that he would say to himself, for example, "Oh, there is magnification again," and that was sufficient to undermine the distortion significantly. Some clients begin to identify distortions in other people's comments, which also aids their awareness of these cognitive styles. One formal way to help clients identify and name their distortions is to add another column to the Thought Record, in which clients can name their distortions.

The other general principle embedded in the evidence-based approach to testing automatic thoughts is the idea that thoughts can be evaluated against the database of experience. Often, experiments or assignments are created in which clients can compare their thoughts to the evidence.

This strategy encourages empirical hypothesis testing, and an approach toward, rather than avoidance of, problem situations.

EXAMINING THE EVIDENCE RELATED TO NEGATIVE THOUGHTS

One of the most straightforward ways to counter distortions is to ask clients about the evidence *they* use (i.e., not how you might view the situation, or how they "should" see it). You can attend to various aspects of the evidence, including its type, quality, and amount. You can contrast these pieces of supportive evidence with data that do not fully support, or that are even inconsistent with the original thought (e.g., "Yes, my boss did criticize me in our sales meeting this week, *but* she did give me a fairly positive appraisal report 5 months ago"). This strategy is most likely to be successful if you have the client provide a complete description of the trigger event, and if you get the disquieting sense that his or her perceptions are dictated more by beliefs than by the event itself.

In some cases, asking for evidence that both supports and refutes the original negative thought reveals that the client does not have all of the information needed to drawn any firm conclusions about the event or situation. In such cases, you can work with the client to see whether the situation is important enough to warrant a homework assignment, to discover the facts of the situation. Setting up this type of homework is sometimes difficult to do, however, because often you are trying to re-create a disturbing situation to see how it can be viewed differently. Sometimes the homework assignment involves having the client ask others how they saw the situation. This strategy is certainly possible, but you need to be sure that the client will accept the information from the people to whom he or she talks, or else the client can potentially distort or discount that information, too. One way to think about this dilemma is to ask yourself and the client, "What evidence or information do you need to convince you that your original automatic thought was not exactly accurate?" If neither you nor the client can generate an answer to that question, or if it is impossible to gather that evidence, then you may want to encourage the client to pay attention to such information in future situations but let the current one go.

IDENTIFYING UNREALISTIC EXPECTATIONS

Many clients not only distort past events but also predict negative futures. Anxious clients are experts in this process, and some are even adept at making their anticipated negative future become a reality. For example, a female client who believes that she is shy and anxious by nature, and who therefore avoids social situations, does not receive any disconfirma-tory evidence for her beliefs. Helping such a client to see the self-fulfill-ing prophecies that she makes, then gathering objective evidence related to her prediction, can be a very powerful way to undercut her negative expectations. When you think it is important to gather evidence related to a negative prediction, you need to engage in several, related therapy activities:

1. Clarify clients' expectations: Get them written down as clearly and fully as possible.

2. Determine what evidence they would use to confirm or discon-firm this prediction. A good idea is to ask clients about the worst case outcome, the best possible outcome, and the most realistic outcome (this process itself sometimes helps to decatastrophize predictions).

3. Have clients identify how they will collect the relevant evidence. This ensures that the information plan actually gathers information that is related to their expectations. If necessary, devise a recording system to reduce the risk of reinterpretation of the event by clients, before the next session.

4. Help clients to commit to a homework assignment in which they can collect the information, if possible. If the ideal homework assignment is not possible (e.g., in an interpersonal situation), recognize the limits of the data that clients collect. Sometimes the act of collecting evidence is as important as the outcome of the situation. The message being sent is that clients can confront, rather than avoid, the situation, and sometimes unanticipated outcomes that occur can then be grist for the mill in future therapy sessions.

5. In the next session, be sure to compare the clients' homework expectations with the actual outcomes. Without overstating the results, and presuming the outcome was not as negative as expected, have the clients engage in several actions:

   a. Give themselves credit for the effort.
   b. Be attentive to and address minimization if it occurs (e.g., "It was not as hard as I thought"; "Anyone could have handled it, after all").
   c. If they tend to predict more negative outcomes in general, have clients question themselves. Have them ask themselves if they are willing to try to be more evidence-related in the future.
   d. Have clients recognize that approaching, rather than avoiding, difficult issues is helpful, because it helps them to get more accu-rate information about the "real" problem.
   e. Help clients learn how to use problem solving (see Chapter 5, this volume) for any issues that emerged from the assignment.

f. (If appropriate) design another prediction-related homework assignment to see whether this process can be repeated in another area.

EXAMINING ATTRIBUTIONAL BIASES

Attributions are the explanations of the causes that people give to events. Three well-recognized dimensions of attributions are locus (internal vs. external), stability (single occurrence/unstable vs. permanent/stable), and specificity (specific to one situation vs. global). It has been shown on the one hand that depression is related to the tendency to make internal, stable, and global attributions for failure (e.g., "I am a failure"), but external, unstable, and specific attributions for success (e.g., "I was lucky that time") (Abramson & Alloy, 2006). On the other hand, clients with anger problems tend to make external, stable, and global attributions for negative outcomes, such as "He meant to insult me, and he'll do it again, if I give him the chance." You should be sensitive to and address attributional biases whenever they appear. One strategy to do so is to ask for more details about the problematical situation, and to expose the tenuous relationship that may exist between the event and the attributions made in the situation. Often, such cases also involve mind reading on the part of the client, so this cognitive distortion may also be identified. In some cases, the evidence-based homework assignment exercise we discussed earlier can be used to expose attributional biases, and to contrast the client's thoughts and the evidence of the situation.

REATTRIBUTING CAUSES USING PIE CHARTS

One specific technique to help with reattribution of causes is the use of pie charts. For example, if a client blames himself fully for an outcome (e.g.,"My wife left me because I was such a critical partner"), it is possible to identify first that this thought treats the client as if he is totally responsible for this outcome. You can then emphasize how anyone would probably feel badly if he was totally responsible for the failure of a marriage. You might draw a pie chart (see Figure 7.3) showing that he is likely 100% to blame. You might then ask about other possible sources for the relationship breakdown. The fact that his wife left him, for example, might be evidence that she had a role in the relationship's failure. You might ask for other information related to the wife's responsibility for this outcome, maybe 30%. It may also become clear that the extended family did not support the relationship, and this might be assigned 10% of the blame. Similarly, work demands and work-related travel outside of the client's control might have been a stressor, as were finances, each

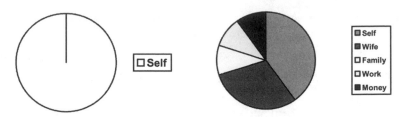

FIGURE 7.3. Original and revised attributions.

of which is given 10% responsibility for the relationship's failure. Taken as a whole, the situation has gone from the one on the left in Figure 7.3, to the one on the right.

The reattribution exercise does not require the use of pie charts. You simply use the percentage metaphor to attribute causes. You might, for another client, simply name the various causes of an outcome, without determining percentage of responsibility. The key to this technique is to ensure that the client is considering all possible sources of the outcome and matching their attributions to the circumstances, as much as possible.

CHANGE LABELING

It is common for people to label themselves or others rather than to focus on the specific actions or attributes that underlie the label. Labeling can be an insidious process, because labels are like permanent attributions that make it hard for people to see how the labeled person can ever change. If your client is engaged in destructive labeling, you can use several interventions to try to reduce this tendency. First, you can point out that the client is using labels and discuss the effects of labels—the way that they constrain future action and actually become self-fulfilling. A very helpful strategy is to have the client specify which specific behaviors or attributes he or she sees that support the label. You might then examine the evidence related to these behaviors and attributes. You may also encourage the client to see the value of focusing on specific concerns that may be modified, as opposed to immutable labels. Then, depending on the specific concerns that have been raised, other techniques, such as problem solving, social skills training, or assertiveness might be considered.

CHANGING DICHOTOMOUS THINKING INTO GRADUATED THINKING

Common cognitive distortions are dichotomous, all-or-nothing, or black-and-white thinking. Dichotomous thinking, a type of attributional bias, can also be addressed by examining evidence related to the thought. Although possible, it is quite unusual for events or experiences to be categorical (e.g., "the *worst* I ever felt," "the *most* difficult person in the world," "a *total* failure"). Listen for terms that express an underlying continuum but in which clients perceive an extreme. In such cases, you can help clients first to recognize that they are using categorical terms, then to contrast the evidence for and against this statement. Another idea is to talk with the clients and see whether they can recognize the underlying continuum. It is then helpful to identify anchors, benchmarks, or exemplars for various places on the continuum, and evaluate whether the original automatic thought fits that continuum or, perhaps, is too extreme. You can also design experiments to determine the validity of the categorical automatic thought by looking for evidence both for and against the original thought. In doing so, you encourage clients to use fewer categorical thoughts and also to recognize more of a range of thoughts. This exercise generally encourages clients to move in the direction of desired change along the identified continuum, rather than forcing them to reject and stop using the underlying categorical ideas, which is much more difficult.

What Are the Alternative Ways to Think in This Situation?

Although evidence-based strategies to evaluate cognitive distortions are effective methods to undermine some negative thoughts, they are only effective when the original thought was itself distorted. In other cases, it becomes clear that a certain thought is negative and leads to emotional distress or dysfunctional behavior, but it is not clear that the thought is actually based on a distortion of the client's environment or circumstances. In other cases, though, although there is a distortion, and one or more of the previous techniques help to address and to modify that distortion, the therapist wants to take the intervention a little further. In such cases, the following methods are recommended.

GENERATING AND EVALUATING ALTERNATIVE THOUGHTS

Sometimes a review of the evidence related to a negative thought indicates that the thought is not sustainable. In other cases, evidence may generally substantiate the thought, but it is clear to you and to the client that the thought is nonetheless unhelpful. In either case, it is possible to ask the client to generate and to consider a novel and more adaptive alternative thought. There are several methods to achieve these goals:

1. Based on a review of the evidence, it may become clear that the original negative thought is out of keeping with the evidence. In such a

case, it can be helpful to explain that the thought makes sense, based on the way the client has been feeling or thinking (i.e., it is in keeping with his or her core beliefs), it would be more helpful to consider alternative, less negative thoughts. If the client concurs, you can ask him or her to generate an alternative that fits the facts and is credible. Make sure to evaluate how the new thought does or does not fit the evidence and, if it is not fully accurate, work with the client to consider other alternatives.

2. If there has not been an evidence review prior to this step, but you and the client agree that his or her negative thought is not helpful, you can also help the client to generate an alternative. In this case, you would not ask for a more evidence-based alternative, but for one that is likely to be more helpful or adaptive. The alternative needs to be one that the client accepts as worthy of consideration, and applicable to his or her life.

3. After you have established a more evidence-based or potentially more adaptive thought, ask the client to identify the advantages and disadvantages of both the original and the revised thought. Make sure that this evaluation is respectful of the original thought (i.e., do not dismiss it as "distorted" or "wrong"), and point out that the alternative thought almost always involves some challenges.

4. One way to take the previously mentioned strategy even further is to develop a point–counterpoint response to negative thoughts. In this method, you and the client work out credible and evidence-based alternatives to the client's various negative automatic thoughts. You might even write these on cue cards, with the original thought on one side and the alternative on the other. Then, state or read the original thoughts and have the client practice saying the alternatives. If appropriate, you might string together a series of negative thoughts in a kind of barrage or courtroom-type summary of negative thoughts, then have the client use the alternatives to respond to the arguments. Even further, you might use a "devil's advocate" approach, in which you not only repeat the original negative thoughts but also actually amplify them in ways that challenge the client.

5. Another technique for challenging negative thoughts is called the Rational Role Play. The negative thoughts and their alternatives are verbalized as a kind of role play between negative and more adaptive thinking. Ideally, the client verbalizes the more adaptive thoughts, but if necessary, you can reverse the role play for a while, so that the client observes verbalization of the adaptive thoughts, before he or she has an opportunity to practice. The goal of these various strategies is to help the client to become fluent in his or her responses to negative thinking.

6. Ideally, you develop a homework assignment in which the client can try out his or her new way of thinking. It may be practiced within in the therapy session, for example, by generating one or more hypotheti-

cal and challenging situations, to see whether the client can use the more adaptive, less dysfunctional way of thinking. Together with the client, you might take a specific from the Thought Record, and generate alternative thoughts and discuss the benefits of that new way of thinking. A common technique is to add two new columns to the Thought Record (see Figure 7.4), one in which the alternative thought is written, and a final one in which the emotional and behavioral consequences of this new alternative thought are examined and recorded (ideally, less negative emotion or more positive emotion, and less dysfunctional behavior).

7. Some clients struggle with the generation of adaptive responses to negative thinking. There are several possible options in such a situation. You might generate the alternative responses to negative thoughts. This option tends to be easy and quick for the therapist, but a few considerations are necessary. Ensure that these alternatives are not presented as the "correct" or "right" way to think, but as possibilities for the client to consider, evaluate, and adopt or not. Often, cognitive-behavioral therapists present these alternatives as choices (e.g., "Do you think that thinking this way would be helpful?") to encourage the client to be an active participant in choosing thoughts that will work in his or her life. Another possible way to generate alternative thoughts is to do a poll to survey opinions on the evidence related to the original negative thought. For example, if the client has a series of thoughts about the "danger" of being in certain places, you could have the client survey his or her friends and colleagues to see whether they share the thoughts. Another possibility is to see whether the client has any experts in his or her life that could provide a fresh perspective on the thoughts. For example, some clients' thoughts have a moral overtone, or one that they believe may be required from certain religious viewpoints. In such cases, a judicious consultation with a clergy member about the viewpoint a client is entertaining may help to ascertain the consistency of these thoughts with moral or religious doctrine, or how much latitude the client may have in modifying that thought.

8. A fairly dramatic, and potentially powerful, way to shift negative thinking is through the use of humor. Almost by definition, humor involves a creative and sometimes bizarre shift of perspective that makes a previous idea or statement seem "silly" or "funny" from the new viewpoint. Dr. Albert Ellis had a famous statement in which he argued that if Martians ever come to visit Earth, they will die of laughter due to all of the irrational thoughts humans hold (Heery, 2001). Such a statement made in therapy can encourage clients to view their thoughts from a different perspective, and potentially to see their thinking as truly worth a laugh. However, if you use humor, do it in such a way that clients see that the thought is funny, and not them. Also, ensure that clients see the

Situation (date, time, event)	Automatic Thoughts	Emotions (list type and rate intensity 0–100)	Behaviors or Action Tendencies	Alternative Thoughts	Consequences

FIGURE 7.4. Dobson Adapted Thought Record, with additional columns for alternative thoughts and consequences.

humor as good-natured, rather than as a sarcastic or insulting dig about their thinking. Our perspective is that humor is likely a better strategy somewhat later in therapy, once you and the client have established a positive working relationship and the client's initial distress is somewhat less than when he or she first came for therapy. Humorous self-disclosure may also be useful, so that the client appreciates that the therapist makes mistakes or finds him- or herself in amusing situations (see Chapter 4, this volume, for further discussion of self-disclosure).

9. Yet another way to evaluate alternative thoughts is through the question of how useful or helpful it is to entertain the negative thought, as opposed to an alternative option. Even clients who do not particularly believe an alternative thought sometimes accept that the original negative thought is not useful to them. In such a case, they may be willing to use it less often, or at the least acknowledge when it does occur that the thought rather than the event is causing distress. In some cases, you can help clients to consider how they might counsel a friend with this type of thinking. Clients are often more considerate toward others than toward themselves; consequently, you can encourage clients to direct this compassion for others toward themselves. It may be useful to have clients rehearse what they would say to a person they care about who finds him- or herself in the same situation. Alternatively, you could encourage a cost–benefit analysis of the original thought and the alternative to evaluate the relative utility of each way of thinking.

10. Sometimes, clients become aware of contradictory thoughts. This can happen, for example, when clients with low self-esteem see

themselves as ineffective but also hold themselves responsible for things that happen around them. How can someone be both ineffective and have such a strong effect on others? If your client engages in contradictory thinking, it can sometimes be helpful to point out this contradiction, and help the client come to a more adaptive, and maybe more evidence-based middle ground.

11. One particular type of cognitive distortion is called *emotional reasoning*, which occurs when clients use the emotions that they feel after a certain negative thought as evidence that the thought itself is valid. This distortion is a logical error (a consequential outcome cannot affirm an antecedent condition), that you can discuss with clients. You may also generate alternative thoughts as thought experiments to help you demonstrate that "thoughts are not facts" or "thoughts are just opinions."

12. Another specific thought intervention has been called TIC–TOC, an acronym that refers to the sound of a clock's pendulum and stands for Task-Interfering Cognitions–Task-Orienting Cognitions. This method can be used if the client has a series of repetitive thoughts that interfere with a particular task or set of tasks (e.g., "I can't do it"). The intervention comprises having a credible, quick alternative thought that the client can use to replace the negative thought (e.g., "I don't have to do it all right now; every little bit helps"). Then, whenever the negative thought emerges, the alternative is supplied automatically, just as a pendulum swings back and forth.

CULTIVATING POSITIVE THOUGHTS

Whereas all of these techniques focus on the modification of negative thoughts, it is also possible to promote and encourage positive thoughts as a way to reduce distress. Three techniques warrant some discussion in this context:

1. Sometimes discussion of a negative thought demonstrates that although the thought has negative consequences, it is actually based on a positive underlying concern. For example, the mother who is always worried about the welfare of her children does so because she is a concerned and responsible parent. A person who feels aggrieved by the criticism of a friend only feels such a response to the extent that he or she cares about the other person. In these and other cases, it is sometimes possible to see the positive aspects of negative thoughts, and to reframe or restate the thought from this perspective (e.g., "I worry about my children because I care about them"). Sometimes such positive reframing helps clients to see the positive aspects of their thoughts and behaviors, and can be used by you to encourage other positive thoughts and actions. If you use this

method, ensure that the positive reframe is credible to the client, and that he or she is willing to consider its broader use. It may undermine the therapy relationship if you try to encourage a client to shift his or her thinking toward content that is not believable to them, and the client thinks you are actually out of step with his or her worldview. It is crucial not to minimize the client's distress when you work with his or her thoughts, and being unrealistically positive can do so.

2. It is also possible to encourage the client to entertain and use functional thoughts to increase positive affect. You can contrast negative and positive thoughts, for example, and see whether a client is willing to increase the frequency of more positive thoughts. You may also pay attention to changes in thinking over the course of therapy, highlighting positive changes, and their emotional and behavioral consequences for the client. Alternatively, if you see a positive shift in affect in the therapy session itself, such as a client's sudden smile or laugh, you can highlight this phenomenon and encourage the client to reproduce it at other times in therapy or in real life. For example, a client of one of us (K. S. D.), who had a history of depression, began to feel less depressed and started to take more interest in his appearance. The therapist noted this shift, and in subsequent sessions, therapist and client had a kind of "game" in which the therapist guessed what changes the client had made that day.

3. A common and, in our opinion, simplistic expression about cognitive-behavioral therapy is that the strategy largely consists of replacing negative thoughts with positive ones. Some authors have encouraged the use of positive affirmations as a way to practice positive self-statements (McMullin, 2000). Our experience in general does not support the use of positive self-statements or affirmations. We find that clients struggle to believe them, and that unless they occur in a situational context, they have no framework to "hang on to" or to incorporate into developing a more positive self-image. Thus, although we do not categorically reject the use of affirmations, we instead encourage the use of more contextualized changes from negative to positive thinking. If self-statements are used, it is critical that the client have at least some belief in them.

What Are the Implications of Thinking This Way?

The third question identified as a way to respond to negative thoughts explores the conceptual implications of these thoughts. You can also think of this last question as "So what?," as in "So what if the negative thought is true? What does that mean about you or the world you live in?" When clients are asked to examine this question, they spontaneously begin to consider the broader conceptual implications of the thoughts.

A common method for asking about the implications of specific thoughts is known as the *downward arrow* (Burns, 1989, 1999; J. S. Beck, 1995). In this method, rather than challenge the original automatic thought, the therapist for the moment considers the thought to be true. The client is then asked what the implication of that "fact" is. The client's response is accepted at face value, and its inference is examined, and so on, until the client reaches, as he or she quickly does, an inference at a very broad and irrevocable level, beyond which other inferences are not possible. Typically, these broad inferences reflect core beliefs or schemas about the self or the world. Table 7.3 provides an example of the kind of dialogue that reflects the downward arrow technique, showing through a fairly simple set of questions how the client's core belief is accessed (in this case, that being socially judged and rejected is metaphorically equivalent to death).

The downward arrow can be used at almost any point in therapy to discover the broader meanings a client attaches to a specific thought. It is also possible, of course, to ask questions related to the inferences attached to thoughts, without going to the broadest and deepest level. The method carries some risks that the therapist needs to keep in mind. As can be seen in Table 7.3, the method typically leads the client to a deep and dark place, associated with more permanent and fixed schemas and beliefs. Asking about these thoughts early in the course of therapy may expose these raw ideas, but in a client who does not yet have the skills or progress in therapy to counter or respond to them. Thus, although this method may be extremely helpful in developing the case formulation, ensure that you start the method with the qualification that you do not yet accept the thoughts at face value, and you want to come back later potentially to challenge them. Also, end with a supportive statement about what the downward arrow has taught you, how the client's distress in the moment makes sense in the context of his or her core beliefs, and how important it is to address these beliefs in therapy. For strategies such as the downward arrow that expose core beliefs, it is particularly important to have a solid, trusting therapeutic relationship.

In essence, the "So what?" question encourages the identification of core beliefs. Core beliefs or schemas are differentiated from automatic thoughts, in that whereas the former are broad, stable, and core aspects of clients' ways of thinking about themselves or the world, the latter are spontaneous thoughts that emerge in specific situations. By definition, automatic thoughts reflect core beliefs, and sometimes they even have the same grammatical expression (e.g., "I'm stupid," "People are always against me"). Also, automatic thoughts that are tied to a core belief often emerge if the appropriate triggers are present, and their frequency may confuse some therapists into thinking they are beliefs. It is important to be clear in your mind whether you are hearing an automatic, situation-

TABLE 7.3. The Downward Arrow Technique

Socially anxious client's statement	Therapist's response
"It happened again last week. We were in a team meeting at work, and my supervisor put me on the spot. She looked directly at me and asked the question we were all dreading. I couldn't speak. I froze."	"And what thoughts or ideas went through your mind, do you think, just before you froze?"
"I thought, 'Oh, no, not me! Don't ask me. I am going to look like a fool.'"	"And just for the moment—not that I necessarily agree that your idea was actually true; we can come back and look at that—what if we imagine that you looked like a fool? What would that mean to you?"
"My incompetence and anxiety would be laid bare to everyone. I would be embarrassed."	"And if you were embarrassed because everyone saw your incompetence and anxiety? What would that mean?"
"It would mean I should be fired; just go away and hide. No one could accept me."	"And what if that was true—that you could not be accepted by others?"
"I might as well crumple up and die. What would be the point in living?"	"And as horrible as that would be, can you imagine anything more—something that having no point in living would mean to you?"
"I'm not sure. Nothing comes to mind. What could be worse than that?"	

based thought or a core belief, because the method for intervening with each is somewhat different, as is their likely timing in therapy.

Other Ways to Address Negative Thinking

In Chapter 8, this volume, we discuss moving from the work with negative automatic thoughts to the deeper level of work with core beliefs. Before doing so, though, two important issues in working with automatic thoughts—addressing realistic negative thinking and problems that occur in cognitive restructuring—are briefly discussed.

Realistic Negative Thinking

One of the potential consequences of reviewing the evidence in support of negative thinking is that it may be realistic, and that there are clearly no better or more credible alternatives. We encourage you to resist draw-ing such conclusions prematurely and potentially "buying into" your client's negative thinking, although we recognize that some distressing situations are likely associated with emotional and/or behavioral prob-lems in anyone. It can be very helpful for clients to realize that their thoughts and reactions make sense under the circumstances. One of us (D. D.) has sometimes said to clients that their response is "normal in an abnormal situation." For example, a client faced with a difficult divorce, an economic downturn, and a new, single life is likely to feel sad and anxious. Thoughts such as "This situation is tough and unfair" may be quite realistic. In such a situation, you may choose to move toward a more behavioral and action-oriented strategy that involves helping the client to change what he or she can, problem-solve the consequences of the situation, and accept what he or she must. Several techniques are pos-sible in this context.

One strategy for dealing with difficult situations is the encourage-ment of optimal coping skills (see Chapter 6, this volume). It is help-ful to encourage the client to increase his or her self-care activities to ensure optimal resiliency. You might encourage your client to maintain or enhance positive life skills (e.g., regular and healthy nutrition, regular sleep, exercise, body awareness and nurturance). Encourage him or her to enlist available social resources and supports. You might recruit new resources, including other social agencies and health services, as appro-priate.

Sometimes negative thoughts seem to have a life of their own, and are not particularly tied to events. Repetitive worry, ruminative thinking, or even some degree of obsessional thinking can fit into this category of thinking. All of these thoughts may be relatively realistic, but their frequency and repetitive nature can be distressing and disruptive for the client. One technique developed for such thinking is *worry time*, in which the clients restrict their worry to certain prescribed times of the day or week. Some clients report that having a dedicated time helps them to worry less at other times. Other clients report that having a dedicated worry time (e.g., 15 minutes every other day) can lead to awareness that worry is unproductive, or even boring, when utilized in a focused way. It can also be useful to have clients engage in problem solving during the worry time, so that they not only worry but also try to resolve whatever is worrying them.

Another method for dealing with repetitive thinking is *distraction*, or temporarily shifting the focus of attention away from the thoughts. Whereas cognitive-behavioral therapists typically focus on the thought's content and try to modify the thought directly, in clients with repeti-tive worry or rumination, therapists help clients to develop a strategy of identifying the thought, recognizing it as the same repetitive thought, then purposely shifting the focus of their attention to some other issue or concern. This method often helps clients obtain some distance and perspective on the thoughts. They may then be able to find a solution to a problem more proactively, rather than simply to worry about it. This method is different than thought stopping or thought suppression, which we do not recommend. Thought stopping has been shown to be relatively ineffective (Freeston, Ladouceur, Provencher, & Blais, 1995), and thought suppression can have the opposite effect of increasing rather than decreasing thoughts.

A class of interventions that is becoming more popular involves acceptance of negative experience as a normal part of human existence (Wells, 2002; Hayes, Follette, & Linehan, 2004). When clients are more distressed, we generally do not encourage acceptance-oriented methods, because use of such methods implies that we cannot address clients' concerns more directly. Thus, whereas acceptance of a problem (but not resignation) fundamentally shifts clients' attitudes toward their problems, such a shift often involves development of a new belief, or the radical modification of the belief or schema that led to clients' problems in the first place. We discuss this approach in more detail in Chapter 8, this volume.

Problems in Cognitive Restructuring

A number of common problems emerge when therapists do cognitive restructuring (J. S. Beck, 2005). Some of these are related to problems in the therapy relationship or resistance on the part of the client (Leahy, 2001; see Chapter 10, this volume, for discussion of these issues). Here we discuss some common issues that occur, as well as how to deal with them.

It can be very difficult to determine the thoughts on which to focus. Certainly, it is most useful to focus on thoughts that appear to be related to distressed affect or dysfunctional behavior. The case conceptualization, theoretically, should guide your choices and be revised as necessary. Be on the lookout for thoughts that occur frequently, because they are being activated by underlying schemas or triggers in the environment. Sometimes, in the case of thoughts that do not occur often but are clearly deeply important, you have to focus on "targets of opportunity." Generally, though, our sense is that thoughts that are important and related to the client's distress will reemerge. So, even if you miss an opportunity, a significant "hot cognition" will recur. Also, you can even use interventions that fall flat or are not very helpful as part of your case conceptualization information, because they tell you what is *not* related to the client's problems.

At times, a client will report that the Thought Record or the interventions you try are not helpful. Listen carefully to the client's concerns, which often will help you to refocus the interventions, so that they are more helpful. Certainly, if you are not responsive to the client's feedback, in addition to the lack of efficacy, the therapeutic alliance may be damaged. Go back and ensure that the client is using the Thought Record properly, because ineffective methods often can be traced back to inadequate assessment. Ensure that the client understands how to use the methods by practicing them with him or her within the session. Sometimes ineffectiveness is related to sloppy application of methods by the therapist. Consult with a colleague to provide a different perspective, to ensure that you are optimizing the likelihood of success. But not all methods work for all clients, so if a method is truly not helpful, back up and try another approach. Flexibility and persistence on the part of the therapist provide a good model for clients.

Some clients tell you that although they see what you mean and accept your intervention intellectually, it does not "feel real" to them. This point has sometimes been described as a conflict between the "head" and the "heart" (J. S. Beck, 1995), or as intellectual understanding versus emotional experience. When you hear this concern, be aware that it usually reflects a conflict between two different beliefs. The intellectual thought is usually related to a nondysfunctional belief, and to the alternative perspective you are trying to help the client to develop; the emotional experience is tied to the original core belief. Help the client to name and to recognize these competing beliefs. This conflict can be a developmental phase that occurs as the client begins to entertain and to try out the new way of thinking. Sometimes, though, this issue reflects the fact that the client still retains old ways of thinking, so you need to identify more strongly and work to modify these beliefs.

One strategy to deal with this conflict between intellectual understanding and lived experience is to ask clients what evidence it would take for them not only to believe intellectually but also really to feel the alternative thoughts with which they are wrestling. Then design the needed experiments to make the alternative a truly lived experience rather than something that clients know only as a more productive way to think. For example, a perfectionistic client might say that, for most people, doing their best is enough, that being perfect is not a reasonable goal. The client may even be willing to experiment with some relatively "safe" assignments of doing less than he or she might previously have done. Although such assignments may reduce the intensity of the original thoughts, they are unlikely in the end to really undercut the core belief, and the thoughts that emanate from it. In such cases, it may be worthwhile to ask clients what evidence it would take for them really to accept that their prior thought is dysfunctional, and to let it go. Gathering such evidence, almost by necessity, moves clients out of their comfort zones and requires an experience that is so inconsistent with the clients' previous ways of thinking that the previous thought becomes untenable.

One issue that can arise as you work with a negative thought for a while is to find that your interventions are ineffective. The client may have come to accept this negative thinking as just a part of his or her life. Be aware that such an issue might arise when you are addressing long-standing, deeply held beliefs. Be careful not to accept a client's negative predictions, negative worldviews, or beliefs without careful review and lots of supportive evidence. Certainly, do not join the client in making negative statements about others (e.g., "No wonder your husband acts that way; all men are selfish"; "Yes, supervisors are often critical"). Be aware that such acceptance of negative ideas may reflect your own worldviews, and that therapy is not about the validation of your belief system, but about helping the client to solve his or her problems. There may be times when you find yourself feeling helpless or hopeless about the client's problems. If this occurs, seek out consultation to get a fresh perspective on the client's problems and/or consider referring the client to another therapist.

One relatively uncommon phenomenon is the overzealous client. We have had clients take to cognitive interventions so strongly that it becomes almost impossible to move them away from this approach. For example, we have had clients generate their own computer spread sheets to track negative thoughts, develop personal device assistant (PDA) software to track their thoughts, and become "super sleuths" in naming their own (and other people's) cognitive distortions. Some clients become quite adept at talking about, rather than changing, their negative thinking. This pattern can reflect an underlying obsessive–compulsive personality disorder and clients' need to organize even this part of their lives. Sometimes it reflects a desire to understand, but not necessarily change, negative thinking. A focus on tracking and understanding can interfere with efforts to change, because it can be indicative of cognitive avoidance. Either way, when we see this type of pattern, we typically shift from a focus on negative thinking to a behavioral and experiential focus. Such a shift helps to focus the therapy on the client's distress and problems, and encourages action rather than intellectualism. In general, as we stated earlier, we discourage cognitive assessment or intervention for its own sake. The goal of cognitive-behavioral therapy is to solve real-world problems in their natural environment.

The Case of Anna C, continued

The fifth scheduled session with Anna C was cancelled on the day of the appointment, because her son had come home from school feeling ill, and she "had to" stay home with him. The appointment was rescheduled for the following week, and when she came in, the therapist used the cancellation as an opportunity to discuss whether it represented another example of putting her own needs after the needs of other people in her life. Anna agreed that it was, but she also indicated that she rarely saw any alternative. She also acknowledged that such an event typically would heighten her anxiety about other people's health.

The therapist introduced the idea of cognitive distortions and provided a definition of some of the distortions Anna was likely using. The client was somewhat resistant to the idea of these as distortions, since she viewed her thoughts as "realistic." But the therapist and Anna agreed that it would be good to monitor these thoughts in any event, so the therapist demonstrated how to use the Thought Record to find out when the thoughts occurred and their effects on Anna.

Anna returned to the next session with five Thought Records, mostly related to health and family concerns. Her observation was that she often worried, and that it did not take much to start her worrying. Typically, the worry increased her distress but did not lead to productive problem solving. For example, any media item about cancer stimulated worry and sadness about Anna's mother, but was usually followed by no particular change in Anna's coping behavior. Together the therapist and Anna discussed the content of the worry, and identified some possible distortions that were related. Anna agreed to continue with the Thought Record, and the therapist worked with her in the next two sessions to become more aware of her negative thinking, and to begin to question it when it occurred.

While reviewing the Thought Records, the therapist noticed another pattern emerging, in addition to those related to self-sacrifice and health worries. This was the fairly frequent use of the word *should*, and Anna's often high expectations for herself. Through questioning, it became clear to the therapist and Anna often held standards that put extra pressure on herself, and to which she would not hold other people. The therapist and Anna agreed that it would be good to discern the areas in which she had these high expectations, so that they could later be reviewed for reconsideration and possible adjustment. Anna also continued to schedule activities and practice being more assertive, when the opportunity arose. Her mood was generally improving. Although she continued to have significant concern about her mother's deteriorating health, she found herself engaging more positive activities. The relationship between the therapist and Anna, by all appearances, was both congenial and productive.

Chapter 8

Assessing and Modifying Core Beliefs and Schemas

The cognitive-behavioral model assumes that clinical problems represent the combined effects of core beliefs or schemas, and some environmental trigger or event that activates these beliefs. It is this interaction between beliefs and environmental triggers that elicits situation-specific thinking, which in turn leads to adaptive or maladaptive emotional and behavioral consequences. In this chapter we address what is arguably the "heart" of the problem, which is the negative beliefs or schemas themselves. We provide a description of ways to assess core beliefs or schemas, then some evidence-based and logical strategies to help clients change these beliefs and schemas, if appropriate. We also discuss when not to do this work, and when to shift to acceptance of such enduring aspects of the self.

We have discussed strategies to conceptualize the process of how negative thinking and behaviors are related to your clients' problems. We have also discussed strategies to intervene with the functional/behavioral aspects of problems in coping, and in Chapter 7, this volume, presented a variety of ways to address negative situation-specific thinking. Here, we present strategies to assess and to intervene with negative core beliefs or schemas, which are hypothesized to be partly responsible for the development of your client's problems. You may wonder why we did not begin at this level, if negative core beliefs are so central to the process of disturbance.

We have several reasons for placing this chapter later in the book. In part, these issues are usually addressed in the latter phases of therapy, so we are mirroring the typical sequence of treatment. As we noted earlier, clients most often come to therapy when their attempts to cope or to deal with a problematical situations have moved beyond their ability to cope. Most clients also come into therapy with emotional and behavioral complaints, because these are theoretically the end products of negative cognitive-behavioral processes. Some clients are aware of their thinking patterns prior to the onset of therapy, because of past treatment, psychological mindedness or through reading about cognitive-behavioral therapy. Although these clients may be aware of the harm their thoughts do to their emotions and behaviors, they are likely far less aware of how to change these patterns. Regardless, it would still be quite unusual to start treatment at the level of directly identifying and changing core beliefs due to client distress and other, more immediate concerns.

After a certain point in therapy, however, when you and your client have been able to address some of the immediate treatment issues, and have established a good working alliance, and when he or she has learned some methods to combat negative thinking, the cognitive patterns become increasingly clear. It is at this point in therapy that you can potentially shift, to deal more directly with these patterns.

The shift toward schema-focused work occurs for some clients. But other clients may end treatment after their distress is reduced and some of the problems have been resolved. Also, in some cases, clients may not have the energy or interest in beginning this process, or they may simply run out of the financial resources or health benefits to engage in ongoing treatment. Because schema-focused work tends to follow symptom improvement and to focus on underlying factors, it typically takes longer than other types of cognitive-behavioral interventions. Later in this chapter, we address the issue of how to respect a client's choice not to pursue schema-related treatment.

Consider schema therapy for the following:

- Clients whose underlying beliefs or schemas create risk for relapse.
- Clients whose immediate symptoms or problems have been markedly reduced.
- Clients who are able to engage in more abstract discussions.
- Clients who are not at risk of current psychotic disorder.
- Clients who have the resources and interest to remain in longer-term treatment.

DEFINING SCHEMAS

One question that arises is why different terms are used to talk about the broad, enduring cognitive patterns that are the focus of cognitive-behavioral therapy. These terms include *attitudes, values, assumptions, beliefs,* and *schemas.* But does it really matter what term is used? Our position is that it probably does not matter too much. Attitudes and values are often conceptualized as long-standing opinions about a topic, object, or person; they usually involve some emotional valence. We often think about positive or negative attitudes (although attitudes can also be neutral), and we often focus on valuing or devaluing certain people, ideas, or objects. Assumptions, in contrast, are often long-standing ideas about the relationships among various concepts or people. We might assume, for example, that "bad people" will somehow be punished, that people who work hard will achieve career advancement, or that because "I am unlovable, no one will ever care about me." These statements by definition fall into an "if–then" form of logical relationship. As such, they come closer to what might be useful in cognitive-behavioral therapy, which also uses a model that examine how clients react to different situations and allows you as the therapist to use a variety of techniques, including those that focus on changing the situation, or that involve changing the client's response to the situation.

Beliefs and schemas are relatively permanent notions about objects, people, or concepts, and the relationships among them. Just like the previous concepts, they likely form as a result of a complex set of developmental processes. Some of the influences on a child's developing schemas include ideas that are imparted from the world (defined broadly as parents, immediate and extended family, friends, the media, music, and educational and other influences). As the child grows, personal experiences in the world create ideas, and actions that reify, reinforce, or challenge these ideas shape the form these schemas take over time. Beliefs and schemas may be categorical (e.g., "All men are selfish"), or relational (e.g., "Most attractive people end up with other attractive people"). They can also be directed toward the self, others, and the world in general. Beliefs and schemas may also may be historical and specific (e.g., "I was happy and carefree as a child"), or futuristic and general (e.g., "I will never get ahead"). People within a society often orient their beliefs along common axes or themes that are relevant to self-esteem, such as social orientation, intelligence, or popularity, but beliefs and schemas can also be highly idiosyncratic, based on unique developmental processes.

Schemas are potentially similar to personality traits, in that they are long-term aspects of the self, but they are different in the sense that traits typically are only seen as aspects of the self. Unfortunately, personality research and theory have also become associated with the concept of personality disorders (A. T. Beck, Freeman, & Davis, 2004; Widiger & Frances, 1994). In fact, personality theories provide many more constructs than have been used in diagnostic formulations (cf. Murray, 1938; Jackson, 1967; Widiger & Simonsen, 2005), but within clinical psychology and psychiatry, our focus has often been on problematical patterns of thought, behavior, or emotion, rather than on the full range of these constructs. Also, the concept of personality often leads to a focus within the individual and tends to deemphasize environmental or situational factors that either encourage or inhibit the expression of these factors. For these reasons, we tend to discourage an emphasis on personality factors in case conceptualizations within cognitive-behavioral therapy.

Based on this discussion, we present strategies to assess, evaluate, and modify either beliefs or schemas. These terms are used interchangeably, because the differences in meaning are relatively minor. As we conceptualize these concepts, beliefs and schemas are relatively permanent aspects of the way that we construct the world and make sense of experiences around us. A useful definition is that "the schema concept refers to cognitive structures of organized prior knowledge, abstracted from experience with specific instances; schemas guide the processing of new information and the retrieval of stored information" (Kovacs & Beck, 1978, p. 527). This definition highlights cognitive processes that are affected by schemas, including memory biases that help to reinforce existing schemas. But also highlighted are future-oriented biases, such as the tendency to pay attention to information that is consistent with existing schemas, and the corollary bias, which means paying less attention to inconsistent or schema-irrelevant information (Mahoney, 1991). These cognitive biases help to explain the durability of schemas, because they have a self-perpetuating aspect.

Young, Klosko, and Weishaar (2003) have discussed the ways that schemas tend to persist over time. Some people engage in *schema maintenance* behaviors, actions that are consistent with and reinforce an individual's self-belief. For example, for a client who believes that she is unlovable and never engages in intimate relationships as a consequence, this absence of intimacy perpetuates the belief of being unlovable. Some clients who believe they are unlovable might focus all of their attention, time, and energy on actions unrelated to intimacy. This *schema avoidance* behavior, while not directly maintaining the schema of unlovability, nonetheless does not allow for the provision of any evidence or experience contrary to the schema, and in this sense maintains the schema. Finally, some clients engage in *schema compensation* behaviors, behaving in ways that overcompensate for the schema. A client with an unlovability schema, for example, might become sexually promiscuous and have many men around her. But these relationships are not truly intimate and caring, and at some level they again reinforce or support the client's belief that she is an unlovable person at core. Young et al. have described the development, maintenance, and treatment of these schema behaviors for clients with interpersonal and other problems.

As we implied earlier, schemas are ubiquitous. All humans have schemas, and about lots of topics. In cognitive-behavioral therapy, we tend to focus on schemas about the self and interpersonal relationships, because these are the ones that typically are associated with distress and therapeutic goals. In the sections that follow, we first discuss how to identify and assess these schemas, then how we approach them from a change or acceptance perspective.

DISCOVERING BELIEFS AND SCHEMAS

Beliefs and schemas are identified in therapy in a number of ways. As described earlier, part of the case conceptualization process in cognitive-behavioral therapy involves speculation about the core beliefs or schemas that make clients susceptible to the problems with which they present. Many of the articles about specific disorders include a description of the most common schemas seen in these disorders (cf. Riso, du Toit, Stein, & Young, 2007).

As noted in Chapter 7, this volume, we make a distinction between situation-specific thoughts and more stable core beliefs or schemas. Almost by definition, if you hear a thought expressed by your client that is not specific to a moment or situation in time, but is more thematic or stable, then it is more likely to be a core belief. As a therapist looking for these themes, you will likely hear them and fold them into your case conceptualization. Even if what you hear confirms your hypotheses, remain aware of disconfirmatory evidence, and do not make assumptions about your client's schemas prematurely. Keep in mind, though, that patterns of emotions and behavior also may reflect a core belief. The client who is typically angry, or who is often socially avoidant, likely has some beliefs that precipitate these reactions. Also, clients who often find themselves in similar situations (e.g., with people who are irritated with them) are often doing things based on their schemas that in turn engender common reactions in others.

Searching for Themes

As you look for common themes across time, the patterns occasionally emerge, without the need for any specific assessment. As a therapist, you may have an understanding of the patterns and describe them to your client at a certain point in treatment. Our advice, in the first instance, is to describe what you have observed in therapy and see whether the client agrees that this is a pattern. If possible, have the client provide a name or label for this pattern, then evaluate the client's way of understanding it. If the description is not presented in a confrontational manner, but more as something you have observed and wonder about, the client is more likely to participate in this process. In contrast, we discourage labeling the schema as something you have identified, then explaining to the client how it functions or the problems that you see tied to it.

Some clients develop awareness of their own patterns and may come to therapy ready to discuss them. Other clients start therapy with this understanding, particularly if they have been in other types of therapy prior to cognitive-behavioral therapy, if they have been reading about their problems, or if they are psychologically minded. Our suggestion, again, is to ask clients what evidence or experiences they have noticed that are part of this process. Here, there may be a decision point, about whether the time is right in therapy to focus on core beliefs. Our perspective is that some concrete problems should be solved in therapy first, and you also need to have enough experience with the client to see the schema in operation before you start to intervene. Engaging in this process too early can lead to misguided interventions or, even worse, set up a confrontation between your ideas for change and the client's schemas. For example, if one of your client's schemas is about being undervalued or not appreciated, and you are encouraging change, that very act of intervention might lead the client to conclude that you also do not care for or value the person that he or she is. On the other hand, if the client has recognized the negative influences of certain core beliefs, then this is the point in therapy at least to understand this process better, if not intervene. In the previous example, you might discuss your idea that, on the one hand, you would like the client to look at his or her sense of being undervalued, but your concern is that it might make him or her feel unappreciated. By doing this, you begin to name the belief and assess the client's readiness to examine these processes.

Recurrent Experience

Another type of response that may indicate that you are close to the identification of a core schema occurs when the client expresses the idea that the current experience reminds him or her of an earlier experience in life. Recurrent experiences, especially if they are "felt" as similar, are a good indication that the client has had a schema triggered or activated by this memory. A good strategy is to probe further regarding the prior situation(s), and to ask the client what it is that draws the situations together. Again, try to work out how these situations fit into the cognitive-behavioral case conceptualization.

Downward Arrow

As we described in Chapter 7, this volume, a specific technique for assessing core beliefs, the downward arrow, can be used to "drill" all the way down to the central beliefs, or to examine the inferences your client attaches to various events or thoughts, or experiences in multiple situations. Over time, assessment of inference chaining helps you to identify your client's core beliefs. Even if you do not use the entire downward arrow method, you get a sense of the inferences your client is making, and what meaning is attached.

Sharing Case Conceptualization

Another commonly used strategy to assess and clarify the role of schemas is to share the case conceptualization with the client. We have suggested that a case conceptualization may be developed following the first session, and it naturally evolves and becomes more complete and detailed over the course of treatment. When you and the client are ready to discuss the schema, you may use one of a number of various formats for discussing it. One of us (K. S. D.) tends to use the format presented in Figure 3.2 to describe the relationships among schemas, activating situations, automatic thoughts, and behavioral and emotional consequences. The way that the case formulation is shared with the client depends on the client. You might use the forms developed by Persons (1989) or J. S. Beck (1995) as a basis for discussion. With any of these techniques, rather than encouraging the client to examine his or her schemas away from their immediate effects, you are encouraging a metacognitive appraisal of the schema and its effects.

Behavioral Assignments

Schemas can also be assessed through behavioral assignments. For example, you and a client might hypothesize that she has a general belief that others will reject her if she is open and honest. Such an assumption is generally based on a deeper belief about being socially undesirable, which you could hypothesize with the client. To test out this prediction, though, you and the client could set up an assignment in which she purposely is more self-disclosing than she would typically be to test whether this assumption becomes activated. Note that this homework assignment also potentially provides disconfirmatory evidence for the belief, but the key part of the assessment is to see whether the situation itself provokes the expected automatic thoughts based on the case formulation.

Hypothetical Situations

A somewhat less demanding alternative to the previous method is to construct hypothetical events and see how the client thinks he or she would respond in those situations. These predictions are likely to come close to the actual responses (but be mindful of possible biases in predictions), and one of the virtues of using hypothetical situations is that they are relatively easy to create and to modify in determining what parameters of the situation are most associated with negative responses. Hypothetical evaluations are also useful if the triggers are unusual or difficult to set up in a homework assignment. But be mindful that these are thought experiments that may or may not reflect the actual experience of your client in a real-life situation. Also, be mindful that some clients will be happy to talk about how they think they would respond, if that satisfies you, because it may allow them to avoid actually testing out the predictions. Try, if you can, to develop an *in vivo* assessment of core beliefs rather than relying on hypothetical events.

Historical Perspective

Another strategy to help with assessing schemas is to ask about their historical bases. Generally, our perspective is that schemas develop when they serve a useful purpose, either to make sense of the world or to help the client adapt to the current situation. Developing a belief that he is somehow flawed, for example, may be a very adaptive way for a teenager to make sense of being socially rejected. If you can identify the approximate period in his life when the schema first developed, and understand how that schema was adaptive *at that time*, it might provide further evidence that you have accurately identified an early schema that has maintained itself over time and is now causing distress or disturbance.

Emotional Prime

Yet another strategy for assessing schemas is to employ emotive techniques to trigger or to activate these schemas. For example, your client may have come into therapy because of depression and other concerns. By the time you begin to address the schemas openly in therapy, the client's depression level may be quite reduced, so it may be more difficult for him or her to remain aware of the schema and its consequences. In such cases, you could do an evaluation in which you encourage the client to recall a sad time in his or her life, and to try genuinely to feel the experience as if it were occurring in the current moment, to see whether that emotional prime can activate beliefs that were present in the past. In some cases, this type of emotional priming can be helpful to demonstrate to the client that the schema or belief is still present, but less active due to treatment success.

Reading Materials

Some clients benefit from readings about core beliefs and schemas. We are quite prepared, if the client expresses a desire, and if he or she seems to have the reading and intellectual ability, to recommend chapters, books, or other materials to help the client better understand the model and how his or her problems are related to dysfunctional beliefs. Good sources include selected chapters from *The Feeling Good Handbook* (Burns, 1989, 1999), *Reinventing Your Life* (Young & Klosko, 1994), or *Mind over Mood* (Greenberger & Padesky, 1995). We have had clients read therapist manuals in some cases to get their sense of how well the model for a specific disorder fits their sense of self. Also, although we tend to recommend materials that have a cognitive-behavioral emphasis, we may instead recommend readings from other models, if they are relevant to the case at hand.

Formal Assessment

A formal way to assess schemas is through the use of questionnaires. Two measures that are relevant to depression in particular are the Dysfunctional Attitude Scale (DAS; Weissman & Beck, 1980) and the Sociotropy–Autonomy Scale (SAS; Bieling, Beck, & Brown, 2000; D. A. Clark & Beck, 1991). Both measures ask clients to read a series of statements that reflect potentially dysfunctional beliefs and to rate the degree to which they endorse each statement. The DAS was originally written with 100 items, but two similar 40-item versions have been developed. Form A, which is the more commonly used scale (Nezu et al., 2000) has been factor-analyzed into two scales, which are the same scales on the SAS. These scales reflect either sociotropy or autonomy. *Sociotropy* has been defined (A. T. Beck, 1993) as the tendency to draw meaning and validation from social relationships; sociotropic people are vulnerable to anxiety, if they fear the loss of relationships or social contact, and to depression, if these negative events actually occur. *Autonomy* is related to concerns about independence and recognition. Autonomous persons are vulnerable to anxiety, if these concerns are threatened, and to depression, if there is a loss of independence, lack of recognition for success, or failure. Studies have generally confirmed that higher scores on sociotropy scales in particular predict future depression, if the triggers are established; the predictions about autonomy have been more elusive in research (D. A. Clark, Beck, & Alford, 1999).

The other scale that is available to measure schemas is the Young Schema Questionnaire (YSQ; *www.schematherapy.com/id55.htm*), a 205-item self-report scale. The YSQ provides statements that reflect various possible schemas, which the client is asked to endorse. There are 11 rationally devised negative schemas on the YSQ, based on the work of Young (see Table 8.1). The YSQ has been factor-analyzed, and the theoretical structure has been supported by that work (Lee, Taylor, & Dunn, 1999). It is relatively lengthy and requires scoring time, but the scale does yield a profile of various schemas that may be present in your clients. Strengths of the YSQ are that the authors have described in detail the phenotype of each schema, a prototypical description of the schemas' development and operation, as well as potential interventions for these schemas (Young et al., 2003).

One of the questions that emerges with questionnaire assessments of schemas is when to use them in treatment. If these scales are completed at the outset of treatment, the scores can be inflated by the current distress of the client. If they are completed too late in treatment, the schemas may already be shifting, and getting a measure of their effect may be more difficult. Our recommendation is to wait to do the assessment until the point in therapy when a number of the client's initial problems have been somewhat improved, but the client is still wrestling with negative thoughts. In this way, the schemas are still active and amenable to assessment but less likely to be inflated by distress. The scale can be introduced as a way better to understand the client's thinking. When you present the results to the client is also be a good time to describe the case conceptualization and get the client's responses. Ideally, the scales confirm your clinical case conceptualization and may be offered to the client as another independent validation of the way that you have come to think about his or her problems. Many clients find feedback from the YSQ and other measures, with follow-up discussion regarding their schemas, very useful.

CHANGING SCHEMAS

You have reached the point in therapy at which the client's day-to-day functioning has improved. You have determined which of his or her core beliefs contributed to the initial problems and have likely discussed with the client some of the historical bases for these schemas, and how they

TABLE 8.1. Early Maladaptive Schemas Identified by the Young Schema Questionnaire

1. Abandonment/instability
2. Mistrust/abuse
3. Emotional deprivation
4. Defectiveness/shame
5. Social isolation/alienation
6. Dependence/incompetence
7. Vulnerability to harm or illness
8. Enmeshment/undeveloped self
9. Failure
10. Entitlement/grandiosity
11. Insufficient self-control/self-discipline
12. Subjugation
13. Self-sacrifice
14. Approval seeking/recognition seeking
15. Negativity/pessimism
16. Emotional inhibition
17. Unrelenting standards/hypercriticalness
18. Punitiveness

Note. From Young, Klosko, and Weishaar (2003). Copyright 2003 by The Guilford Press. Reprinted by permission.

made sense at the time of schema development. You may have used questionnaires to evaluate the presence of various schemas, but you would certainly have developed and shared with the client an idiographic description of the case conceptualization, and have achieved some consensus about it. You are potentially ready to engage in schema change, not so much to solve current problems, but possibly to reduce the risk of relapse or future setbacks.

We urge you to pause for a moment before plunging into schema change interventions. Although it may make logical sense that changing dysfunctional schemas reduces vulnerability to future distress, and you and your client may agree, modifying schemas is difficult work. The client will be asked, in essence, to challenge some of the key ways that he or she has construed him- or herself and made sense of the world. Changing schemas may involve the client's need to modify social circles, to confront people from the past, and even to face rejection from others, if he or she is perceived as changing "too much." This work is likely to lead to some destabilization of identity and may in the short term actually increase rather than decrease distress.

Furthermore, the evidence in support of schema change is relatively weak. In a component analysis of cognitive therapy for depression, the addition of either cognitive restructuring or schema-focused interventions to behavioral activation therapy methods did not improve clinical outcomes in the acute treatment of depression (Jacobson et al., 1996). More to the current point, however, adding these interventions to behavioral activation therapy did not reduce the risk of relapse over a 2-year follow-up (Gortner, Gollan, Dobson, & Jacobson, 1998; see also Dimidjian et al., 2006). So, at least in the treatment of depression, the evidence for additional benefit of schema work is limited. Recent work has shown that schema therapy in the context of borderline personality disorder does reduce both short- and long-term distress (Giesen-Bloo et al., 2006). To our knowledge, otherwise, only cases studies and uncontrolled trials support the value of schema-based interventions. Certainly, much anecdotal evidence gained through informal discussion with therapists supports the use of Young and his colleague's (2003) work, but more research is needed.

These considerations suggest to us that before we embark on this voyage with clients, we all need genuinely to believe that the benefits will outweigh the associated costs of time, money, and likely emotional distress. Also, because clients almost never come to therapy with a treatment goal for this type of change, because awareness of underlying dysfunctional schemas emerges over the course of therapy, we believe we have an ethical obligation to obtain the client's explicit consent for this work before going too far down this road. One of the first things that needs to done in this context is to talk with clients about the implications and potential consequences of making schema changes, so that they understand their commitment. We also respect the right of our clients not to provide this consent, at which point we shift to a termination and relapse planning mode (see Chapter 9, this volume). Also, and even though we recognize that the data are equivocal on this issue, the cognitive model predicts that clients who do not make schema changes have an increased likelihood of relapse. Therefore, it is good practice to offer an "open door," so that clients can return to therapy quickly in the future, possibly to address this change at that time. It is also quite likely that clients gradually change their schemas without direct interventions, by behaving and thinking differently over time. If they continue to do so after treatment is over, it is quite possible that their schemas may change because of their different experiences, without benefit of formal schema therapy.

SCHEMA CHANGE METHODS

Predicated on the assumption that you and your client accept the clinical utility of schema change, and that the client has consented to this work, there are two broad strategies for doing this work. These are evidence-based and logical change methods, and each is described in turn here.

Evidence-Based Change Methods

A number of strategies exist to help your clients modify their core beliefs or schemas. Typically, these interventions begin with the identification of the existing or "old" schema, which is then contrasted with a preferred or "new" schema. From a purely practical perspective, we often begin with a logical discussion of the costs and benefits of the old and the new schemas, to help clients accept in principle that schema change is a good idea (see extended discussion below), then use evidence-based ideas to emphasize the value of change.

Recognizing Continua

One strategy used in schema work is changing schemas from categorical traits to a more specific continuum, or set of continua. For example, a client may have the existing schema of being "distrusting." This schema may have developed from a series of life experiences, including disengaged parents, several social rejections, or even abusive relationships. But mistrust might now be associated with being alone, rejecting any social approaches, being fearful of others, wondering about other people's motivations, and even mind reading about what those motivations might be. Rather than trying to modify the overall schema of being mistrusting, it may be easier to identify the key behavioral or emotional markers of the schema and move to change these. For example, it is easier to recognize, assess, and restructure mind reading than to change a more global construct, such as distrust. But by changing the key elements, the larger construct will shift over time.

Positive Data Log

Another evidence-based strategy for modifying schemas also rests on identifying key markers of the new and desired schema. Having done so, the task for the client, then, is to begin to notice and write down in log form evidence that supports development of the new schema. In doing so, the focus of attention shifts to positive evidence, and fosters other positive actions or cognitions that support the more positive belief. For example, a mother who always worries about her adult children, which could lead her to intrude into their lives, might instead try to develop a schema of being "caring and concerned," and develop several ways to demonstrate this new schema, which could then be tracked and/or augmented using a Positive Data Log. In practice, these logs usually have two columns. At the top of the page, the titles of the old and new schemas are written, then data consistent with the new schema are written in one column.

The other column is used to track evidence that is consistent with the old schema, but with a more positive and therapeutic reinterpretation.

Evidence for the Old and New Schemas

As the client's schemas start to change, an extension of the Positive Data Log is to develop a form to record evidence that supports the existence and effects of the old and new schemas. Initially, it may be that evidence strongly indicates that the old belief system is dominant, but as change starts to happen (we hope the client is making changes), evidence for the new belief becomes stronger and more credible.

What Would It Take to Change the Belief?

Tracking more objective information about old and new beliefs can lead to a discussion of the types of evidence the client requires to believe fully that the new schema has "taken root" and is starting to guide his or her behavioral choices and interpretation of situations. This discussion can be very helpful, clarifying the client's beliefs regarding the nature of change, the extent of possible change, and the criteria he or she employs to recognize change in this area. Some clients set the standard so high that it is very unlikely that they will ever believe they have truly changed. Other clients may see a single setback as evidence that they have failed in the goal of schema change. Anticipating these obstacles with clients and setting concrete, objective markers for change help to reduce the risk of these difficulties.

The question of what it would take to change the belief helps you, as therapist, to evaluate the realistic prospects of a client's internalized, felt change. For example, if a client who struggles with lack of trust says that she needs to be trusting and calm with everyone she meets to really believe the schema has changed, she is likely to be discouraged and potentially to perceive herself as failing with this treatment goal. A more realistic new schema might be to give others a chance to prove themselves. Another possibility might be to learn some signs of judging who might be trustworthy and who might not. Again, movement toward the new schema is more likely than through setting impossible standards or goals through discussion with the client and establishment of some realistic benchmarks.

Therapy Role Plays

Another strategy to modify schemas is by using therapy time to practice. For example, if the client's old schema was "incompetent" and the new one is to be "assured and competent," then you can help the client practice acting assuredly and competently in the therapy session. Some clients may need behavioral instruction or some of the other methods discussed in Chapter 6, this volume, to make behavioral changes, especially if their childhood backgrounds were impoverished or failed to provide the key skills in this domain. These skills can be communicated and practiced in the therapy session, so that clients have the chance to maximize their chances of success. Ideally, you can even develop some demanding role plays, in which you increasingly challenge the new and more positive schema that is being developed. You might even present yourself as a "devil's advocate," using the same information the client used in the past to berate or criticize him- or herself, to see how the client deals with this evidence as the new schema develops.

Therapy "Confrontation"

As discussed by Young and colleagues (2003), it is very helpful to use the therapy relationship itself to promote schema change. For example, if you have a client who is socially dependent or demanding, perhaps because his schema is one of ineptitude or inability to foster change, you and he can discuss how his schema affects the therapy relationship. You can identify signs that indicate the schema is changing within the treatment relationship, and you can encourage such change through your own comments and actions. Ideally, when you see these signs, you can provide positive feedback to the client that you have noticed these changes. In this way, the therapeutic relationship itself can become a vehicle for providing evidence that the schemas are shifting.

> You have been seeing John for some time. He initially presented with generalized worry and depressive symptoms. Over time, you have noticed that he looks for reassurance and tends to be deferential in therapy. Once his symptoms improved, he expressed interest in schema change therapy. When you and he reconceptualized his case, schemas related to dependence on trusted others and fear of failure were apparent. In therapy sessions, you point out times where he looks to you for guidance and minimizes his own efforts at change. You note that you are likely to make mistakes in providing advice for his life. You encourage him to take risks in the sessions and make choices for himself. Together, you and John appraise therapy progress, encouraging genuine feedback in the process.

Behavioral Assignments

One of the common and more effective strategies to generate evidence to support the utility of a new schema is that of behavioral assignments.

This strategy consists of discussing with the client how they would act, think and feel if they truly internalized the new schema. You and the client can then devise a behavioral assignment in which some aspect of the new schema gets acted out. For example, a quiet and passive female client who adopts a martyr role at work, and regularly stays late to do extra work to "save" her ineffective boss could purposely decide to be more assertive and not to stay late. The direct experience provided by the adoption of the actions associated with the new schema will provide experiential learning with this new way to think and act. Hopefully, when the homework is reviewed, the client will perceive more advantages than disadvantages associated with the new schema, and will be encouraged to take further steps in this new direction.

> John, the client discussed previously, continues to seek reassurance from you and is reluctant to take risks. After reidentifying the dependence and fear of failure schema, and discussing how it is interfering with change, a collaborative behavioral assignment is proposed for homework. He agrees to behaving "as if" he were not so dependent on the approval of others whom he respects. John tends to be very agreeable when his partner makes suggestions regarding weekend activities. He proposes suggesting activities he is interested in, but has no idea whether she enjoys them. In addition, both you and John agree that he will do an additional experiment that he decides would be useful, but is not discussed in session.

Acting "As If"

A similar but extended behavioral assignment is to try to act as if the new schema actually has been fully incorporated into the client's schema system. This method has also been referred to as "faking it till you make it," but this language has a negative connotation that is unfortunate. What we imagine is a thorough discussion of how clients think, feel, and act with the old schema, and contrasting that with how they would function using the new schema. This discussion can even extend to clothing or lifestyles, career paths, and social networks. Having discussed these considerations, you then can ask clients how far they are willing to extend this idea of acting as if they really believe the new schema, then organize this experiment with them. With some creativity, imagination, and an open mind, this type of behavioral assignment extension could also be fun and liberating for clients.

Typically, the acting "as if" technique involves several areas of functioning. It may be so dramatic to other people in the client's social sphere that some planning is needed. For example, the client should be warned to expect others to comment or potentially even to react negatively to the perceived changes, and there may be social pressure to shift back to the old way of being. These responses can be used to indicate who in the client's world is supportive of his or her positive changes, and who is not. On the other hand, the client could also be warned that other people may not notice, which may also be very useful information. The client him- or herself may feel quite uncomfortable with the new way of behaving, and may be inclined to shift back to old patterns. The extent of the impulse to give up or to shift back, of course, is itself an index of the strength of the old schema.

As an example, one of us (K. S. D.) was treating a client for depression. Part of the client's problems was that she had low self-esteem in intimate relationships, yet felt that she needed the love of a man to provide a sense of validation. Despite being a successful working woman, she often reacted positively to men's sexual advances and not infrequently ended up in sexual situations that later left her feeling regretful and degraded. Yet, due to her schemas, she experienced a kind of quiet desperation as each weekend approached, because she felt the need to attract a partner. Paradoxically, her pattern of temporarily accepting unacceptable partners ultimately was not satisfying to her. Having identified this pattern, and the schemas that drove it, the therapist discussed how the client might behave differently if she did not have these schemas. Changes in her social actions, the people with whom she spoke, her manner of dress, and even some of her usual social companions were identified. Alternative behaviors to going to the bar and attracting men were identified, including doing some painting in her apartment to make it more her own space, and resuming an enjoyable hobby that she had neglected. She agreed to try the experiment of living for a month "as if" she did not need the love of a man to be complete. She changed her social activities and patterns (and endured some negative feedback from others). She painted several rooms in her apartment, about which she felt very positively, and began a course related to her hobby. She was lonely at times, and once was sorely tempted to quit the experiment, but she persevered. By the end of the month, the client was proud of her own persistence and reported feeling more rounded and self-considerate. She did want to be in an intimate relationship, but she came to realize that she was not likely to achieve that outcome with her previous strategy. Further therapy was needed, of course, to further redefine the emerging schema and plan how to put it into operation, but the monthlong acting "as if" experiment was an important part of the shift in this self-schema.

Confronting the Past

Yet another method that examines evidence related to schemas is to determine the history of their emergence and potentially to confront the past in therapy. This method is useful when the client expresses conflicted feelings or thoughts about past events. For example, a client may discuss parenting that was ineffective, neglectful or even abusive, but have a generally positive appraisal of his upbringing. Even though his schemas may be related to the parenting he experienced, he may have a difficult time discussing this because of ambivalent feelings about his parents. In such cases, you can have the client recall in detail some of his early experiences, and try to reexperience fully these events through the use of imagery. Often, such reliving helps to demonstrate that the parents were the primary source of problems when he was a child, because children are relatively impotent in affecting overall family functioning. Such reexperiencing may even help the client to reexplain events in his life that are inconsistent with his negative schemas, and in such a way that permits change. Use of this method in therapy is likely to generate strong and conflicted emotions. Some clients feel emotions, such as intense guilt or shame, when recalling early experiences. Others, particularly those who have had past trauma, may have dissociative experiences. Although these intense emotional reactions are quite common, you likely know your client quite well by this point in therapy and are aware of the reduction in the distress that brought him or her into therapy. The "hot" cognitions evidenced during the emotional reactions are likely very useful in schema change.

In some cases, the client's memory of the past is too indistinct or emotionally laden to confront or to change past impressions effectively. In some cases, clients may still have people from their past available to them, so that they can actually confront people from their past in reality. For example, a client might talk to her mother about parenting actions to see whether her own perceptions and memories correspond with her mother's recollections. Talking to siblings about shared experiences can similarly be used to reexamine the family's role in schema development, as well as to obtain multiple perspectives on events. The goal of these questions should be to examine and challenge the schema rather than to determine whose memories are accurate.

Although, confrontation of the past at times, can generate important new information to help clients reevaluate their development and their need for schemas, the method involves some significant risks. One of the risks associated with this method is that the client's own schemas may bias the memory and recall of these events, making a fresh look at them very difficult, if not impossible. Also, confronting people involved in the development of schemas runs the very real risk of also needing to understand and appreciate the role of other people's schemas in how they discuss these events. Other people may not be open to the discussion or may disagree with the client about the benefits of reviewing past events. If this strategy is used, it is helpful to plan carefully and perhaps use role-play practice to rehearse the conversations with the other people. Some discussion of these limitations is warranted prior to your client undertaking historical reconstruction of schemas. Finally, reexamining the early experiences associated with schema development cannot be a goal in and of itself, because the information gleaned from this exercise would then need to be incorporated into other schema change exercises.

Logical Change Methods

All of these methods involve obtaining and examining evidence related to old and new schemas. They provide powerful methods for schema change. If the work is done carefully and collaboratively, then the client begins to experience the new schema as something more positive and adaptive than its precursor. Often, these evidence-based strategies are used in concert with more logical or inductive methods of schema change discussed here. Thus, you might begin schema change with a logical discussion of the idea, generate an early experiential exercise to examine the influence of the schema, promote further logical discussion that might then prompt a new evidence-based exercise, and so forth, until the client actually has begun to shift beliefs and schemas.

Imaging the New Self

As described earlier, a necessary part of schema change is contrasting the old schema and its influences with the new, emerging schema and its effects. To do so, the new self needs to be identified as clearly as possible, so that the client can imagine its effects as fully and vividly as possible. Even the process of imagining the new schema may have the effect of "loosening up" clients' commitment to their old ways of thinking and being, allowing greater flexibility in their thought process.

One of the most straightforward ways to help clients imagine ways that they might change is to ask questions about the areas of their lives with which they are dissatisfied and might seek change. Try to connect these ideas to the problematical situations you have seen in therapy, and help the client to think these changes through. Ideally, clients will come up with these ideas themselves, but if not, you can encourage them to get ideas from a number of sources, including books (e.g., biographies) or movies. You might assign readings that discuss these issues (e.g., the final chapters in *Feeling Good* [Burns, 1999] or *Reinventing Your Life* [Young & Klosko, 1994]). You might employ parables from either classic writings, such as *Aesop's Fables*, or other cases you have treated. If appropriate, you might self-disclose, discussing changes you have made in your own life (be sure not to disclose in such a way that you represent yourself as an ideal model to follow). If these ideas fail, you can consider making suggestions to the client, but ensure that you respect the client's right to choose his or her own path. For example, the client might read the biography of Christopher Reeve, a person who did remarkable things despite a life-changing accident, or the biography of Mark Tewksbury, a person who ultimately overcame shame and stigma to be true to his real self.

Soliciting Social Support and Consensus

In conjunction with imagining his or her new self, you could encourage clients to obtain ideas and reactions from others in their social sphere about their intended changes. In this exercise, you can have clients plan what they want to reveal to others, and what types of reactions they want from these people. Such feedback can help you and your clients predict what types of social reactions the clients will face if they start to make choices, and may have an effect on the nature of the changes themselves. For example, a client who finds that her plans to make modest changes are not only welcome, but, even more, would be acceptable to friends and family, may be encouraged to make even more changes in her life. Also, the act of having these discussions with others helps to prepare them for whatever changes ensue. Make sure that clients seek out social support or information from people they trust and with whom they are willing to discuss these ideas. It is not likely to be helpful to get reactions from people who are not important to clients, or whose feedback they will dismiss.

Discussing the Advantages and Disadvantages (Short and Long Term) of Old and New Schemas

One of the more formal, classic methods used to evaluate the potential utility and effects of adopting a new schema is to examine it from a variety of angles. This usually includes the advantages and disadvantages of the old and the new schema. By the time your client is ready to entertain the adoption of a new schema, he or she likely has seen the disadvantages of the old schema and views the alternative as an ideal. We suggest that you stop for a moment, though, and explore more fully all aspects of the old and new schema. According to the model, schemas develop based on past experiences, and they help people make sense of their world. Thus, even the most crippling and apparently dysfunctional schema likely "made sense" or was adaptive at the time of its development. It is also not too difficult to imagine the "benefits" associated with negative beliefs. For example, a client who believes she is unlovable does not need to try to find a meaningful relationship and risk being hurt. A client who thinks he is "flawed" can make sense of repeated rejection. A perfectionist can appreciate why she is always frustrated with others, and why they always let her down. On the other hand, even the most attractive alternative belief comes at a cost. The unlovable client who begins to challenge this belief needs to risk being hurt in relationships. The flawed client needs to learn that perhaps he has some positive attributes, and that he has to take responsibility for his part of the success (or failure) of social relations. Part of overcoming perfectionism is learning to tolerate imperfection in the self and in others. All of these changes are stressful and difficult for these respective clients. You can point out to clients, however, that any change involves risk taking, with potentially positive results.

We also recognize that some of the advantages and disadvantages of the old and the new schemas have different time frames. Thus, the "advantages" of the old schemas have likely occurred in the more distant past, but they largely have negative consequences in recent history or in the present. In contrast, new and more adaptive schemas likely have some short-term disadvantages, but more positive long-term advantages. Table 8.2 provides an example of this type of analysis, in the hypothetical case of a client with a dysfunctional schema about being flawed. Note that this type of analysis likely takes some time to develop, and that therapist and client can work on it together, using a combination of reflection, logical analysis, and behavioral experiments.

Time Projection

Yet another logical strategy to shift core beliefs is to encourage the client to assume that his or her new schema is in place, and to project him- or herself forward in time to imagine the person he or she wants to be. Some strategies of this type include writing new personal scripts. Such scripts might be narrative documents, similar to a short story or a novel. They might alternatively be lists of developing attributes, notes to oneself, or even index cards for the client to remind him- or herself of the type of schema he or she is trying to develop. Note that these are not the same as simple affirmations, such as "Every day in every way I am getting better and better." Rather, these are goal-oriented change reminders, with a concrete and specific set of criteria for recognizing success. For example, a client who is trying to modify her self-expression, to appear more warm

TABLE 8.2. Contrasting Old and New Schemas

Areas to evaluate	Old schema: "I am flawed at the core."	New schema: "I am basically 'OK'; and doing the best I can."
Advantages Short-term	"I don't need to expect much." "I don't need to try too hard."	"I can expect more positive outcomes in my life." "I can expect more from others. This belief allows me to grow and develop."
Long-term	"It explains why my father beat me as a child."	"A chance to be happy." "A chance for new relationships and intimacy." "The chance to work toward a goal that I believe in."
Disadvantages Short-term	"Limited personal and career success."	"Confusion about my real worth." "Some people may not know how to react to me." "It will be hard work to change my negative belief."
Long-term	"Low self-esteem." "Depression." "Lack of social relationships." "Lots of lonely nights." "Limited risk taking."	"I need to take risks to grow, which is fraught with the possibility of failure."

and welcoming to others, might place a cue card on her dresser mirror that reminds her to "dress the way you want to feel."

A particular type of time projection, of a bit more macabre form, involves having the clients imagine themselves at the end of their lives, and how they would like to be remembered. Various ways to formalize this type of time projection might include writing an idealized personal memoir, or writing the funerary eulogy or personal epitaph for a client after he or she has died. Obviously, some discretion is needed in using this method. Ensure that your client is not prone to hopelessness and/or suicide. This exercise, however, can help some clients focus on what is most important to them and lead to more focus within their lives, as well as shifts in their schemas.

ACCEPTANCE-BASED INTERVENTIONS

Cognitive-behavioral therapy is generally oriented toward change, and the previously discussed methods are related either to evidence-based or logical analysis in service of change. In some instances, clients choose not to change their schemas, perhaps because of the perceived energy, time, and resources it might take, or because of fears about potential social or other consequences of making these changes. They may also believe that this change is not possible or totally desirable. Some clients who reach the point in therapy that they have made some positive changes, and generally feel better about themselves and their situation, choose to take a break from therapy. One of the important skills for a cognitive-behavioral therapist is to know when change is possible, and when to urge the client to continue in this direction, or when it may be more appropriate to shift to a stance of awareness and acceptance as the final goal of treatment.

What we are discussing here is not capitulation or giving up on schema change. Rather, we are referring to a conscious, and joint, decision not to pursue schema change at a given point in time. Ultimately, this decision is the client's to make, and your job is to help him or her make the best choice under the circumstances. If the client decides to terminate treatment without making significant schema change, there are several strategies that you can pursue:

1. Help clients to recognize and accept that their decision is a sound one for them at the current point in time. This attitude helps them to revisit their decision in the future, to recognize that it can potentially be changed, and to realize that they can come back into therapy to discuss the decision with you again.

2. Discuss the potential effect of their decision, particularly with respect to the risk of relapse (see Chapter 9, this volume). Although not engaging in deliberate schema change treatment may theoretically increase the risk of relapse, there is little evidence to support this prediction.

3. Undertake interventions that make clients resilient to relapse, even in the absence of schema change. Such interventions include the following:

   a. Learning how to predict, recognize, and tolerate stress that emanates from unchanged schemas. For example, someone with a "martyr complex" can learn to recognize the ways that she thinks and behaves as a martyr, and can come to expect the negative outcomes associated with this pattern. Sometimes predicting and naming a pattern can reduce distress, even if the pattern itself is not modified. Over time, and with awareness, the schema may gradually shift without treatment.

b. Develop other competencies to offset the stress associated with the schema. For example, a perfectionist who has extremely high standards and causes himself a lot of personal distress can perhaps increase social skills and activities, as a way to reduce distress associated with perfectionism.

c. Develop compensatory strategies. Young and colleagues (2003) have written extensively about schema compensation, and they typify such strategies as negative. For example, they discuss most forms of avoidance of schema-related topics as maladaptive, and they are, in the sense that they maintain the schema. However, if the goal is not to modify schemas, but to learn to tolerate and live with them, then avoidance can serve an adaptive function. For example, if, due to his sense of defectiveness and shame, a male client is repetitively drawn to women who are psychologically abusive, he might purposely choose not to engage with this type of woman. This schema avoidance is not likely to undermine the schema, but at least the negative experiences associated with the schema are minimized.

d. If the schema patterns have been fully elucidated, then the triggers or stimuli that activate the schema should become apparent. With this knowledge, the client can choose to reduce the exposure to these triggers. For example, if the client has in the past chosen to confront her partner when he drinks too much, and this pattern has led to abuse and later self-denigration on her part, she can instead choose to withdraw from her partner when he drinks. This withdrawal reduces the likelihood of any blow-up, and the negative pattern of self-denigration that ensues.

e. Schedule a follow-up session. Although clients may be unwilling to accept the need for schema change at the first instance of seeing the pattern, they might be willing to do so some months down the road. Assuming that your setting allows such a decision, it can be very helpful to schedule a 6-month checkup, just to check in and to remind clients that you are available, if they are now ready to take the next step in therapy.

f. Engage in acceptance interventions. Although we do not focus on this topic too much here, there has been a recent emphasis in cognitive-behavioral therapy on the importance of acceptance of negative experience as a normal part of the human experience (Hayes et al., 2004). From this perspective, the goal is not so much to change or reduce distress as to be aware of it, to be mindful of the extent and nature of the experience, and to accept it as a normal and even healthy response to a negative situation. This attitude of mindfulness and acceptance is especially appropriate when clients experience chronic or residual symptoms, since it may indeed by unrealistic to expect change on these dimensions. Mindfulness and acceptance are not the same as tolerance or merely or putting up with a problem, and they are not easy to achieve. Treatment programs that have been developed to promote an attitude of acceptance (Hayes et al., 2004; Segal et al., 2002) are often presented as stand-alone treatments.

In a paradoxical sense, development of mindfulness and acceptance itself constitutes change. It requires that clients reflect on their own experience and way of approaching different situations, or what has been called *metacognition* (Wells, 2002). Metacognitions about experience may be negative, in which case clients typically appraise negative experience in a negative way and want to avoid or eliminate such experience. Acceptance, in contrast, reflects a neutral stance toward negative experience, in which clients are aware of the experience but chooses not to resist or fight against it. Thus, a shift of perspective needs to be achieved. Techniques that have been used to achieve this shift of perspective include attention to sensory experience, meditation, body awareness methods, yogic methods, and discussion of the "letting go" of control (Hayes et al., 2004; Kabat-Zinn, 1994; Segal et al., 2002).

The Case of Anna C, continued

Anna C canceled her ninth therapy session, due this time to her mother's declining health. In the phone call canceling the session, Anna advised the therapist that her mother was being moved to hospice care, and that she likely only had weeks to live. Anna was conflicted about this move. Although it meant that her mother would have better and more consistent care, Anna felt guilty about not being the person to provide that care.

Anna was fairly distraught at the next session, mostly due to her mother's health. Her daughter also had engaged in some recent acting-out behavior, and her husband was still working long hours and feeling quite a bit of stress. Fortunately, Anna had recognized the role of her own thinking in augmenting personal distress, and she was able to catch and to challenge some of her negative thoughts. She also was developing a self-care routine of daily walks and formal lunch breaks, which she said helped to calm her and reinforce her own importance to herself. Anna was thinking more about how she had adopted what she called a demanding "martyr" role in her life, and was realizing how unhealthy this was for herself, as well as for others around her, who were not as competent as they could be, because she tended to do their work for them. She gave as an example how she had actually completed her daughter's homework one night, because the daughter had been sent to bed early for misbehavior but had an assignment due the next day at school.

Anna's coping and mood continued to be better for the next two sessions, and she found that having her mother in hospice care actually provided her with the time to do things she had let slip. She indicated to the therapist a desire to take a break from therapy in session 11, mostly because she was expecting her mother's death, and stated that she needed the time to take care of family business. The therapist supported her in this request, and pointed out that sometimes taking time away for therapy was itself a sign of self-care. They agreed to two further sessions, both to review what Anna had learned in therapy and to plan against potential relapse.

Chapter 9

Completion of Treatment and Prevention of Relapse

All therapy comes to an end—we hope, after the achievement of the initial goals that were set, and significant improvement in the problems that brought the client into treatment. Relapse prevention typically is the last phase of a successful cognitive behavioral treatment, although, by definition, it cannot occur until at least a partial remission of symptoms has been achieved. What about the client who does not recover? What if your client drops out of treatment or has an inconsistent course of improvement? What if your client only has insurance coverage for eight sessions or you work in a setting with strict limitations on the length of treatment? Many variations of improvement occur on a case-by-case basis, and they are difficult to predict. In this chapter, we discuss clinical realities in the completion of treatment, including relapse prevention strategies.

In an ideal world, cognitive-behavioral therapy would lead to a "cure," and clients would continue to use methods they have learned in therapy, without the need for future or ongoing treatment. We often say to clients that the goal for therapists is to work themselves out of a job, by teaching clients to be their own therapists. In cognitive-behavioral therapy, we teach a methodology and "mind-set" to clients, so that they can utilize the techniques for themselves when problems arise, even long after therapy is completed. When you read treatment studies and textbooks, it is easy to get the impression that therapy completion and relapse prevention are easy and smooth processes. In most of the case vignettes and examples in texts, the client recovers and, even with challenges, the therapist and the therapy prevail.

In clinical reality, clients often present with complex and chronic problems that may be improved but not eliminated in a short period of time. Cognitive-behavioral therapists in clinical practice report that they see some clients for a long time, or have "intermittent" therapy, in which they focus on new concerns in clients' lives. These clients may present with one problem that responds to treatment, then return a few months or years later with similar or different concerns. Therapists who see clients for lengthy periods of time sometimes feel guilt and a sense of inadequacy, because their clients do not improve as quickly as those in the textbooks, or they keep returning for more help. In addition, after working hard to establish a therapeutic alliance and a good collaborative relationship with your client, both you and the client may be reluctant to say good-bye. In most clinical settings, therapists and their clients often find ending therapy a difficult process. Clients often have residual symptoms or problems and, in some cases, the end of treatment is abrupt and may not provide the chance to do the relapse prevention work that might be ideal.

The first portion of this chapter addresses different issues and concepts related to the completion of therapy, both for clients who respond and for those who do not respond as expected. In the second portion of the chapter, we discuss the questions that arise when treatment ends and provide practical suggestions to address them. We also discuss system constraints in treatment. Finally, we discuss the concepts and practice of relapse prevention.

CONCEPTS AND SYSTEM FACTORS
RELATED TO THERAPY COMPLETION

The cognitive-behavioral therapy literature tends to be very optimistic about change, and the outcome literature generally supports this positive attitude. Yet it is important for clinicians to remember that not all clients improve, even in outcome trials with optimal results, and not all improved clients recover to a degree that may be satisfactory or that leads them to function effectively in their lives. The old adage regarding the difference between clinical and statistical significance stands true; however, most recent randomized clinical trials assess remission, as well as response rates, to a certain intervention (e.g., Dimidjian et al., 2006; Dobson et al., 2008). Definitions (Bieling & Antony, 2003) used in the relapse literature include the following:

- *Remission*—either full or partial improvement of symptoms, to the degree that diagnostic criteria are no longer met.
- *Recovery*—remission lasting more than a prespecified period of time (e.g., 6 months).
- *Lapse or "slip"*—short-term, temporary, or minor recurrence of symptoms or problem behavior.
- *Relapse*—recurrence of symptoms or problem behavior following remission, to the degree that diagnostic criteria are met.
- *Recurrence*—occurrence of symptoms or problem behavior following recovery, including the presence of a new episode of a diagnosable problem.

All of these terms apply to Axis I or episodic problems or conditions. They may also be used for problems such as low self-esteem, poor communication skills, or marital distress; however, there are no standardized methods to assess remission or recovery from these nondiagnosed problems. It is also much more difficult to measure improvement when the focus of treatment is long-term behavioral or interpersonal patterns or core schemas. Consequently, *relapse prevention* interventions apply primarily to Axis I problems or when the goal of treatment is to eliminate a problem rather than to increase skills, knowledge, or positive function.

Even if Axis I symptoms dissipate, some clients continue to request therapy, particularly if they have other ongoing problems in their lives that may be underlying precipitants of future symptoms or life dissatisfaction. Indeed, work on a long-standing problem may actually be more effective when a client does not have acute symptoms, because the client may be less distressed and more able to focus on these concerns. For example, a client may present with depression, few social supports, and work dissatisfaction. Cognitive-behavioral interventions that include relapse prevention may alleviate the symptoms, as well as the client's fears about relapse. The client may be left, however, in a life situation comparable to the one that triggered some of the concerns in the first place. It may be in a client's best interests to address these concerns fully once the initial problems are resolved. This point also underscores the importance of the timing of different interventions. Remain aware that most clients come for help at the height of their problems, so often they are very distressed. The distress itself can make it difficult to resolve underlying problems, even though problem resolution would likely alleviate future distress.

Cognitive-behavioral therapists are influenced by not only the research and literature in the field, but also other concepts, models, and systems within which they practice. In addition to positive beliefs about change that emanate from the research literature, there are common beliefs and influences from other models of treatment and traditional practice. Negative beliefs about change may also exist, particularly in hospital or institutional systems. For example, in a setting in which clients with severe or persistent symptoms are treated, the focus may be more on "management of illness" than on "recovery from a disorder." The term *mental illness*, as opposed to *mental disorder* is commonly used in many settings. In settings with a biological focus, some disorders are likely to be perceived as permanent problems to be managed for the person's lifetime. Some clients you may see have been influenced by these beliefs, and you may need to address these beliefs in treatment. It is important, however, to be clear with clients that, in most cases, cognitive-behavioral therapy is intended to be relatively short term, with a focus on long-term change. In general, we encourage cognitive-behavioral therapists to use terms that are consistent with such a perspective, such as *disorder, symptom,* or *problem,* rather than terms such as *illness* or *disease,* because the latter tend to promote both a more chronic and a more biological orientation to mental health problems.

Two terms that originated in psychodynamic therapy but are frequently used in many systems by therapists of all theoretical backgrounds are *dependence* and *termination.* These terms have a significant impact on both practice and on the way our clients' problems are viewed. *Dependence* by the client on the therapist or therapy process is typically seen as negative and pathological, an indication of the client's inability to form healthy relationships outside of therapy. Because independence is highly valued in Western society, it is often viewed as a goal to be aspired to both in therapy and in life in general. Yet clients sometimes persist with therapy over a long time period because they simply have not recovered sufficiently or do not have the confidence to "do it on their own." It can be very difficult for a therapist to differentiate between overdependence that is due to interpersonal problems and dependence that is due to high distress or genuine fear of relapse. Certainly, sometimes clients meet criteria for dependent personality disorder, and may require specific interventions for this problem, but at other times, negative beliefs in the systems culture regarding dependence can make it difficult both the therapist and the client to manage this issue.

With some clients, however, overdependence on a therapist can be a poor prognostic sign. For example, the client may not attribute change to her own efforts, and she may have a difficult time generalizing change to situations beyond therapy sessions. The client may question how she will be able to maintain improvement once she has completed treatment. Although it is difficult to predict whether clients are likely to have problems ending therapy, certain clues may guide therapeutic decision making. See Table 9.1 for some ways to identify and manage dependence in cognitive-behavioral treatment.

TABLE 9.1. Strategies to Identify and Manage Dependence Issues with Clients

1. Encourage clients to take responsibility for their treatment. Strategies can include ensuring that they decide on their own homework and create their own relapse prevention plans. Ensure that they (not someone else in their lives) take responsibility for treatment. For example, some young adults rely on parents to book appointments or bring them to sessions. Phase such actions out over the course of treatment, using graduated exposure or contingency management.

2. Many clients make external attributions for change during treatment, giving credit "away" to therapist efforts, medications, or changes in their environment. Point out frequently, and have clients recognize, how their own efforts led them to change, including the decision to take medication and to tolerate side effects, to go for therapy, and doing homework and engaging in the sometimes difficult work of treatment. It can be helpful to have clients create a list of tasks that they have completed in treatment, including ideas or strategies that they thought of independently.

3. Be aware of some clients' tendencies to seek reassurance from the therapist. This tendency is particularly true for clients who lack self-efficacy or are unsure of themselves, or anxious. It can be helpful to identify this tendency formally as a problem in the clinical case formulation and work toward its reduction.

4. In general, the more dependent clients tend to be, the more important it is to have them be in charge of the treatment. This control may include more structuring of the therapy sessions, and developing homework and relapse plans. It may also include learning ways to manage crises or problems other than contacting a therapist. If clients successfully manage crises on their own, then their confidence is likely to increase.

5. Utilize resources in addition to individual cognitive-behavioral therapy. Clients ideally depend on multiple resources, including ones that may be relatively separate from the mental health system. These resources may include vocational counseling or employment services, recreational and leisure services, and nutritional counseling or other modalities of treatment, such as group treatments or family therapy. Through this process, clients learn how to access ongoing community resources and reduce their dependence on psychotherapy.

6. Gradually "wean" clients from therapy, reducing the frequency of sessions, as well as the way that the sessions are conducted. If clients are highly anxious about not having regular sessions, encourage them to see this as an experiment in independence, and schedule a follow-up session to review the experiment. The use of brief telephone or e-mail check-ins can aid this process. Clients often feel more comfortable reducing session frequency if they are provided with information about "what to do if ... ?" This information may include community crisis lines, emergency contacts, or a crisis intervention plan.

7. Agree to take a temporary break from treatment, with a scheduled follow-up session to assess the client's response to lack of treatment. Discourage the person from engaging in another form of treatment if the goal of the break is to experiment with independence.

8. Agree to disagree. If you think that it is a good idea to end treatment and your client does not agree, tell him or her so. If you believe that further treatment may be not only unhelpful but also detrimental in the sense of promoting dependence, be frank about this concern and encourage your client to take a break from therapy. In some cases, it may be appropriate to refer your client to another type of service or to a community support group.

One of us (D. D.) had a client, Don, who presented with profound depressive symptoms and was desperately afraid that he would not recover from his problems. Prior to the onset of his symptoms, he had been a competent professional man, but he was unable to function on his own either at home or work when treatment began. He had been referred for outpatient treatment after a hospital admission for depression.

The possibility of dependence was noted on the referral information. Don's symptoms were very slow to respond to treatment, and he engaged in frequent encouragement seeking, asking questions such as "Do you think I'll ever get better?" and "What is going to happen to me without therapy?" Due to suicidal ideation and intense distress, he was initially seen twice per week. Don's family was very concerned about potential risk of self-injury and his slow response to treatment.

Don began to improve slightly and was then seen once per week. He had several setbacks and was sensitive to any perceived stress or threat to regular therapy sessions, such as therapist holidays. His therapy was longer than average in duration (e.g., more than 30 sessions), and Don seemed to develop self-efficacy more slowly than was usual. The therapist wondered how the end of treatment would transpire and questioned whether Don met criteria for dependent personality disorder. As Don's symptoms began to remit, however, a whole other side to his personality was seen. He gradually began to have confidence in his improvements and ability to maintain progress. Don was engaging, humorous, and quite eager to move on in his life. What initially appeared to be dependence symptoms were reinterpreted as signs of his distress and feelings of vulnerability.

Termination in psychodynamic therapy, the final phase in the treatment process, occurs after the "engagement" and "working through" of the transference relationship with the therapist (Ellman, 2008). A successful termination of the therapeutic relationship is a necessary step toward the successful completion of therapy. This concept does not transfer well to cognitive-behavioral therapy, yet the term is used in many settings and applied to other types of therapy. We do not use the term *termination* in this text (cf. O'Donohue & Cucciare, 2008); in our opinion, *completion of therapy* (reaching goals or solving problems) is a more accurate term. Ideally, treatment ends when goals that were initially established are achieved. This ending may be temporary, because other problems or symptoms may arise in the future and the client may return for help. From our perspective, termination is not the goal of therapy; the goal of therapy is the resolution of the problems that brought the client into treatment.

Toward the end of a treatment, maintenance or occasional booster sessions are often useful for clients as they attempt to practice strategies relatively independently of the therapist. For example, the client may be seen once a week, then biweekly, monthly, and even quarterly or bian-nually. This type of care, which helps to foster independence without cutting off the process of therapy, can stretch the treatment period out for quite some time. In some settings, this type of practice may be viewed negatively. It may be seen as encouraging dependence on the therapist or the therapy. In other instances, it may be impossible, because some settings actively discourage maintenance therapy or limit the length of treatment. The amount of coverage available to the client may make maintenance treatment impossible. As noted earlier, at times, a pejora-tive attitude toward client dependence, and commensurate pressure for termination, can permeate interdisciplinary teams that comprise practi-tioners from different theoretical backgrounds, particularly if practitio-ners do not understand the different concepts from cognitive-behavioral theory (see Chapter 12, this volume). We encourage you think about your own ideas about termination and the process of ending treatment, to see whether your own beliefs might be antithetical to maintenance and booster sessions.

Certainly, it is important for all cognitive-behavioral therapists to ensure that their clients generalize the changes made in treatment, hone their skills on their own, and make internal attributions for change. It is often unrealistic, however, to expect people with ongoing mental health problems never to require therapy again after they complete 10–20 ses-sions focused on specific problems. You will notice in your practice that many new clients have had assessments and different types of interven-tions in the past. Many of these interventions were successful for a period of time, but then the problems recurred, or other stressors arose in these people's lives. Recurrence of problems does not mean that past treatment failed.

A major influence on treatment planning that has not been explored to any extent in the literature is the setting or system in which thera-pists work. The amount of treatment available or the limits of the setting within which you practice can have as great an effect on the length of treatment as the presenting problem or the client's preference. In this regard, we believe that mental health systems would benefit from a new model of treatment completion. For example, most of us do not worry about dependence on our dentist, and most systems recommend and pro-mote twice-yearly dental checkups! Similarly, we believe that biannual maintenance sessions or assessments could help people monitor their own mental health, and that mental health checkups could be promoted by health systems or organizations. This practice has not yet been advocated as a preventive measure by health care or mental health organizations, but it could be a useful addition to health care, especially for vulnerable or high-risk individuals.

We now turn to practical aspects of therapy completion, then review ways to work toward relapse prevention with your clients. We discuss treatment guidelines gleaned from research results, as well as when and how to engage in "maintenance" therapy. Throughout the remainder of the chapter, we explore some of the clashes between current systems of care and "ideal" treatment.

First, it is useful to differentiate between two different models of practice that are implicit to this discussion thus far: a *family practice* versus a *specialty clinic* model. *Family practice* (R. Wilson, personal communication, April 10, 1985) refers to a clinical setting in which clients can access treatment without referral and are likely to see the same practitioner across different problems or times in their lives. The client may come for treatment for a specific problem, not be seen for several years, then be seen again for a different concern at a transition point in his or her life. A client in such a setting is comfortable contacting the clinic or therapist when she has questions about herself or her family members. She may refer herself for assistance with a crisis, help with emotional responses, relationship concerns, or other problems. The term *family practice* is used because the cognitive-behavioral therapist serves as a generalist practitioner, similar to a family physician. This type of model works well for private practice, community mental health clinics, or some outpatient settings. The client may require referral for specialized services, if problems arise that are beyond the competence of the therapist or the clinic within which he or she practices.

In contrast, the *specialty clinic* typically focuses on a single disorder or group of related disorders, or on a particular treatment modality, and is more likely to be located in a hospital, outpatient clinic, or research or university setting. Examples of such specialty services include early psychosis treatment, dialectical behavior therapy, and bipolar or addictions services. Specialty clinics vary, based on either the type of problem on which they focus (e.g., eating disorders) or the type of intervention (e.g., mindfulness meditation) offered. The availability of such specialty services varies considerably across locations. A referral is typically required for specialty services. Specialty resources may be limited, and treatment may follow certain protocols, such as that in a research setting. It is typically difficult for the therapist to continue to see clients after the completion of treatment, because clients more often are referred back to the original provider or clinic for follow-up. Clients must be "discharged" from the clinic, so that new clients can be "admitted." Such practices, however, make maintenance therapy, booster sessions, or easy return to treatment somewhat problematic. Instead, recommendations regarding the type of follow-up are sometimes made to original clinicians, so that they can work with the clients to maintain treatment gains.

COMPLETION OF THERAPY

How Much Therapy Is Enough?

It is virtually impossible to answer the question: How much therapy is enough? Every client who presents for treatment has a unique set of problems and circumstances. Cognitive-behavioral therapy is intended to be a relatively short-term treatment, typically ranging between six and 20 sessions for most Axis I or episodic problems. In clinical trials, treatment for depression often lasts between 16 and 20 sessions. For most anxiety disorders, treatment lasts between eight and 12 sessions, although specific phobias or a crisis may be treated in fewer sessions. On the other hand, most treatment guidelines suggest that therapy for clients with comorbid conditions or significant interpersonal problems needs to last longer and be more intensive (Whisman, 2008). The client may require several sessions per week, or other components of treatment may be added to the plan. For example, dialectical behavior therapy for borderline personality disorder typically includes both a skills training group and individual therapy lasting at least 1 year (Linehan, 1993). Clients who are suicidal, who function poorly in their lives, or who are acutely distressed may require inpatient or day hospital program admission.

Many problems that clients experience may be recurrent or chronic in nature, particularly if they are untreated. Approximately 10–20% of people with depression have chronic symptoms (Bockting et al., 2005), and the chance of a person with depression maintaining recovery without treatment is approximately 20% (Keller, 1994). Increased severity and recurrent episodes of depression lead to a greater chance of relapse. Even with treatment, 30% of clients in one study who had completed cognitive-behavioral therapy for panic disorder and agoraphobia did not meet the study criteria for "high end-state functioning" (D. M. Clark et al., 1994). In generalized anxiety disorder, one of the most common problems that people have, estimated rates of clinical improvement range from a low of 38% to a high of 63% (Waters & Craske, 2005). Other problems, such as substance abuse or eating disorders, have notoriously high rates of relapse (McFarlane, Carter, & Olmstead, 2005; Rotgers & Sharp, 2005) and may be very difficult to treat successfully. Many clients have residual symptoms at the end of a *successful* therapy, and there has been limited follow-up data for any problems after 2 years. Residual symptoms are predictive of relapse for some problems, particularly depression (Rowa, Bieling, & Segal, 2005). On average, the more severe or chronic a person's problems, the more likely that he or she will relapse. Consequently, it is not realistic to expect that a brief course of cognitive-behavioral therapy in a specialty clinic will lead to long-term recovery for a client with such problems. Follow-up with a clinician who can see the client in a family practice model is very useful.

On a more positive note, some research has shown that cognitive-behavioral therapy leads to lower rates of relapse compared to treatment as usual or medication (Hollon, Stewart, & Strunk, 2006). In a recent comparison of relapse rates for clients who were treated successfully for depression, approximately one-third of clients treated with either behavioral activation or cognitive therapy had relapsed by the 2-year follow-up. By comparison, over three-fourths of clients previously treated with antidepressant medication had relapsed (Dobson et al., 2008). In another recent study, Strunk et al. (2007) found that the development and independent utilization of cognitive therapy competencies in a sample of moderately to severely depressed clients predicted reduced risk for relapse. These clients were all successfully treated and followed up for 1 year. This study links not only reduced rates of relapse in clients treated with cognitive therapy but also their competent use of strategies. Consequently, this finding provides support for the claim that it is the strategies themselves that lead to improvement rather than some other factor.

Some interventions that have been developed specifically target relapse, and others have successfully improved long-term outcomes. Group cognitive therapy used specifically for relapse prevention (Bockting et al., 2005), mindfulness-based cognitive therapy (Teasdale et al., 2000; Ma & Teasdale, 2004), continuation phase cognitive therapy, and booster sessions have all been found to be helpful, primarily for clients with depression. Anxious clients who are treated successfully often continue to improve after the completion of treatment, and relapse rates may be relatively low (Dugas, Radomsky, & Brillon, 2004). Avoidance and difficulty with generalization of changed behavior are good predictors of relapse for social anxiety disorder (Ledley & Heimberg, 2005); consequently, they are good areas to target.

Overall, we recommend the following for the cognitive-behavioral therapist based on the relapse prevention, in clinical practice:

- Build a relapse prevention phase into therapy.
- Work toward complete rather than partial reduction of problems.
- Try to eliminate any residual symptom(s).
- Work to minimize or eliminate dysfunctional avoidant patterns for any disorder or problems.
- Actively encourage generalization of change.

- Work toward change in a number of modalities, including behavioral, cognitive, emotional, and social areas of functioning.
- Help the client to utilize internal attributions for change.
- Gradually reduce the frequency of sessions once the client has recovered, working toward independence from therapy.
- Use booster or maintenance sessions during the relapse prevention phase, as needed.
- Use cognitive-behavioral therapy during medication discontinuation.

More severe problems require more therapy. Some problems (e.g., psychotic disorders or personality disorders) may require maintenance treatment over lengthy periods of time. Although clients may require ongoing treatment, the frequency of sessions may ebb and flow, depending upon the severity of the disorder and needs of the client.

Clinical Realities versus Ideal Treatment

No health care or funding system is ideal. Clients do not have endless funds with which to cover their own mental health treatment. Many clients have insufficient coverage or funding even for the recommended amount of treatment for their particular problems. Clients may have funding for very few sessions. You may have to submit applications to third parties to extend funding. Clients may not have the resources to pay for further sessions, even if they clearly need more help and are in full agreement with treatment continuation. Even though cognitive-behavioral therapy is of relatively brief duration, limitations to coverage affect clinicians who work in many systems. Clients must sometimes make difficult choices between funds for the necessities of life and ongoing treatment. You may not be in a position to provide more than the basics of cognitive-behavioral therapy. On the positive side, there are times when a limited number of sessions encourages both client and therapist to work more efficiently than they otherwise might work. Make the best of the amount of treatment available, and access whatever resources may be available in your community. For tips regarding making the best use of scarce resources, see Table 9.2.

The goals of treatment often differ from the perspectives of the *client*, the *therapist*, and the *system*. Clients' preferences obviously are central and typically focus on symptom reduction, elimination of distress, greater general satisfaction with their circumstances, and improved quality of life. Usually clients come to treatment with a desire to feel better rather than to recover from a particular disorder. Therapists' preferences are typically similar to those of clients; however, they are often more

TABLE 9.2. Making the Best Use of Limited Resources

1. Be straightforward with your clients. If your setting has a limited number of sessions available for all clients, plan your time carefully.

2. Use sessions wisely, always using the structure of cognitive-behavioral therapy. Set the agenda and stick to it.

3. Set appropriate goals that are likely to be met with the resources available. See Chapter 4, this volume, for more discussion on goal setting. Setting and achieving specific goals can be very helpful for clients. Your clients should be able to also learn to apply this methodology to other problems in their lives.

4. If clients' problems are mild, consider the use of less resource-intense interventions, such as bibliotherapy, web-based interventions, or psychoeducational sessions that may be available in your community.

5. If appropriate for your clients, schedule less frequent or shorter sessions. Many clients' coverage is for a certain number of sessions or treatment hours annually, and renewed each year. The *year* is not necessarily the regular calendar year; it may follow the financial year end for the third-party payer.

6. Check into the specifics of your clients' coverage, because it can be categorized in a number of different ways, such as by the client or by the problem. For example, some insurance programs provide clients with six sessions per year *per problem*, whereas another payer may provide eight sessions for the client per year plus the same for each family member.

7. If coverage is limited and a client appears to have problems that are not likely to respond quickly, start to investigate other options after the first session or two. Keep updated information in your files about available community resources.

8. Use cognitive-behavioral group treatments where available. A group that teaches the basic components of cognitive-behavioral therapy is cost-effective and efficient.

---

focused on remission or recovery from a disorder, and on the achievement of therapeutic goals. Obviously, as clinicians, we gain a sense of gratification when our clients have lower Global Assessment of Functioning (GAF) scores upon completion of therapy and are discharged "in remission." We also appreciate their satisfaction with treatment, as well as their positive comments to others about services they received. Often, though, therapists impose on the treatment process the idea of solving the underlying or causal process that resulted in the initial problems. In the context of cognitive-behavioral therapy, such an idea might include identifying and modifying dysfunctional core beliefs or schemas (see Chapter 8, this volume). The system may be a clinic, group practice, or a larger health care system, such as an HMO, hospital, or regional health system. Generally, the goals for systems are more population based than focused upon individual clients. Consequently, the system's aim may be to assess and treat the greatest number of clients for the least cost and system impact (e.g., hospital admission or length of stay, complaint). Obviously, improvement in clients' problems is important for health care systems; however, clients' satisfaction with the services they receive is likely equally important. Systems that routinely use satisfaction surveys often mistakenly equate satisfaction with improvement, when, in fact, there is no correlation between these two variables for clients (Pekarik & Wolff, 1996; but note that there was a modest correlation between clinician ratings of outcome and satisfaction in this study).

It is also crucial to remember that some clients do not recover, even if provided optimal cognitive-behavioral therapy. If two-thirds of clients recover in a carefully conducted randomized trial with exclusion criteria, fewer clients are likely to recover in most "real-world" settings. Furthermore, a certain percentage of these clients likely experience lapses, relapses, or recurrence over time, depending on the problems and the life circumstances that they encounter. Some clients may solve some problems but not others, especially those that are outside of their control. These clients may return to see you in the future, which is likely a sign that they trust you and feel comfortable contacting you for further help.

The Decision to End Treatment

Clinical case conceptualizations guide your treatment toward its endpoint, but there is considerable variability in how therapists approach the completion of treatment. It is wise to discuss the length of treatment and the process of ending therapy from the beginning of treatment, even if it is difficult to make these predictions. Time-limited therapy can make the issue of termination very straightforward: If the maximum is eight sessions, for example, make your client aware of this limit up front. Plan accordingly in your clinical case conceptualization, which may necessitate focusing only on the most pressing problems. Remind your client regularly about the number of remaining sessions. Decision making is also straightforward when you follow a manualized program or a time-limited group therapy. Once you have completed a time-limited treatment protocol or the client has reached the maximum number of appointments available, it is necessary to complete a follow-up assessment and refer clients who have not improved to follow-up treatment.

The following steps may be considered in decision making, depending on your setting, your client's preference, and your own clinical judgment.

- *End therapy when the crisis or problem that brought the client in to see you has resolved.* Many clients seek help when they experience a personal crisis, life transition, or a specific problem, rather than for any diagnosable condition. For example, a client may present for assistance as he attempts to make an important decision in his life, or when he is distressed about a relationship breakup. If the client does not have a serious psychological disorder (or sometimes even if he does), the crisis may resolve fairly quickly with minimal intervention on the therapist's part. For the client to gain perspective, engage in problem solving, and learn to approach rather than to avoid the problem, a few cognitive-behavioral sessions may be of significant help. With such a client, however, you may recognize the possibility of relapse, unless he makes other changes in his life. In these circumstances, it may be wise to offer brief (one to two sessions) relapse prevention, focusing on the future and on ways to manage potential problems. Be frank with the client about your rationale for suggesting relapse prevention. A short intervention may be all that is required to resolve a crisis. In some cases, the client may end therapy even though you recommend against it, particularly if the crisis has resolved and he feels less distressed. Another strategy is to book a follow-up appointment within a relatively short period of time, at which point you and the client can reevaluate the need for further intervention.

• *End therapy when the Axis I symptoms decrease or are eliminated.* This goal for ending therapy is common in many outpatient clinics or mental health settings. Most clients who come for treatment desire to feel better and to be less distressed, and they feel ready to end therapy when this change occurs. Again, it is prudent to offer relapse prevention as part of this therapy to reduce the likelihood of symptom recurrence. Just like clients who end treatment when the immediate crisis resolves, clients who end therapy when the symptoms abate may have future relapses or recurrences, if they do not learn how to recognize recurrence, develop strategies to prevent its likelihood, or identify the triggers that caused the problem in the first place. Many clients feel relief early in therapy, simply because they have made a decision to see someone, and they feel supported and have a chance to voice their concerns. The benefit of having a neutral party to listen to one's problems is no doubt an important part of the positive changes associated with therapy. These improvements are likely, however, to be short lived. One of us (D. D.) saw a client who initially had very high distress, including scores on the BDI and BAI that indicated severe levels of symptoms. Only 2 weeks later, with basic interventions such as self-monitoring and activity scheduling, this client had scores in the normal range. Neither her automatic thoughts nor her very low self-efficacy had been addressed, however. If therapy had ended at that time, she would likely have been at high risk for relapse, because her symptom reduction seemed primarily to be the consequence of support rather than any specific interventions.

• *End therapy when the therapy goals are achieved, regardless of symptom change.* At times, the therapy goal may be *not* to focus on current symptoms, or you may work in a system that does not use DSM diagnoses. Typically, distress or symptoms decrease as behaviors or cognitions change; however, symptom reduction does not always occur. For example, a client may have a treatment goal to improve her problematical relationships. Such a client may actually experience an increase in distress as she tackles issues with the people in her life—issues that she has been avoiding for years. Symptom improvement may not be relevant in all cases; some clients may address their psychological disorder with another professional, and choose to see you for cognitive-behavioral help with other concerns. For example, a client with schizophrenia may request help to improve his relationships, while he continues to receive symptom-focused psychiatric treatment elsewhere. Other clients may achieve their treatment goals but continue to experience symptoms that they have not addressed, or that have not responded to previous work. In these circumstances, it is preferable either to consider other therapy goals and revise the clinical case formulation, or to make a referral for these residual problems (e.g., to a specialty clinic). Recall our hypothesis that certain types of changes may lead to improvement, but we may sometimes be wrong.

• *End therapy when symptom change and goals are both achieved.* This set of outcomes is preferred, because the goals have been achieved, and the symptoms have been reduced or eliminated. Relapse prevention has occurred, and both therapist and client feel comfortable saying goodbye. There is no apparent need for further treatment, unless underlying causative factors are judged to increase the chances for relapse significantly. These are ideal cases in which to review the strategies learned in therapy, to emphasize the importance of healthy thinking and behavior, and to maintain treatment gains.

• *End therapy when the hypothesized underlying causative factors have changed (e.g., beliefs, schemas, or precipitating situations, such as family or work stress).* All schema therapies and some other types of interventions fall into this category, particularly any therapy that aims for long-term change of Axis II problems. It is difficult to make judgments about how much change is sufficient here, because both therapist and client may want to ensure core schema change or environmental shifts. It is easy for therapists trained to look for psychological disorders to see problems as opposed to strengths or positive areas of function. Some therapists are likely to recommend more treatment than others. We have both participated in cognitive-behavioral case conferences at which the predicted type and length of treatment differed considerably among therapists, despite similar training. Remember, however, that there are limited data to support the use of longer-term schema therapy except for clients with Axis II problems (see Chapter 8, this volume).

• *Other ends to treatment.* Other scenarios can and do occur in treatment. Some clients drop out of therapy without explanation. There may be little the therapist can do in these cases, other than attempt to follow-up with a telephone call or letter to obtain some closure or explanation. Always document efforts at follow-up with such clients, and communicate to them as best you can your decision to close the file, depending on your organization's policies and practices. In the absence of a formal case closure, you may have legal liability for the client in some circumstances.

At times, therapy does not appear to be effective, or client and therapist may have different opinions regarding treatment outcomes. Although it is best to respect the client's opinions, it is wise to obtain clear indications about why the client sees treatment as effective, if you do not. The client may find the support and opportunity to talk to a neutral person helpful but not be engaged in efforts toward active change. At other times, crises arise or problems persist despite appropriate interventions and real efforts on both the therapist's and client's parts. For more discussion about some of the challenges in cognitive-behavioral therapy, see Chapter 10, this volume. Overall, it is important for both client and therapist to learn to settle for imperfect or average outcomes.

Perhaps one of the most distressing types of endings is when a "therapeutic rupture" occurs. Such problems can arise for a number of unforeseen reasons, such as when the client has a crisis that does not quickly resolve, the therapist gets frustrated with the pace of change and makes a negative comment to the client, the client rejects the methods that the therapist has proposed, or some other problematical relationship issues arise. In such cases, the client may "fire" the therapist abruptly, without the chance for an adequate end to therapy. Our best advice here is to be as nondefensive as possible and to appraise honestly what happened in this case, so that you can better serve a comparable client who might come along. Supervision, or a confidential discussion with a trusted colleague, may help you to figure out what occurred, and how you might handle such an issue differently in the future.

RELAPSE PREVENTION

Relapse prevention is the final phase of most cognitive-behavioral treatments, although implementing it requires improvement of the client's problems or symptoms. Relapse prevention includes a review of treatment, creation of a plan for the future, and a discussion of both the client's and the therapist's feelings about therapy completion (Antony, Ledley, & Heimberg, 2005). In some cases, relapse prevention is an integral part of the therapy, particularly when the clinical problem is chronic or recurrent. In most cases, however, relapse prevention takes place over the last two to three sessions. Clients who have been in treatment for longer periods of time, due to the chronic or complex nature of their problems, may require more help during this phase. What follows are some practical suggestions and guidelines for helping with this phase of therapy (see Table 9.3 for a summary of major methods).

Ideally, both parties finish therapy with a sense of closure to treatment. Thus, although it may sound paradoxical, it is often helpful near the completion of treatment to predict setbacks. This prediction encourages realism and a discussion about how to manage future problems. Whenever setbacks occur in therapy, use them as an opportunity for new learning. Warn clients that they may feel a desire to take a break from the work they have been doing after the completion of regular sessions. Generally, this is not a wise decision, because clients may not have fully incorporated these strategies into their lives. Breaks may also reflect a subtle type of avoidance. Discuss ways that clients may balance the use of therapeutic strategies, along with other goals and desires in their lives.

TABLE 9.3. Relapse Prevention Strategies to Consider Near the Completion of Therapy

1. As therapy progresses, gradually give more responsibility to clients for issues such as the setting agenda, scheduling sessions, and determining homework. This step is especially important for clients who are uncomfortable about ending therapy.

2. Experiment with client-led sessions, even switching chairs to create a more realistic effect. This step can be effective in teaching clients to be their own therapist.

3. Some clients take notes on sessions throughout treatment. If they have not done so, ask them to create summary notes of sessions, or to use their therapy notebook to review work.

4. Ensure that clients make internal attributions for success throughout treatment. This step is particularly important for clients to develop confidence in their own abilities to cope after the end of therapy.

5. Frame lapses as opportunities to learn, while the clients are still in treatment. Help clients anticipate and prepare for lapses following therapy completion.

6. Schedule less frequent sessions, once clients' symptoms are reduced and they are actively using cognitive-behavioral strategies. Review and reinforce their skills during the next session.

7. Review and have clients record, or you record, what therapy strategies have been most helpful.

8. Provide frequent feedback about changes you have seen, and what work may need to be continued following therapy.

9. Develop an individualized summary of the therapy, with the client's help. If you have not already done so, ask the client to create a therapy binder. All therapy handouts, including a summary of treatment and the relapse prevention plan may be placed in this binder.

All clients have triggers or eliciting events that lead to negative reactions. By definition, they have had difficulty in managing these triggers before treatment. Most clients will have identified their personal triggers in therapy. Discuss how clients can cope differently, if or when these triggers recur after the completion of therapy. Encourage them to try to cope with these triggers on their own, which will enhance their confidence and self-efficacy. It is important, however, to determine with clients what the "early warning signs" of a relapse look like, and what they can do if these signs occur. For some clients, symptoms such as sleep disruption, agitation, or suicidal thoughts are signs that they need to get help. One strategy is to write out a personal list of warning signs or symptoms, and strategies to cope with these signs and symptoms, based on the completed therapy work. This list can be kept by clients in places that they can recall and access, if needed.

If at all possible, perform a posttherapy assessment upon completion of the working part of treatment. Many therapists do an excellent job of the initial assessment but are less thorough in their follow-up assessments. Repeat measures that you had the client complete at the beginning of treatment. Provide information to the client about the results of the posttherapy assessment, and compare the client's symptoms at posttest to pretherapy results. It is very helpful to create a graph or chart of the results to give to the client as a visual summary. This chart might include pre- to posttreatment symptom measures, behavioral checklists, or any other measures that are sensitive to change and reflect the work you accomplished together. Be honest about areas of lack of change, because these same areas may reflect dimensions on which the client is more sensitive to relapse. Discuss how the client can continue to address these problems on his or her own, or through other types of intervention.

Teach clients how to do their own self-assessments. For some clients, it is helpful to provide written checklists of the typical symptoms of the disorders they have experienced. Clients can then keep these checklists on hand, to help them decide when to access help in the future. Recommend that a client hold therapy sessions with herself, following the completion of therapy with you. These self-sessions can mimic the process of cognitive-behavioral therapy: The client can establish an agenda of current issues, go through each problem areas using the techniques she learned in therapy, and assign homework to herself to deal directly with the negative thoughts or behaviors tied to each problem area. She can experiment with starting these self-sessions in the final weeks of therapy and discuss any concerns during the next scheduled session. These sessions can be scheduled at the same time that the client comes in for her therapy sessions. One idea is to make yourself available for consultation—either by a brief phone call or e-mail—in the first few weeks that the client is trying out these self-sessions, to deal with any problems right at the outset.

Although you may be in the final stages of working with a client, help him set goals to achieve after therapy is over. Discuss methods and time lines by which he will work toward these goals. "Normalize" your client's fears about lapses or relapse, but be realistic in your discussions regarding risk. Make the client aware that relapses occur, even with interventions, so that he does not blame himself if he has problems. Help him to determine the difference between normal negative emotions and symptoms of a disorder or significant problem. Many clients have difficulty with this distinction and may have reduced tolerance to normal distress. Encourage them to struggle with their problems for a while, but then let them know that it is okay to make future contact with you, if that is necessary.

Work with your clients to create a written Relapse Prevention Plan, which includes a summary of the most helpful strategies they have learned in treatment, their goals after treatment is over, recommendations for follow-up work, and how to access future help if needed. Begin this plan, using the clinical case conceptualization and your treatment notes, in which you have listed interventions you used and client responses to them. This plan can serve as a stepping-stone to discussing the plan in the last few treatment sessions. Some clients like to have handouts, other types of psychoeducational information, symptom or strategy checklists, or pictorial reminders, which they put together to create a relapse prevention kit or binder.

Ramon had been in therapy for 22 sessions, over approximately a 6-month period. As he came to the end of treatment, he and the therapist agreed to develop a relapse prevention kit. Ramon accepted the homework of reviewing all of the Thought Records he had completed over the course of therapy and also the other forms he had filled out. He also had been keeping a personal diary, which he agreed to review. The relapse prevention kit developed over the last three sessions included the following:

- A list of his previous symptoms, and possible symptoms that could indicate relapse.
- A blank symptom questionnaire, to measure his status at any given point in time.
- A summary of the major techniques used in therapy, in words that Ramon understood.
- A blank copy of the therapy forms that Ramon had found most helpful.
- Contact information for the therapist, and instructions about how to access further help, if needed.

Although cognitive-behavioral therapy is generally based on the premise of change, and on the direct confrontation of problems in one's life, acceptance-based interventions, such as mindfulness training, may be considered during the relapse prevention portion of treatment or as a follow-up to treatment. Some of these interventions have empirical support either as an adjunctive or as a separate relapse prevention component for some disorders after remission has occurred (e.g., Segal, Williams, & Teasdale, 2001). If you want to incorporate these ideas into your treatment plan, we recommend that you either obtain specific training in mindfulness-based treatments or refer your client to an appropriate service provider. Although this idea remains an untested assumption, proponents of mindfulness approaches generally advise that therapists should themselves practice the strategies on a daily basis, for optimal results in their work with clients. Consider a referral to a mindfulness meditation training group or program, if you are not able to provide this approach.

Most clients who have had a positive experience in therapy express anxiety about therapy completion and some degree of sadness about not having the opportunity to discuss their concerns with their therapists. It is also common for therapists to feel some sadness about completion of therapy, as well as some "healthy maternalism" about the future welfare of their clients. Let your clients know that most people feel this way, and that it is healthy to express and to discuss these feelings. If it is appropriate, you can provide feedback to a client about positive changes that you think she has made, and what you may have learned from working with her. Client change is the major focus for cognitive-behavioral interventions, but just as we have an effect on our clients, our clients have a lasting effect on us. Although client gifts to the therapist are neither expected nor an inherent part of cognitive-behavioral therapy, we certainly do not discourage or reject small gifts or cards if they are meaningful to the client as an expression of thanks or indication of some lesson learned in therapy.

Discuss how clients can access help in the future, if needed. During the course of treatment, clients may have worked to increase their social support system. Ensure that this social support exists and is likely to continue for your clients. A referral to an ongoing support or self-help group may be useful for clients who continue to be socially isolated. Encourage all clients to engage in appropriate self-care and lifestyle balance. What lifestyle balance includes will vary from person to person, so determine what it includes for each individual client.

The Case of Anna C, continued

Although Anna's file had been closed, based on her wish to end treatment, and just over 6 months had passed since her last appointment, the therapist was not entirely surprised when she called. Anna told the therapist that her mother had died about 5 months previously, and that although she had coped quite well with that stress, she now realized she was falling back into some old habits.

When she met the therapist for an appointment, Anna relayed how her worry about her son was getting worse, and that she found herself increasingly taking care of family members. She realized that this pattern reflected her "martyr" schema, which she had learned about previously in therapy, but she did not know exactly how to change this pattern. After agreeing that making this change would be helpful, the therapist and Anna contracted to meet for six sessions to work on this issue.

Treatment techniques for Anna included setting limits, learning how to vocalize her needs, and saying "no" to unreasonable requests. Anna realized that, in her mind, the opposite of being selfless and caring for others was being "selfish," and the implications of this dichotomous thinking were explored. It was agreed that Anna would experiment with being selfish, to see what it felt like. She chose to take a trip away from Toronto to see extended family members in Chicago. While there, Anna was taken care of, and was able to attend to her own needs and wishes. This "as if" exercise proved to be quite powerful. Anna recognized her latent ability to enjoy experiences, and to "let go" of the burdens she had accepted. This trip also enabled her family members to experience responsibility, and to see Anna in a new light. When Anna returned home, she was ready to renegotiate her roles. She talked with Luka about the extra help she wanted, and he supported this request. Together they renegotiated duties for the children. Anna and Luka registered for an evening dance course at a local community center that forced them to get out of the house and be together, which she appreciated. Importantly, Anna sought and obtained a better position, with increased salary and benefits, in the law firm where she worked.

An interesting part of the therapy during this time was that the relationship between the therapist and Anna notably "matured." Anna was more forthright in her expression of ideas and more active in assigning herself tasks between sessions. The therapist noticed and commented on these changes, which Anna acknowledged. Anna went further, though, and said that when she first came for therapy, she was perhaps overly compliant with the therapist at times, based on her previous self-beliefs. This discussion led to a deeper understanding of the therapy process for both therapist and client, and was interpreted as further evidence of Anna's changing belief system.

At the end of the six sessions, Anna said that she felt more ready to proceed on her own, because her worries and sense of martyrdom had decreased. The therapist and Anna spent a seventh session reviewing what Anna had learned during her earlier therapy, and the more recent effects of becoming a "selfish" and caring woman and mother. Anna noticed that she was seeing herself in a more complex way than before, in a way that she respected and liked. She made a personal commitment to continue to travel down this road.

Chapter 10

Challenges in Conducting
Cognitive-Behavioral Therapy

This chapter reviews some of the challenges that can occur in cognitive-behavioral therapy. Although the word challenges is negative in tone, demands on the therapist are partly what make the work of a cognitive-behavioral therapist interesting and rewarding. This review is limited in scope; we have chosen some of the most common challenges rather than attempt to be comprehensive. Various challenges have been reviewed in other texts; if you want to read more on this topic, please see Dattilio and Freeman (2000), J. S. Beck (2005), A. T. Beck et al. (2004), Linehan (1993), and Young et al. (2003).

The definition of a *challenge* varies among clinicians, although there are situations that are difficult for most practitioners. In this chapter, we define *challenging elements* as situations that are more demanding and difficult to deal with than the therapist's current level of competence. Thus, what is challenging differs from therapist to therapist, or even for an individual therapist over time. These challenges can be categorized as those that originate with the client, with the therapist, within the therapy itself, and from outside the therapy. Although these distinctions are somewhat artificial, and likely overlap and interact with each other, it is helpful to differentiate the sources of the challenges to discuss them. We describe some of the common challenges within each of these areas, discuss relevant research where possible, then suggest practical solutions for your practice. Our goal in this chapter is to help you learn how to identify challenges in cognitive-behavioral therapy and develop strategies to overcome them.

CHALLENGES THAT ORIGINATE WITH THE CLIENT

Lack of Adherence to Treatment

Client problems with adherence can range from not attending sessions and being late for appointments to not completing homework or struggling with the structure of cognitive-behavioral therapy itself. Although avoidance in cognitive-behavioral therapy is a problem in and of itself, it is not discussed in detail in this chapter (see Chapter 6, this volume). Obviously, attendance is a prerequisite for change in any type of intervention! Clients who set clear goals and do their homework are more likely to achieve good outcomes than clients who do not (Burns & Spangler, 2000; Helbig & Fehm, 2004; Rees, McEvoy, & Nathan, 2005).

If you are working with a client who does not adhere to some aspect of treatment, the first step is to identify and describe his or her behavior prior to determining any reasons for the problem. Try simply to note the pattern, before taking any steps. Some clients' problems may result from a struggle with the structure of cognitive-behavioral therapy. Other clients may bring up many related and unrelated topics during the therapy session, and overwhelm themselves. Some clients are disorganized and may lose or forget their homework. Other clients may leave therapy with the best intentions and a clear idea of what to do, then "lose their nerve" at home. Still others may almost never do an assigned homework task, instead doing some other activity they have come up with themselves. Different types of nonadherence may well have different bases.

If you suspect a pattern in clients' nonadherence, take an observer stance and try not to react negatively or personalize a client's behavior as some kind of reaction to you or defiance. Gather data over time and present the pattern to your client in an uncritical and straightforward way. See whether you and the client together can identify this pattern as a problem that might interfere with successful treatment. Ask the client questions about what you both see.

Once you have identified any existing patterns, look for the simplest explanation first. Therapists may be prone to develop elaborate hypotheses regarding clients' behavior. Initially, it is wise to avoid interpretations about why clients have not completed homework or otherwise adhered to plans. Many therapists have speculated on client reactance (sometimes called *resistance*) and have been proven wrong (Leahy, 2001). For example, during the supervision of a predoctoral intern doing therapy, one of us (D. D.) noted that the supervisee habitually neglected to bring the file of one of her clients to supervision sessions. This pattern was noted over several weeks and the supervisor began to formulate hypotheses about why the supervisee was avoiding discussion of this client. Following one such discussion, the supervisee noticed that the missed client's records were in a different colored folder than those of her other clients. Most likely, she had neglected to bring the folder because of this color difference, not due to any complex avoidance or "countertransference"! The problem was easily solved by the substitution of a folder of the same color as those of the other clients.

The cancellation of an appointment following a challenging session presents a certain temptation to speculate. Many therapists may "jump to conclusions" and think that the client reacted negatively to the session, did not do his or her homework, is avoiding this difficult part of therapy, or may be thinking about termination. Although such ideas may be valid, always remember that the client may just have a cold! At the next session, inquire first about the missed session, before making any assumptions about the cancellation. It would be unfortunate if the client felt accused, or had to defend him- or herself against your unwarranted suspicion, which could lead to a rupture of the therapeutic alliance.

It is important to assess the potential relationships among problems with attendance or homework completion and clients' presenting problems. What is perceived by a therapist as nonadherence may be due to symptoms of a psychological disorder. If clients struggle to function with completion of their day-to-day activities, then this struggle is likely to carry over into the therapy. Lack of motivation, low energy, fatigue, or poor problem-solving skills are all likely to interfere with clients' ability to follow through with tasks. Cognitive problems, such as poor concentration, may cause clients to forget the homework shortly after the session, without a memory aid. Demoralization and discouragement occur frequently in clients with mood-related problems. Fear of encountering overwhelming situations outside of the session leads some clients to avoid homework. Anxiety about social judgment may translate into not completing homework for fear of negative evaluation. Anxious clients may be self-focused, which causes them to appear inattentive during the session. Learn to be an astute observer of clients' in-session behaviors. All of these problems should become clear when you complete your case formulation. Make predictions and revisit your case formulation as necessary.

Ask yourself whether there is anything about *your* behavior that might have a negative effect on your clients. It is important to follow the basic tenets of cognitive-behavioral therapy and to be a good role model. Adherence on your part goes a long way to prevent the development of problems. Set and follow an agenda every session.

Make sure that you include sufficient time to make decisions about appropriate homework. Many nonadherence problems may be solved by providing clear written homework for clients to take away with them. Consider using a standard homework form, similar to a prescription pad. Most clients are used to medical prescriptions, so one of us (D. D.) developed a Prescription for Change form (see Figure 5.1), which is approximately the same size as a medical prescription form. These prescription forms include the homework, as well as the next appointment and the therapist's contact information. One of us (K. S. D.) has developed a standard way of using a therapy notebook, in which all homework assignments are written, and activity logs and other forms are also kept. Having a single source for therapy materials can work well for clients (although it does tend to break down, if they lose or forget the notebook). Having a duplicate copy in clients' files can help resolve some of these problems.

> Roger was working with his new client Paul. Although Roger had done a good job of developing with Paul a set of reasonable homework activities, and provided Paul with forms to track the homework, Paul lost the forms on every occasion. Paul indicated that he worked with computers all day but rarely thought about paper. He suggested the idea of using his cell phone to send himself a text message from therapy about the homework assignment, which he could later transferred to his computer's appointment program. He also set up a spreadsheet to track his homework assignments, which he printed off before each session. Although Roger initially thought this process was much more complex than simply using a written form, it worked better for Paul's technical approach to life, and was adopted with success.

Always ask about homework assignments at the next session, and discuss the results seriously and carefully. Plan to spend some portion of the therapy session doing this work, especially in the first few sessions, which is when you set the tone for treatment. Discuss any problems, including noncompletion, openly and frankly with your clients. We suggest you use therapy nonadherence as a chance to evaluate clients' problem-solving abilities. See what has gotten in the way, and try to effectively solve it with clients; if the homework is still important, reassign it. If the homework is not done a second time, spend even more time going over it. Advise clients that this part of therapy is essential, and that they have to find a way to translate in-session discussions into real-life practice. You might tell them that "what goes on in your life between our sessions is much more important than what we talk about during our appointments," to relay this message.

Homework assignments should be assigned with an eye toward maximizing the likelihood of success and building clients' self-efficacy. Try to ensure early success, and if clients are successful, assist them in giving themselves credit for their efforts. You can also give praise, as long as it is measured against the degree of success actually achieved and not clinically contraindicated. However, do not give praise if clients do not perceive the homework as a success. Rather, use this mismatch of perceptions to better understand clients' perspectives and help to build your case conceptualization.

Have clients keep written records regarding homework completion and outcomes. In addition, build in a margin of error for unrealistic expectations or perfectionism in homework. Be realistic in your expectations of clients. For example, an assignment with the goal of doing a given behavior every day is less likely to lead to success than an assignment of the same behavior for 4–5 days a week, allowing for some days off. Clients are more likely to continue successful behaviors than to continue unsuccessful ones. If they feel discouraged following homework "failures," they are less likely to attempt additional homework, which can lead to reduced self-efficacy. For a list of questions regarding adherence and possible solutions, see Tables 10.1 and 10.2, respectively. The solutions for nonadherence obviously depend on the cause of the problem.

Occasionally, despite your best efforts, clients do not follow through on a homework assignment, even when they continue to insist that they truly want to make changes. Contingency contracting can be extremely effective for clients whose nonadherence patterns persist over time and interfere with therapy. One of us (D. D.) was a therapist in an outcome

TABLE 10.1. Questions to Consider Regarding Adherence Problems

1. Is the problem a one-time occurrence or part of a pattern?
2. Does the client have a similar pattern outside of therapy sessions, or is the problem unique to therapy?
3. Has the client participated in other types of therapy that have not used structure and homework?
4. Does the client struggle with the structure of therapy?
5. Does the client understand the importance of following through with homework?
6. Does the client react to some aspect of either the therapy or the therapist's style?
7. Has a collaborative relationship developed?
8. Does the client have the skills and/or resources to follow through?
9. Does the client understand how to go about doing the homework?
10. How organized is the client? Does he or she seem to have difficulty generally with organizing his or her time, paperwork, or activities?
11. Were clear, concrete, written plans provided to the client to take home?
12. Are any symptoms (e.g., poor concentration, motivation, anxiety) that your client experiences interfering with his or her adherence?
13. Have you been clear in the discussion about adherence and/or homework?
14. Have you avoided bringing up difficult issues with your client?
15. Have you done anything to subtly undermine the homework, such as forget to ask about it or to reinforce the client's attempts?
16. Have you adhered to the goals and plans of cognitive-behavioral therapy with the client?

TABLE 10.2. Methods to Facilitate Adherence in Treatment

1. Ensure that clients understand and accept the treatment rationale.
2. Ensure that any homework assignments make sense to clients and that they understand how each step is related to their overall goals in treatment.
3. Have clients write down main points, summaries, and suggestions during sessions. If they ask to tape record sessions, say "Yes."
4. Repeat things more than you think you need to, and use language that clients understand.
5. Anticipate problems. Ask questions such as "What are the chances you will successfully complete this homework assignment?" If client response is less than about a 60 or 70% chance, change the assignment or make it easier.
6. Always be collaborative and ensure that clients have a great deal of input into the goals, methods, and process of therapy, including the homework.
7. Always make sure to ask about homework in detail. Reinforce any homework efforts. If homework has not been completed, discuss the obstacles that got in the way. If homework has not been completed for several sessions in a row, change it. Some clients seem to manage to improve, despite not being very good at doing homework.
8. Be creative in the use of homework. Some clients struggle with written homework but do well with other types of assignments, such as watching videos, obtaining feedback from other people, doing computer research, or engaging in behavioral experiments. Even though most therapists like to read, remember that not all clients like to do so.
9. Do not underestimate client anxiety about trying new behaviors or doing outside session exposure on their own. After anticipating problems with homework, if fears seem likely to reduce the chances of clients doing homework, rehearse it within the session.
10. Make sure the homework is not too inconvenient for clients. For example, signing up for membership at a local gym is likely to have better success than signing up at one having a discount sale across the city.
11. Consider any possible barriers that clients may not want to mention (e.g., cost, literacy levels, unsupportive people in their lives). Ensure that clients have the skills and resources to carry out the plan.
12. Always write the homework down or have your clients write it down. One of us (D. D.) has developed Prescription for Change pads (see Figure 5.1), which are similar to a physician prescription form. The homework is written on this sheet, along with clients' next appointment time and therapist contact information.
13. Some clients like to use a therapy binder to record homework progress across time.
14. Stick to time limits. If a client is late, do not extend the session, even if you can.
15. Assign homework to yourself at times (e.g., finding an article for a client). Follow through with your homework and talk about the results at the next session.
16. It may sound simplistic, but the four P's can be helpful: Persistence, Patience, and Pacing = Progress! Don't give up. Your determination can help clients be more determined.

study in which lack of homework completion was automatic grounds for cancellation of the next session. The protocol allowed the therapist to spend 10 minutes discussing the reasons for the lack of adherence, then reassign the homework, but the rest of the session was canceled. All participants knew this rule in advance. There was only one breach early in therapy, and the therapist found it difficult to follow through with this "tough" agreement. However, following the agreed-upon consequences homework completion improved considerably.

In another setting, a young adult male client was habitually at least 10 minutes late for his sessions. He had developed a pattern of sleeping in and not allowing sufficient time to organize himself to come to the session. After identifying the problem, therapist and client agreed that if the client was more than a certain number of minutes late, the session would be canceled and rescheduled for the next week. This agreement was remarkably effective. Such consequences communicate the message to the clients that not only is homework taken very seriously but also the therapist's time is important and to be respected. Note that this type of intervention is only effective if the client values therapy and has a good therapeutic alliance. Payment issues also must be worked out in advance, because a client may resent paying for a session that did not occur.

One of us (K. S. D.) has sometimes suggested "three strikes," which is the idea that you consider termination if a client cannot or will not do assignments, and if the same important homework does not get completed despite good work on your part and on that of the client, and having problem-solved nonadherence in previous sessions. In many ways, as a therapist, your hands are tied if a client will not or cannot implement therapy assignments. Maybe your time would be better spent with clients who are ready to make that commitment. If you are sure that you are not simply being punitive with a struggling client, then delaying or terminating treatment may be a responsible decision. Also, if you use any of these contingency contracting or consequence systems, then it is absolutely crucial that you follow through with the agreed-upon consequences. The only exception is when there is imminent risk to the client or other people, or some other type of emergency situation.

Finally, it is important to identify whether a pattern of nonadherence appears to be part of a significant interpersonal problem, such as an Axis II disorder. These problems may not be immediately apparent, but over time, you may start to suspect them. Although some challenges are related to clients' long-standing interpersonal styles or cognitive schemas, it is not our intention to cover Axis II problems in this text. For information on psychological treatment for clients with personality disorders, see the texts referred to earlier (A. T. Beck et al., 2004; Young et al., 2003). For a comprehensive review of resistance in cognitive therapy, see Leahy (2001). For a list of clinical clues to Axis II disorders, please see Table 10.3.

Clients Who Are Overly Compliant

Some clients do not struggle at all with adherence but are instead extremely compliant. Although compliant clients can be a pleasure to work with,

TABLE 10.3. Clinical Clues for Axis II Problems

1. The problems appear to be long-term, based on the reports of the client, significant others, and other professionals.
2. The client's history of treatment noncompliance includes past treatments.
3. Treatment seems to have a "start" and "stop" pattern, sometimes coming to a halt for no apparent reason.
4. The client does not seem to be aware of his or her effect on other people and may blame others for his or her problems.
5. Other professionals have questioned the client's motivation for treatment.
6. The client talks about the importance of treatment, but there are no or few observable or measurable changes. If improvements occur, they are not sustained.
7. Psychoactive medications do not appear to have been helpful.
8. The client talks about problems as being a "core" part of him- or herself. There is an "egosyntonic" nature to the problems.
9. You notice that frequent crises occur, and treatment seems like a series of "brushfires." You find yourself worrying about the client after sessions.
10. Extensive records provided with the referral indicate numerous previous treatments. The client may have a history of emergency room visits, hospital admissions, and past treatment "failures," including lack of response to medications. Professionals (including yourself) have had negative reactions to the client, which include becoming angry or frustrated. There may be disagreements in case conferences about how to manage the situation or the treatment.
11. The client does things that you cannot understand right away, that seem out of character or self-defeating.

Note. Based on data in Freeman and Leaf (1989). Adapted with permission from Arthur Freeman.

this tendency can sometimes be challenging and impede progress. You may gradually notice that such clients are not only very compliant but also very passive and eager to please you. They do not ask many questions, but they frequently request your suggestions and support. They never arrive late; in fact, they are more likely to be early and may sometimes be found reviewing their homework in the waiting room. They do not tend to cancel sessions; instead, they may come in even when they are obviously sick. They may not only do an Activity Log but also may create a special form on their computer, which they fill in with additional of data, then bring in to the session for your approval. These are the clients who may bring small gifts on holiday occasions. They express concern about the end of therapy.

Although working with these clients can be very gratifying for therapists, it is important to ensure that true collaboration is occurring. Ideally, clients not only value the therapist's input but also take a collaborative role in therapy. A goal of cognitive-behavioral therapy is to help clients "become their own therapists." Some clients may be very compliant because that it their typical pattern, and it serves them well; other clients may be "going through the motions" and not really expressing their thoughts and opinions to the therapist.

Once you have identified this pattern as a problem, the first step is to discuss it openly with clients and try to determine their thoughts that underlie it. These beliefs can then become part of the agreed-upon goals for change. Try to have such clients assign their own homework, if possible. Or, if you assign the homework, ensure that you obtain the clients' input. They may have automatic thoughts, such as "The therapist knows best"; "My opinions are not as valid as my therapist's"; "Pleasing other people is more important than saying what I want"; or "My therapist will become angry if I do_____." You may want to address these automatic thoughts directly, and advise clients that you would rather have their honest disagreement and ideas than their ongoing compliance.

You may notice perfectionism in the cognitive and behavioral patterns of overly complaint clients. If their compliance is to please you rather than to make changes for themselves, set up behavioral experiments in which they can deliberately try to displease you. These experiments might include canceling a session without good cause, being a few minutes late, or not doing the homework properly. It can be difficult, but very helpful for conscientious, perfectionist clients, to try this type of experiment. One of us (D. D.) had an overly punctual client try a homework assignment of being 5 minutes late (with the agreement of both parties). He was observed virtually waiting around the corner to ensure that he would not be more than the precise number of minutes late! Discussing the results of these experiments in the session can be very helpful. The client can learn other people's responses through such experiments and, we hope, learn to meet his own needs rather than acquiesce to his perceptions of other people's needs. In a paradoxical fashion, evidence of nonadherence in some clients may be a sign of independent thinking and increased self-sufficiency.

Clients Who Are Demanding, Aggressive, or Very Angry

Angry and aggressive clients are very different than overly compliant client. They expect a great deal of the therapist and become irritated when their expectations are not met. They may express blame toward you when they are disappointed. These patterns may not be apparent at the time of the assessment, but become clear only under certain circumstances. For example, if you change an appointment, are late yourself for a session, or appear distracted, demanding clients may become irritated. If a homework assignment does not turn out as planned, they may blame you for the outcome. If these clients call the clinic during the week, they may expect you to take time out of your schedule to talk to them about minor concerns. For example, one of us (D. D.) had a client periodically show up at the clinic at times other than her appointment time. She would make demands of the receptionist, and request to see the therapist or to use the telephone. She behaved as though she believed her problems were more important than the problems of other clients.

It is important not to avoid these topics, but to label them as "problems" for you or for the organization in which you work. As with any problem, it is important to have frank discussions with clients and to gain an understanding of their beliefs underlying the behavior. Provide feedback. People who express anger are probably least likely to receive feedback from the people in their lives. Others are more likely to acquiesce to these clients' demands or, over time, learn to avoid them altogether rather than give feedback. You want to ensure that you do not simply repeat this pattern. Being given feedback may be a real service to them, because it may help them become more aware of their effect on others. In these cases, it is important to have a solid therapeutic alliance and to consider the timing of the feedback (ideally, do it right after the aggressive or demanding behavior, to minimize the chances for rerembering or distortions of what happened). It is also useful for therapists to set very clear limits with demanding clients. For example, new therapists' eagerness to please their clients can lead to overflexibility with appointments or outside therapy contacts. A therapist who is eager to please, in combination with a demanding client, can lead to problems. Stick to session time limits and scheduled appointments with *all* clients, except in the case of a true crisis or emergency situation.

Finally, do not tolerate verbal or other forms of abuse from your clients. Our suggestion is to state immediately that this pattern is not acceptable, and advise the abusive client that you will not accept this treatment. Be clear with clients about the behavior you find objectionable and tell them what change you expect. Be sure to document this set of expectations in your therapy notes. In most cases, this confrontation will lead to a change in behavior, but if not, you should advise these clients that you will terminate treatment with them, if the abuse does not stop. If the change does not occur, advise them you are terminating treatment, and offer them a referral to at least two other services or therapists. Document this action and close their files. Having closed their files, do not take phone calls from them or engage in further contact. Even if their lawyers should contact you, you are well within your rights to protect yourself, having taken the previously mentioned steps. Remember that aggressive clients may not easily accept being rejected. Although this may be a difficult period of time, your safety and well-being are of utmost importance.

Clients Who Are Entertaining

Some clients seem to enjoy entertaining their therapists. They may be quite engaging, humorous, particularly interesting to listen to, or self-effacing. It is easy to fall into the habit of being entertained, but this is not an appropriate role for you to play! You need to be able to see humor as a possible problem in the therapy relationship, and as such, to question it. Such clients may be exhibiting an avoidance pattern by being entertainers. For example, it may be difficult for clients to express negative emotions or discuss problems in their lives. This type of avoidance can inhibit change, both within the therapy sessions and during homework. Provide these clients with feedback and limit your own response to their entertaining style.

This "entertaining" pattern may interfere with therapy, although there are times when it can actually be helpful to respond to your client's style. Work to identify when a pattern interferes with, rather than enhances, therapy. Most people may be humorous at times or have unusual interests or quirky habits. When this style is not part of a problematic pattern, your positive response to clients' humor or stories can be very reinforcing to them. Your smiles or enjoyment might even help to build therapeutic alliance. Laughing at a joke told by a depressed client is likely to improve his or her mood and sense of mastery. If you respond to your client as a complex person, and recognize and appreciate his or her diverse array of interests and experiences, this response itself can help to shift the client's self-view.

Clients with Other Difficult Interpersonal Styles

Many other interpersonal patterns exist, including overly dependent and noncommunicative clients, and intrusive, complaining, or negative clients. Rather than review all these patterns in this chapter, we encourage you to identify these interpersonal styles as early as possible in therapy and review your case formulation regularly. What predictions do you make prior to a session? Do you look forward to seeing the client or secretly hope that he or she might cancel the session? Are you glad when the session is over? Do you find yourself irritated with a given client? Do you worry more about certain clients than about others? Work to develop your own self-awareness. Listen to your own automatic thoughts about your clients. Use a Dysfunctional Thoughts Record for your own automatic thoughts. Assess whether your thoughts about clients are distorted or realistic. How do your reactions fit with the original case formulation? Is there any chance that your own reactions are being communicated to clients, so that the pattern has become self-fulfilling? Make modifications in the case formulation as needed. It is generally wise to be open and transparent with your clients, even as you privately consider the therapeutic alliance and your communication style.

Clients Who Have Competing Models for Change

Occasionally, clients never completely "buy into" the cognitive-behavioral model of therapy, despite the best efforts of the therapist to socialize them into the approach. There is no known research on outcomes for clients who accept a cognitive-behavioral model for their problems compared to those who do not. However, common sense suggests that clients who understand and accept the model are more likely to work harder and attribute change to their own work rather than to other factors. They also are likely to leave therapy with a greater sense of self-efficacy that possibly leads to greater efforts in the future and a lower chance of relapse.

Clients' beliefs about the causes of their problems may be treated just like any other beliefs. They may be addressed in therapy with common cognitive strategies, such as cognitive restructuring and behavioral experimentation. For example, if a client believes in a biological cause for her problems, she is less likely to see change as being due to her own efforts. A behavioral experiment could be set up in such a case. The experiment includes self-monitoring and setting up an ABAB experiment, in which the client self-monitors, introduces a behavior, stops it, then starts it again, all the while assessing variables, such as her mood, automatic thoughts, and other consequences. Through this type of experiment, the client learns that she can gain control of her responses, and that biological variables are perhaps only one possible cause of her overall level of functioning.

It can be useful for clients who struggle with beliefs about causality of their problems to start to attribute causes to multiple factors (e.g., Zubin & Spring, 1977). These multiple ideas about causes lead to clients' more complex attributions for change, including their efforts in cognitive-behavioral therapy. We have used an exercise in therapy that asks clients to list all possible causal variables, such as genetic background, early and recent experiences, relationships and other environmental factors, self-control, and "bad luck" or misfortune. They are then asked to ascribe a percentage of "variance accounted for" by each variable. A follow-up exercise might include rating the amount of control clients' have over each variable at the time. Some variables (e.g., genetic background or early experiences) cannot be changed; others (e.g., current environmental factors, relationships, beliefs and attitudes) can be shifted. This exercise can help you to assess clients' causal beliefs and to introduce a multifactorial model of causes. This discussion may also pinpoint ways to change the current problems. The general principle here, though, is that there are many pathways to developing a set of problems, and many pathways (and not always the same ones!) to back out.

Be realistic in your discussion of models of change with your clients, because they also receive different and competing messages from other people and the media. Sometimes a lack of "buy in" can be related to, and influenced by, other people's beliefs, such as those of a partner, parent, or family physician. Family members may give clients the message that they just need to "pull their socks up," "get a backbone," or get a prescription for the right drug. If this type of discrepancy becomes apparent, discuss different types of models with clients and assess their acceptance of these various ideas. You can help clients rehearse what to say to other people in their lives who do not agree with the therapeutic model. Other strategies include written information about cognitive-behavioral therapy for family members, or an invitation to the other person for a psychoeducational session (with the client's permission). If you have a session with a family member, we generally recommend that the client be present.

Check to ensure that clients have not received conflicting messages from other practitioners whom they are seeing. For example, a family physician could refer a client to cognitive-behavioral therapy but undermine the success of the therapy in subtle ways. For example, he might increase the dosage of benzodiazepines for an anxious client. Sometimes, a client might complain to his or her physician rather than to the cognitive-behavioral therapist about a lack of progress. Clients who are not comfortable with direct expression of their concerns about continued problems may do so when asked about progress by another professional. In such cases, the physician might make another referral to a separate service without consultation. Obviously, this type of practice may lead clients either to question the appropriateness of your treatment with them or your competence. The main way to circumvent these problems is to have open and frequent consultations with everyone involved in clients' treatment. These problems also may occur simply due to lack of time, as well as the reality that practitioners often work in different geographic locations and have few opportunities to communicate directly with each other. Be sure to build enough time into your schedule to maintain good lines of communication with other service providers.

The cognitive-behavioral therapist should not make comments that undermine other types of treatments that clients might receive, such as medications. Exceptions to this guideline are treatments that are clearly ineffective, contraindicated, or potentially harmful. During the psychoeducational portion of treatment, you can provide information on treatment outcome studies or clinical practice guidelines. Clients can then come to their own conclusions. Helping clients develop strategies to discuss their concerns with other practitioners is not the same thing as directly criticizing or undermining that treatment. When clients are more committed to another treatment that is not compatible with cognitive-behavioral therapy, it may be advisable to suspend or end therapy. It is generally not good practice for clients to receive concurrent psychological treatments from different practitioners, unless these treatments are closely coordinated and work in harmony with each other toward the same treatment goals. For example, compatible inpatient or residential treatment programs often may be used in concert with outpatient cognitive-behavioral therapy. Sometimes, couple therapy may address relationship issues, even while you work with a client about his or her individual problems.

The concurrent use of medication and cognitive-behavioral therapy is a topic that warrants special consideration. Most clients will have had at least one consultation with a medical practitioner prior to seeing a cognitive-behavioral therapist, and it is possible that a medication prescription will have been written. In some areas, and depending on the severity of the client's problems, the concurrent use of medications and cognitive-behavioral therapy may increase treatment success (Pampollona, Bollini, Tibaldi, Kupelnick, & Munizza, 2004).

In some cases, you may question the added value of medications, or even wonder whether the medications will interfere with your work. For example, the use of anxiolytic medications can become a "safety behavior" for anxious clients, making exposure therapy less effective and ultimately decreasing the efficacy of the treatment. This problem is most likely to occur with anxiolytic medication that is taken on an "as needed" basis, particularly just before or during exposure therapy. Rather than trying to convince a patient to give up medications, we suggest that you communicate with the prescribing physician in order to discuss the medication treatment.

General practitioners are not specialists in cognitive-behavioral therapy and may not be aware of the need for emotional experiences in the treatment. Sometimes, just asking this question will lead to a reevaluation of the value of medications. Generally, we encourage you to ask the prescribing physician to not alter the medication type or dosage for the period of time that you work with the client. If you can keep these things constant, it will be easier for the client to attribute improvements in their life to your work with them, rather than to the medications. As it is common for clients to attribute change to medications rather than to their own efforts, a constant dose of medication makes this attribution less likely. As the client sees improvement in his overall functioning without the need for new or more medications, this information may lead him to question the need for ongoing medications. If he desires such a change, you, the client, and the prescribing physician can together work out a plan to reduce and/or eliminate the medication if appropriate, even while you provide continuing support and assessment, prior to your eventual completion of therapy. Be sure to discuss this issue with your client and the prescribing physician. There may be situations where it is not possible or appropriate to consider discontinuing or reducing medications (e.g., antipsychotic medications) and it is important not to create thoughts about failure for your client if they remain on medications for lengthy periods of time or to create circumstances where they may be at risk for noncompliance with other treatments.

> Frances had for some time taken a low-dose antidepressant medication when she first saw Penny in cognitive-behavioral therapy for problems with low self-esteem and moderate depression. Rather than focus on the issue of medication, Penny and Frances collaboratively worked on the problems that had been brought into treatment, and used a variety of cognitive-behavioral methods to look at and modify Frances's ongoing negative cognitive and behavioral patterns. Over time, it became clear that Frances also had some core beliefs that underpinned these patterns. These beliefs included a general lack of confidence, and reliance on people and other outside supports.
>
> When Frances raised the issue of reliance on medication as one reflection of this belief, Penny explored with Frances her desire to experiment with reducing or eliminating her use of medication. Frances agreed, and together they worked out a strategy to approach the prescribing physician about this issue. Because Frances was largely unsymptomatic at this point, the physician readily agreed with the suggestion. They worked together to reduce, then to eliminate medication use, even while Penny continued in cognitive-behavioral therapy to address her core beliefs. Penny was completely off of medication by the end of treatment and, as a result, reported a greater sense of self-efficacy.

Clients with More and More Problems

Some clients bring in additional problems, after the therapeutic goals and contract have been set. Indeed, clients more commonly have multiple problems than a single, focused problem. Some clients have frequent issues that arise in their lives, which can sidetrack the therapist or even derail therapy in diverse directions. Although these problems are not crises, you may be tempted to deviate from the initial goals, because clients become distressed when these problems occur.

A useful strategy for clients with multiple problems is to stick to the basics of cognitive-behavioral therapy. Always remember to set an agenda for each session. Respect your clients' input if they wish to discuss additional topics, but set a time limit for each one. Provide feedback on deviations from the agenda to ensure that the clients are aware of the pattern. It is your job to provide the structure for each session. A simple strategy is to keep a clock in your office that is behind the client, so that you can discretely remain aware of the time. A "10-minute warning" prior to the end of the therapy session is useful for some clients. Frequent deviation from the agenda should be a signal to reevaluate the initial treatment goals.

Occasionally, clients raise important issues that are not on the agenda, right at the end of the session. This pattern can be termed the "last chance" phenomenon. Experienced therapists of many orientations comment that a lot happens in the last 5 minutes of the session. Whereas cognitive-behavioral therapists work hard to complete their session summary and discuss homework, clients may want to add something not mentioned previously. Significant disclosures can occur just as a client stands up and gathers her coat and bag, or even as she opens the door to exit the interview room. Examples include "When are we going to get to my sexual problems?"; "Did I mention that my partner left me this week?"; or "I'm thinking about trying EMDR" (eye movement desensitization and reprocessing). All of these comments can "hook" the therapist to extend the session to discuss these important topics.

Resist the temptation to prolong a session except in cases of real emergencies! If a crisis or emergency situation exists, then it almost always is apparent during the session. Clients sometimes bring up difficult issues that they do not wish to speak about in depth, but they want the therapist to be aware of them. Thus, a useful response to a "last chance" disclosure is to state that you will make a note of the client's concern or question, and put this item on the agenda for discussion at the beginning of the next session. Some clients may test the limits of therapy and use a "last chance" statement to observe your reactions. For example, if you do not seem shocked or surprised at a revelation regarding sexuality, a client may feel more comfortable discussing it during the following session. It is not appropriate to extend the session, however, because the client has then been reinforced for a late-session disclosure. You also have deviated from the usual cognitive-behavioral therapy session structure, sending the message that the agenda does not really matter. From a practical perspective, you may inconvenience your next client, or limit his or her care, if you extend the session of the client who makes a "last chance" revelation. Even at the end of the day, or when no other client is in the waiting room, extending the session sends the message that it is not important for the client to consider your time and other commitments.

Clients in Crises and Emergencies

Outpatient treatment is most common for all mental health problems, even for clients with severe disorders, frequent crises, and suicidal ideation. Many third-party payers, such as insurance companies and HMOs, impose limits to the length of therapy. Longer-term treatments may be a luxury that is not available to most clients, even when needed or recommended. When inpatient admission occurs, the length of stay is shorter than it was in the past, and clients may not have adequate follow-up from the hospital system. With fewer clients being treated in hospital settings, you are more likely to see outpatients with both acute and chronic suicidality, or other types of crises (Joiner, Walker, Rudd, & Jobes, 1999). Even if crises occur infrequently in your practice, they are typically stressful for all parties involved in the situation. It is imperative emergencies for all cognitive-behavioral therapists to learn how to manage and to treat different types of crises and.

Knowledge about suicide and its management is mandatory for mental health therapists. Between 90 and 93% of adult suicide completers have been found to have a major mental disorder (Kleespies, Deleppo, Gallagher, & Niles, 1999). Also, 30–40% of individuals who completed suicide had been diagnosed with an Axis II disorder (Kleespies et al., 1999). One of the best predictors of suicide risk is a history of suicide attempts; however, approximately 60–70% of suicide attempters commit suicide on the first known attempt (Kleespies et al., 1999). For the purposes of suicide assessment and intervention, it is not sufficient just to know a client's diagnosis or suicide history.

Joiner et al. (1999) describe suicide risk on a continuum from nonexistent to extreme. They discuss specific ways to assess risk. Rudd and Joiner (1998) have further divided factors related to suicide into predisposing factors (e.g., gender, family history of suicide), risk factors (e.g., acute symptoms, current stressors), and protective factors (e.g., social support, problem-solving abilities). Predisposing factors are not changeable, but risk factors may be reduced through short-term interventions, and protective factors may be increased through environmental changes or short-term cognitive-behavioral interventions. Short-term interventions tend to address the current situation rather than the underlying precipitants, such as problems with emotion regulation, skills deficits, or long-term interpersonal difficulties.

Virtually all therapists have training in the assessment and intervention for suicide risk. Suicide risk assessments and interventions are common in many settings, and the onus is on the therapist to learn how to manage this situation safely and effectively. The local laws and regulations vary somewhat from place to place, so you need to learn these statutes and standards in your local jurisdiction to make appropriate clinical decisions. Some settings have protocols to manage this problem. The specifics of suicide assessment and intervention are beyond the scope of this book. A useful text by Simon and Hales (2006) includes discussion of practice guidelines for suicide assessment and treatment. Table 10.4 presents ideas regarding suicide risk management, particularly as they relate to cognitive-behavioral therapy.

It has been suggested that self-harm behaviors, including suicide and parasuicide, may represent an attempt to solve a problem rather than the problem itself. Linehan (1993) has discussed this way of viewing self-harm in her text on borderline personality disorder. For example, self-harm behavior may represent an attempt at emotion regulation, a method of communication to other people, or misguided problem solving. It may not be possible to determine the underlying reasoning when the client is very distressed. If you know the client in advance, however, you may be aware of the problem and try to deal with it more directly over a series of sessions. For example, hopelessness that is driven by negative predictions about the future may lead a person to suicidal behavior. These thoughts can be treated through cognitive restructuring or behavioral interventions within the context of a strong and supportive therapeutic relationship.

Different types of crises and emergencies can and often do occur with clients. Distinguishing a crisis from an emergency is useful. Kleespies et al. (1999) define a *crisis* as an emotionally significant and very distressing event that does not necessarily include serious physical or life-threatening danger. A crisis, however, can contribute to or escalate to an emergency situation, which is a more focused problem that occurs within a discrete period of time. Because a person in crisis is usually in a state of emotional disequilibrium, the crisis can easily worsen. Hence, it is necessary to take some type of action to deescalate the situation. Kleespies et al. state that an *emergency* exists when there is imminent risk of serious harm to self or others in the absence of an intervention. From this perspective, examples of emergencies include high-risk suicidal states, potentially violent states, very impaired judgment, and high risk to a minor or a defenseless individual.

While the most common emergency in clinical practice is suicide, other serious problems may occur. Other possible emergencies include violence or aggression toward other people, including the therapist. Clients may report homicidal ideation, violent fantasies, or make threats toward other people. They may report that a child or minor has been abused or injured.

After completion of a risk assessment, the intervention usually involves increasing the safety of the people involved. Actions may include warning others or calling the police. Other risks involve clients with tem-

TABLE 10.4. Suggestions for Suicide Risk Management

1. Develop a strong alliance with the client, and use the alliance in the treatment plan.
2. The efficacy of relatively short-term, problem-solving and crisis-oriented outpatient treatments for suicidal ideation is well established.
3. Intensive follow-up through telephone contacts or home visits may improve treatment compliance over the short term for lower-risk clients.
4. Improving ease of access (e.g., a clear crisis intervention plan) to emergency services may possibly reduce subsequent suicide attempts and service demand by first-time suicide attempters.
5. Intensity of treatment should vary according to degree of risk.
6. Short-term cognitive-behavioral therapy that integrates problem solving as a core intervention effectively decreases suicide ideation, depression, and hopelessness over periods of up to 1 year. Brief approaches do not appear to be effective over the longer term. For acute crisis, provide a relatively short-term directive approach.
7. For individuals identified as high-risk, intensive follow-up treatment after an attempt is most appropriate. "High-risk" includes people with a history of multiple attempts, psychiatric diagnosis, and comorbid problems.
8. Long-term treatments should address the underlying causes of suicidal behavior, such as emotion regulation problems, impulsivity, and negative self-image or interpersonal problems. For chronic crises (particularly those including Axis II disorders), provide a relatively long-term approach that focuses on the underlying causes.
9. If inpatient hospitalization is available and accessible, high-risk clients can be safely and effectively treated on an outpatient basis.
10. Use of structured follow-up and referral process (e.g., letters or telephone calls) may reduce risk for people who drop out of treatment.
11. Obtain consultation, supervision, and support for clients with difficult problems.

Note. Based on Kleespies, Deleppo, Gallagher, and Niles (1999) and Rudd, Joiner, Jobes, and King (1999).

porarily impaired judgment, which may be caused by a psychotic state (e.g., delusional beliefs, brain injury, or substance abuse). In such cases, both the client and others may need protection. Questions that you should consider include the following:

- Is the client impaired in the session?
- Did she use a substance or take an overdose? What and how much?
- Can he drive safely? If not, how can he get home (if appropriate)?
- Is she having a panic attack?
- Is he dissociating in the session? (Remember that dissociation can occur as a result of high anxiety or other disorders.)
- Is she experiencing serious enough psychotic symptoms to impair her judgment and safety?

- Did he experience a recent trauma?
- Is there risk of self-harm (parasuicide), independent of suicide risk?
- Is there imminent risk to you or others in the current setting?

Fortunately for many therapists, severe client distress is not that common in treatment, but it can happen, and you should be prepared in case it does. During an acute emergency, it may be difficult to differentiate between emotional and physical distress. You may not have experienced a client having dissociative or panic symptoms, and the first time it happens may alarm both the client and the therapist. You may not have worked directly with clients with psychotic symptoms, so you may not know what to expect. See Table 10.5 for guidelines to deal with crises and emergencies in your practice.

Your own safety is paramount, as is the safety of others with whom you work. You cannot be an effective therapist if you are afraid of your clients. Use common sense and good judgment, and trust your intuition. It is generally a poor idea to see clients when you are alone in the office, especially after hours. Some settings go so far as to arrange the therapy offices so that therapists can easily escape if they feel threatened, or to arrange "panic buttons," so that assistance can be obtained quickly. Exercise good self-care, particularly following crisis intervention or when dealing with an emergency situation. Apply psychological first-aid strategies as needed (see Table 10.6).

CHALLENGES THAT ORIGINATE WITH THE THERAPIST

Just as different challenges may arise with clients, they also arise with therapists. We are often deeply affected by our work. We can be changed by the clients we see, even while we try to help them incorporate change into their lives. For an excellent discussion of the joys and challenges of being a therapist, see Kottler (1986). It is necessary and desirable to use cognitive behavioral interventions on yourself at times (Persons, 1989). Supervision and peer support can be useful interventions, as is formal therapy, if needed. Virtually all therapists have crises of confidence at times. Indeed, it might be suspicious behavior never to have self-doubts, because such over confidence might be related to a lack of self-awareness or insufficient knowledge of the limits to competence. In this section we discuss some of the difficult elements of cognitive-behavioral therapy, both for less experienced and more seasoned therapists.

TABLE 10.5. Guidelines for Dealing with Crises and Emergencies

1. Complete the assessment, and determine the severity of the problem and the degree of risk as well as you can.

2. Ways of managing the crisis and preventing an emergency include:
   a. Increase your activity compared to other times during a crisis. The greater the distress or decompensation of the client, the greater the degree of activity or intervention on the part of the therapist. Become more directive than usual. Use closed rather than open-ended questions. Be specific, and do not expect much problem solving from the client. If the client is not able to cope or make decisions due to distress, you may need to intervene temporarily. Remain calm and in control (even if you do not feel calm).
   b. Build in more support for the client. Support may include making yourself more available, with more frequent sessions or telephone contacts. Support may also include access to other services, such as distress centers, crisis teams, or clinics. Other people in the client's life may also be used for support, such as the family physician, the partner, colleagues, or close friends.
   c. Provide clear, written instructions for plans made. Keep wallet-size cards available in your office to give to clients before a crisis escalates. These cards should include local contact information for distress lines, emergency services, and shelters. Make personalized cards for the client to keep with their own emergency contact information. Encourage clients to practice using services when they are distressed but not in crisis, to increase the chances of use during a crisis.
   d. Delaying impulses can help "buy time" and encourage the client to reconsider other options. During these delays, work to restore the client's hope.
   e. Environmental interventions can help delay or prevent a client from acting on impulses. These include having the client or others remove risks (e.g., lethal doses of medications, weapons), increasing social support, and using community resources. Delaying an impulse, and accessing support in the meantime, can cause a change of heart in many clients.
   f. Engage in short-term planning, such as what the client plans to do immediately after the session if you decide that he or she is safe to leave. If the client does not have plans, will be alone, and does not have easy access to social supports, work with him or her to make concrete plans.
   g. Consider asking a colleague who is close by for a second opinion.
   h. Consider whether hospitalization is necessary. If you do not work in an inpatient setting, you may need to arrange a safe method of transportation for the client. If the client agrees and appears to be capable of getting to the hospital, inform the mental health practitioner in the emergency department that your client is coming. Tell the client that you have taken this step as a precaution.
   i. If the client's crisis has escalated to a statement of emergency (e.g., imminent risk to self or others) and the client does not agree to a more intensive intervention, you must involve others, such as the police or security. Keep emergency contact information close at hand.

3. Consult with others. Document what you have done and why you made the decisions you did. Also document any consultations. If needed, inform your supervisor or manager of what has occurred. "The twin pillars of risk management are documentation and consultation" (Kleespies et al., 1999, p. 457).

4. Obtain support for yourself following the event (see Table 10.6).

TABLE 10.6. Cognitive-Behavioral First Aid for the Therapist

After you manage a crisis or emergency, it is common to feel anxious and to worry about your actions. This anxiety is typically related to one or more of the following questions:

- Did I do the right thing?
- Did I miss anything? Could my intervention(s) be improved on?
- Did the intervention lead to increased safety for my client?
- What will the outcome be?
- Will I feel safe in future therapy with this client?
- What are appropriate limits for me to set with my clients?

First-aid measures can include the following:

- Answer the previous questions to the best of your abilities. Examine the evidence that does or does not support negative thinking, and list the pros and cons of your intervention. Bring your thinking into line with the evidence. Use Socratic questioning with yourself.
- Weigh your own needs against the needs of your client or the system in which you work.
- Obtain emotional support from colleagues, family, and others who are close to you.
- Obtain consultation when needed. It is typically reassuring to know that others would have taken the same steps.
- Exercise good self-awareness; we all have emotional reactions to crises.
- Exercise good emotional, cognitive, and physical self-care.
- Consult with colleagues. Document your steps prior to leaving your office to help you leave the situation there.
- Distractions can help. Go for a walk, do some exercise, or do something that consumes your attention after work. If appropriate, plan a holiday from work for a while.

Difficulty with Adherence to the Cognitive-Behavioral Model

Clients are not the only ones who do not adhere to a model of treatment or therapeutic interventions! It is relatively easy to "drift" from any model of treatment, particularly with clients who struggle, do not respond well, are overly effusive, or do not accept the model themselves. If you have had training and supervision in other theoretical orientations, you may be tempted to incorporate other models or tools into therapy, which can confuse both you and your clients, and be less effective in the long run. We have often heard therapists describe their approach as "eclectic." For example, they may use a psychodynamic case formulation but incorporate occasional cognitive-behavioral strategies "as needed." This practice indicates nonadherence to the model and is not an appropriate use of cognitive-behavioral therapy, with its cognitive-behavioral case formulation (see Chapter 3, this volume), and the methods and strategies that follow from that conceptualization.

One of the best ways to check on your adherence is to have a supervisor or colleague observe your work and rate the session with the Cognitive Therapy Scale (Young & Beck, 1980; online at *www.academyofct.org*; see Appendix A and for discussion see Chapter 12 of this volume). Another option is to videotape a session and rate yourself using this scale. If you have the good fortune to supervise student therapists or work in a training setting, it may be feasible to have others observe your sessions, and vice versa. Regular case consultation and peer supervision are useful strategies to ensure that you follow good cognitive-behavioral practices.

Not all therapists "buy into" the cognitive-behavioral model, just as not all clients do. If you are not sure whether or not this model "fits" with your interpersonal and therapeutic style, then consider reading more or participating in workshops, supervision, or other types of training activities. Even though cognitive-behavioral interventions may have more empirical support than other interventions, the onus is on all therapists to find a method and a style of conducting therapy that is effective, as well as authentic and genuine for them.

Therapist "Impostor Syndrome"

It can be upsetting to lack confidence or to doubt your ability to help the people who come to see you for therapy. However, this concern is common in beginning therapists, particularly on the heels of a professional training program and internship or residency that provided supervision and time to read about the problems of clients you were treating. In many busy practices, it can be a challenge to keep up with new research findings. In particular, if you see many clients with many different types of problems, or work in independent practice, it is easy to feel overwhelmed and isolated. Automatic thoughts, such as "I can't really help anyone" or "This client can see right through me and knows that I don't know what I'm doing" may occur.

In some cases, you might be able to catch and to recognize your own distortions about treatment. A completed Dysfunctional Thoughts Record can help you to assess and evaluate such thoughts. If your thoughts are distorted, challenge your own cognitions with available evidence. For example, have you helped others in the past? Be sure to separate unrealistic thoughts from practice that is outside your level of competence. You need to develop the confidence to say "no" to referrals of clients with problems that you do not feel competent to handle. Discussions with other, new therapists can reveal similar thoughts and provide validation of your own insecurities. Clients and therapists alike feel encouraged and less alone when they realize that others share their problems. It is a good idea for all therapists, but particularly inexperienced ones, to obtain peer consultation and supervision.

Therapist Stress and Anxiety

It can be overwhelming to work with clients in distress, especially if you doubt yourself. But even therapists who generally feel competent in their skills experience stress and anxiety. There may be certain types of clients or problems that tend to trigger your feelings of anxiety. Some settings offer more staff support compared to others. Independent practice can be stressful for many new therapists, because there may be limited opportunity to share your anxieties or to obtain consultation from more seasoned therapists.

It is important to monitor your stress levels, to ensure that you are not suffering negative consequences from your work. Table 10.6 provides some therapist first-aid tips that are meant to be used following crisis intervention or when handling an emergency. In addition, general self-care strategies should be developed early and practiced regularly. These strategies include time management, and cognitive, emotional, and behavioral self-care. A focus on the positive aspects of professional life, rather than the negative ones, helps you to be a better role model for your clients. Positive aspects of work include the satisfaction of seeing change in clients, frequent intellectual stimulation, learning about many aspects of behavior disorders and psychotherapy, the intimacy of psychotherapeutic relationships, and being creative with cognitive-behavioral interventions.

Finally, many new therapists engage in cognitive distortions that increase anxiety, such as personalization ("If Jane doesn't improve, it's my fault, and she will be angry at me") or all-or-none thinking ("If Erik continues to experience some symptoms, he hasn't improved at all"). Obviously, it is important to monitor your own thoughts and be aware of your own particular distortions. It is imperative to learn how much responsibility you can assume on behalf of your clients. Leahy (2001) has developed a Therapist's Schema Questionnaire, which describes common schemas, along with the assumptions that accompany them. Such schemas include a need for the approval of your clients, helplessness, and excessive self-sacrifice.

Therapist "Fatigue" or "Burnout"

Some therapists find themselves emotionally drained by their work and start to experience negative thoughts about clients (e.g., persecution or judgmental schemas). They may make negative predictions about their clients, such as the client "is trying to provoke me," "is not motivated to change," "is not working hard enough," or "will not likely be able to change, or is hopeless." Rather than feeling energized following a session, you may feel frustrated and upset. It is normal to experience negative feelings after an occasional session, but if these reactions become part of an ongoing pattern, a cynical attitude may be just around the corner. If you do not exercise good self-care and maintain balance in your life, a large client load over a sustained period of time can lead to mental exhaustion. No one is immune to the development of psychological problems. In addition to monitoring yourself, exercising self-awareness, and using first aid methods after a crisis, it can also be important to obtain help to deal with these problems. A number of preventive measures may be instituted to reduce stress and burnout:

- See clients with a variety of problems, including those with different levels of severity.
- Monitor how you schedule your most difficult clients, so that they are not "back to back" or late in the day, when it can be difficult to access support or consultation.
- Be realistic about the limits of what you can manage.
- Learn to be assertive with supervisors, students, clients, or others who are likely to make demands on your time and energy.
- Be aware of and challenge your own distorted thoughts about clients.
- Make sure that you have a variety of activities in your work week, including scheduled time for paperwork, reading, consulting with colleagues, and going for lunch.
- Ensure that you participate in regular, continuing education activities, such as peer supervision, workshops, and conferences.
- Be assertive with your supervisor or manager about your workload.
- Ensure that you have and use a set of self-care activities, such as regular exercise, personal care, hobbies, social activities, and holidays.

CHALLENGES THAT ORIGINATE
WITH THE THERAPEUTIC RELATIONSHIP

Problems in the therapeutic relationship are related to both clients and therapists. Some of the previously discussed issues can lead to problems in the treatment relationship and therapeutic alliance. For example, if a client consistently does not accept the model or behaves aggressively toward the therapist, the therapist can become frustrated and react negatively toward the client. A rupture in the therapeutic alliance might occur (for a discussion about the therapeutic relationship, see Chapter 4, this volume). It is common for avoidance to be an issue in cognitive behavioral therapy, typically on the part of the client, but sometimes on the part of the therapist as well (see Chapter 5, this volume).

Not all clients recover from their problems, and not all improve, even given a sound course of cognitive-behavioral therapy. Occasionally, a client's problems may even get worse. Many clients attend for only a few sessions and drop out of treatment. If contacted, however, some of these clients express satisfaction with their outcomes. No treatment has 100% success. Although most clients are likely to be satisfied with treatment, not all clients will be.

Positive media coverage and increased empirical support for cognitive-behavioral therapy have led to more positive expectations, for both clients and their therapists. Whereas increased expectations typically lead to better outcomes, these same expectations can be unrealistic at times. All therapists wrestle with their own expectations about themselves, their clients, and the outcomes for therapy. Although it is natural to make predictions, remember that they may be incorrect. It is common for therapists to have higher expectations than do their clients. Remember that the outcome studies only predict results for the average client, or provide percentages of people who show improvements. We can extrapolate from these results for our clients, but these predictions are educated guesses most of the time. It can be humbling to work with clients, particularly if they have multiple problems or live in difficult circumstances. Learn to live with uncertainty and ambiguity.

Clients sometimes return to therapy following either a successful or an unsuccessful outcome. Psychodynamic approaches term the final phase of a successful therapy *termination* (Ellman, 2008). Indeed, most tertiary care systems have historically modeled their treatments on psychodynamic approaches and use the term *termination*. Many systems view readmission to an outpatient or inpatient program as a sign of relapse, and as a cost to the program's funding. Our view is that returning to treatment should not necessarily be viewed as a failure. When asked, many clients who return do so because they found therapy helpful, they felt comfortable with the therapist, and they expect therapy to be helpful again. The return of a "satisfied customer" can easily be viewed as a sign of success rather than failure. See Chapter 9, this volume, for more discussion of therapy completion and relapse prevention.

CHALLENGES THAT ORIGINATE
OUTSIDE OF THERAPY

Therapy exists within the context of clients' and therapists' lives, as well as within an organizational context. Life does not stop when the client is in therapy, and many different stresses can occur that have an effect upon therapy. Partners may leave or die, or your client may lose a job, get into a serious accident, or develop a life-threatening illness. Positive changes that can affect therapy also occur. Sometimes your client may make some of these changes as a result of being in therapy itself.

When major changes happen in your clients' lives, the goals of therapy may change to focus temporarily on these other issues. At times, a referral to another type of intervention, such as grief counseling or family therapy, may be helpful. It is wise for you as an effective cognitive-behavioral therapist to be aware of different types of services in your community. It is a good idea to keep an updated list of emergency community services for ready reference, if needed. These might include food, child care, financial aid, transportation, health care, housing, or crisis intervention services. Obviously, cognitive-behavioral therapy is not helpful if your clients' basic needs are not being met due to some more urgent problem. Sometimes, clients are embarrassed by these life circumstances. If so, do your best to minimize shame, so that your clients can express their concerns, and you can direct them to services where they can access help.

Situations similar to those describe earlier may occur in your own life. The organization or system in which you work may lose its funding or change its mandate. Your parents may become ill and infirm. Your partner may need hospitalization and intensive care. Be open and honest with your clients and those in your work settings about such events; if therapy needs to be altered, suspended, or ended, then try to find a like-minded therapist to whom you can refer clients, and minimize any negative impact on the work you have done to date.

Chapter 11

The Research Context
of Cognitive-Behavioral Therapy

In this chapter, we introduce more formally the idea that cognitive-behavioral therapy is based on a research foundation. We explore the ways that science and practice can be meaningfully linked, then summarize two key ways the research literature relates to practice. The first of these summaries is related to the literature on therapist–client factors and how the therapy relationship contributes to outcomes. The second examines the evidence base related to interventions, and how this relates to outcomes. We argue that both of these issues needs to be optimized to achieve best practice in cognitive-behavioral therapy.

W e used the metaphor of building bridges in Chapter 1. We recognize that psychotherapy is built on both research evidence and knowledge gained from experience, or, as has sometimes been said, it is both an art and a science. Ideally, the bridge would be a multilane, paved highway supported by bedrock, with lots of varied traffic. In some areas, though, the bridge is much more like a rope suspension bridge, with only an occasional foot passenger. Put another way, there are some areas in which the evidence base is strong and sufficient to support practice, and practice feeds back into the research issues being examined. In other areas, practice is loosely built on a research base, and the practice rarely leads to testable research questions.

In this chapter, we summarize what is known about the evidence base for cognitive-behavioral therapy. In doing so, we focus on two broad areas of research. The first is related to the interpersonal aspects of the therapy, and what we have learned about the importance of relationship factors and outcome. The second area of research is the examination of technologies or interventions, and how these relate to outcome. Our attempt is not to be exhaustive, in part because the literature is so large and rapidly growing. Rather, we offer a summary of the research literature, and provide sources of further information for the interested reader.

A GLOBAL PERSPECTIVE ON OUTCOME

There has been a long-standing debate about the percentage of clinical outcomes that can be attributed to various causal factors. This debate centers on interpersonal factors (or what have also been called "nonspecific" factors [DeRubeis, Brotman, & Gibbons, 2005], as they are found in most forms of psychotherapy), and treatment-specific techniques or methods (Wampold, 2005). The widely discrepant estimates of the amount of variance can be attributed to these factors, and this variability should be a clue that the evidence is equivocal and subject to interpretation. In some respects, though, we submit that the debate is moot. It is like a debate about whether it is the skeletal system, the nervous system, or the musculature that permits humans to walk. Each of these factors is necessary but not sufficient. So it is in psychotherapy. Both client and therapist bring their unique attributes and history to the therapy room, where they jointly try to solve problems. That process of solving problems involves client and therapist as individuals, relationship issues, and treatment methods; all are necessary, but none is sufficient. From a practical perspective, cognitive-behavioral therapy involves both a relationship and a set of activities or interventions, and neither can exist without the other.

The significance of this debate is that we need to understand the relative contributions of the client, therapist, relationship, and techniques to clinical outcome. But the situation is more complex than simply determining these characteristics for the average or typical client. Since most clients do not fit the profile of the typical client, there is always the need to translate research findings into case-specific clinical decisions. We return to this issue later in this chapter, but first we discuss what research tells us about each of these four contributing factors (see Figure 11.1).

Client Factors and Outcome

Before we discuss evidence related to the relationship between client variables and clinical outcome, we want to note briefly the methodology that has been used to examine this issue. For the most part, these studies use

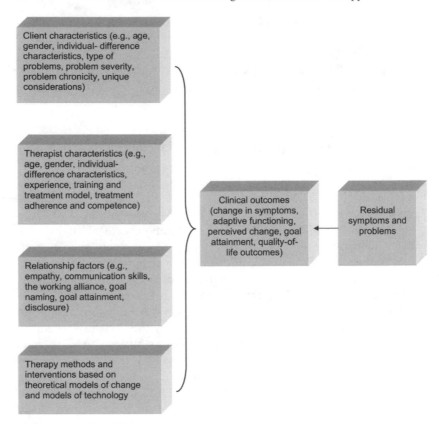

FIGURE 11.1. A conceptual model of clinical outcome.

preexisting client variables or characteristics, then assess the correspondence of these variables with clinical outcomes, often with correlational methods. In some cases, client variables are allowed to range widely, but the possible range of client variables is restricted in many psychotherapy studies. This restriction of range comes about by virtue of the inclusion and exclusion criteria employed in some studies, the use of speciality clinics to conduct psychotherapy research, and even therapist preferences for and selection of certain types of clients. For example, a considerable literature examines the relationships between client variables and clinical outcome in the context of controlled psychotherapy trials, which potentially affect the relationships observed. The effect of all restrictions in client variability is "restriction of range" and increased difficulty in showing relationship between client factors and outcome. To give an extreme example, it would be impossible for you to examine the relationship between religion and treatment outcome, if all of your clients were Christian or any other single faith.

The issue of relating client variables to outcome is complicated even further by the fact that whereas some of these variables are discrete (e.g., gender, marital status, diagnostic status), others are continuous (e.g., age, various personality traits or dimensions), so the statistics to document associations between various characteristics and outcome need to vary. Furthermore, although a considerable amount of the research looks at correlations or relationships between a given client variable and a specific outcome measure, there are much more complicated models to examine. For example, there are statistical methods in which several different client variables can be simultaneously considered as predictors of outcome, or in which outcome is conceptualized as a multidimensional phenomenon. Put another way, the research has really only begun to examine some of the potentially complex ways that client variables might relate to clinical outcomes.

This being said, we are able to offer a few general conclusions about client variables and how they relate to outcome. Haby, Donnelly, Corry, and Vos (2006) conducted a systematic literature review that examined the relations between a number of factors and outcome (defined in various ways) in cognitive-behavioral therapy for major depressive disorder, panic disorder, and generalized anxiety disorder. Based on 33 controlled clinical studies, they determined that the type of disorder was not related to outcome, because outcomes were roughly the same across different problems. However, two other client variables were related to outcome: (1) nationality of the study; that is, studies in English-speaking countries had somewhat stronger effects that those in non-English-speaking countries (however, note that this is not just a client variable, and that the number of non-English-language studies was small); (2) the relationship between higher levels of initial client problem severity and poorer outcomes in treatments.

In a more focused review of client predictors of outcome in cognitive-behavioral therapy for depression, Hamilton and Dobson (2001) found that client problem severity predicted outcome, but they also reported that clients with more episodes of depression (increased chronicity) also tended to have worse outcomes than clients with fewer episodes of depression. Saatsi, Hardy, and Cahill (2007) have reported that clients with more secure attachment styles tend to have better outcomes in cognitive-behavioral therapy for depression.

In a major review of client variables that predict outcome, although not specific to cognitive-behavioral therapy, Castonguay and Beutler (2006) identified a number of client variables associated with poorer treatment outcome. These variables were higher levels of client impairment, the presence of a personality disorder, and the occurrence of financial and/or occupational difficulties. Furthermore, they noted that increased client age and ethnic/minority or racial status were associated with worse outcome in the treatment of dysphoric disorders. They also noted that a match of therapist and client ethnic/minority or racial status was associated with reduced dropout and improved outcome in treating clients with dysphoria and that treatments that did not induce client resistance (or were collaborative) had better outcomes.

Table 11.1 summarizes what appear to be fairly consistent client predictors of positive outcome in cognitive-behavioral therapy. These include lower client problem severity and chronicity, the absence of a personality disorder, and positive attitudes or expectancies about treatment. Although the first three factors may be considered selection factors, in that they are characteristics for which you might select, you cannot really change these factors before treatment. In contrast, client attitudes or expectancies are probably a combination of general positive or negative attitudes, plus specific knowledge about and attitudes toward you as a therapist and the therapy you offer. These are issues that you can modify, in the way you begin to work with the client and introduce the cognitive-behavioral model (see Chapter 4, this volume).

Therapist Factors and Outcome

Therapist factors have been an understudied phenomenon in cognitive-behavioral therapy. When writing this chapter, we could not find a single review article that tried to examine this issue in depth, or as a specific topic. The Haby et al. (2006) review of predictors of outcome did examine some predictors, however. They reported that cognitive-behavioral therapy provided by "psychologists" had better outcomes than that provided by "therapists," but warned that the number of studies with more generic therapists was relatively small, and the pre-

TABLE 11.1. Client Variables Related to Better Treatment Outcome

General	Specific
• Lower problem severity	• Younger age (for dysphoric disorders)
• Lower problem chronicity	• Lack of racial or ethnic/minority group membership (for dysphoric disorders)
• Absence of a personality disorder	• A match between client and therapist on racial or ethnic status (for dysphoric disorders)
• Positive expectations about treatment	• Assignment to treatments that reduce patient resistance (for dysphoric disorders)

cise training or background of the therapists in these studies often was not described.

Perhaps surprisingly, Haby et al. (2006) reported in their review that the amount of therapist training was not related to outcome. This result is similar to results reported elsewhere (e.g., Jacobson et al., 1996), in that there is often no strong relationship between therapist training and competence, and clinical outcomes. This result is less surprising, however, when one considers again that much of the data are collected in randomized clinical trials. The therapists in such trials are generally well-trained, -supervised and -monitored, so although the average level of competence is high, the range of competence is fairly restricted, which makes establishing a correlation with outcome more difficult, than if there were more range in these variables.

As noted by Lambert (2005), relatively few studies have systematically studied the outcomes of novice versus experienced therapists, the effects of training on outcome, or even the relative importance of treatment adherence and competence for therapy outcomes (see also McGlinchey & Dobson, 2003). In an exception, Bright, Baker, and Neimeyer (1999) compared professionals and paraprofessionals doing either cognitive-behavioral therapy or mutual support group therapy for clients with depression. Although the immediate outcomes for the two therapist groups in the cognitive-behavioral therapy condition did not significantly differ with traditional statistical analyses, the clinical significance results favored the professional therapists. More research is warranted in this area.

Relationship Factors That Work in Cognitive-Behavioral Therapy

A plethora of research has examined aspects of the therapist–client relationship and treatment processes. Much of this literature relates to the context of treatment models that emphasize interactional processes as key aspects of the treatment, such as psychodynamic or experiential therapies (e.g., Norcross, 2002; Teyber, 2000; Yalom & Leszcz, 2005). A commensurate myth sometimes perpetuated is that cognitive-behavioral therapists do not pay attention to these factors, and that their sole focus of attention is on treatment techniques (see Chapter 12, this volume, for a further discussion of myths). The truth lies in between. Cognitive-behavioral therapists are acutely aware that psychotherapy takes place in an interpersonal crucible, but they also believe that the techniques employed in that forum make an important contribution to treatment outcome.

Most treatment manuals in cognitive-behavioral therapy address the nature of the optimal psychotherapy relationship. Often these manuals suggest that therapists need to be compassionate, empathic, caring, and respectful, and to have good social skills, including the ability to engage the client in therapy, to establish and work toward mutual goals, to provide needed feedback to the client, to teach skills, and to anticipate and deal with relationship difficulties. The fact that researchers within the cognitive-behavioral movement have focused relatively more time on the establishment of treatment efficacy for various disorders, and relatively less time examining relationship factors, does not indicate an absolute disregard for the latter. For example, in the Cognitive Therapy Scale (Young & Beck, 1980), which is the most commonly used measure of therapy competence in the field, several items relate directly to relationship and therapist characteristics that affect the quality of the relationship.

Again, the research methods used to establish relationship factors in psychotherapy are worthy of discussion. In some instances, the methodology is very much like that examining client variables, in that some attribute of the therapist is measured before the beginning of treatment, then it is correlated or otherwise examined with respect to some aspect of treatment outcome. In this way, variables such as therapist age or years of experience can be correlated with outcome. In other studies, though, ratings made by therapists and/or clients during the course of therapy are related to outcome. This type of study is more complex, because early changes experienced in therapy may "confound" or confuse therapist or client perceptions of therapy or of the other person. This potential problem becomes more acute if the therapist and client ratings are collected later on in treatment. For example, if you ask a therapist about the probable outcome of a specific case after the first session of therapy, he or she largely has to make an educated guess about what will transpire. If you ask the same question after the fifth session, however, the therapist already has the experience of several sessions, as well as any early benefit observed in therapy, on which to base his or her prediction of outcome.

To get away from the potential confusion between outcome and therapist–client perceptions of process, some psychotherapy process researchers have moved to external ratings of therapy sessions. This strategy removes the potential biases of the therapist and client, but it has its own problems. For one, the therapy rating process within a single session requires expertise, so that the rater knows what to look for and recognizes it when it occurs. Agreement among independent raters is one way to show that consistent ratings are possible, the interrater reliability in some of these studies has been difficult to obtain. This fact suggests that some of the constructs being studied are elusive, or at least difficult to recognize. Another problem, which is no doubt related to rater consistency, is that rating sessions in the absence of the other parts of treatment decontextualize the session. It is difficult as a rater to know what came before, or what general tack is being taken in therapy, so the rater has to make assumptions or fill in the gaps of his or her knowledge of the case.

Another issue in independent rating of sessions regards the content of what is being rated. Some researchers are interested in specific behaviors. Generally, the rating of a specific behavior (e.g., how many times did the therapist say "I agree"?) is easier than the rating of categories or induced characteristics of the therapy (e.g., how empathic is the therapist?). Also, some researchers are interested in the process of therapy and focus on issues such as empathy, collaboration, response to disruptions in the relationship, and so on.

Other researchers, interested in the treatment dimensions themselves, focus on the assessment of *treatment integrity* (McGlinchey & Dobson, 2003). Treatment integrity itself comprises two aspects: *treatment adherence* and *treatment competence*. Adherence is the extent to which a therapist adheres to a particular model of therapy, and performs interventions consistent with that approach, while not using methods from other models. Competence builds on adherence, and refers to the skillful and timely deployment of adhered to interventions, using an algorithm that determines optimal methods to use for a given client and stage of therapy. Consequently, a therapist might have good adherence and not be particularly competent, or a therapist might have both poor adherence and poor competence. Again, it has been shown that achieving interrater reliability is easier with respect to adherence than with respect to competence.

It is also worth noting that the lens through which researchers examine the therapy process reflects in part their belief about the key aspects of therapy, and tends to reinforce these schemas. Researchers who focus on nonspecific or common aspects of the therapy process tend to support eclectic therapy practice, and tend to believe that the majority of outcome in psychotherapy can be found in these aspects of treatment (Lambert & Barley, 2002; Teyber, 2000). Researchers who emphasize specific treatment components tend to study aspects of treatment integrity, and tend to believe these aspects of therapy are more critical for optimal outcome (DeRubeis, Brotman, et al., 2005). The latter group is also more likely to conduct randomized clinical trials, in which one specific therapy is "pitted" against another to determine the better or optimal treatment for a given disorder, where the "better" treatment is defined by outcomes on clinical or symptom dimensions.

Evidence-Based Process Variables

The previous discussion reveals how complex the study of therapy process can be, how it can be approached from various angles and methodologies, and how the research process itself can reinforce beliefs about which aspects are more important for treatment outcome. If we accept that these issues are important for psychotherapy, then what does the literature tell us? In general, it says that therapist characteristics most associated with positive outcome include higher levels of empathy, authenticity, caring, and warmth (Castonguay & Beutler, 2006; see Table 11.2; see also Josefowitz & Myran, 2005). Therapists with better outcomes also tend to have a more secure attachment style in their relationships with others and are able to demonstrate positive regard toward their clients, even if they need to confront or challenge certain thoughts or behaviors. There is also evidence that more successful therapists are able to engage in appropriate self-disclosure, although therapists tend not to disclose very often in therapy in any event (Goldfried, Burckell, & Eubanks-Carter, 2003; Hill & Knox, 2002).

There is also literature that has addressed the various interpersonal aspects of therapy process and linked these aspects to clinical outcomes (see Table 11.2). Irrespective of the therapy model, it appears that outcomes are enhanced when there is therapeutic collaboration, or what has also been termed a strong *therapeutic alliance*. The concept of *collaborative empiricism*, which has been described as a goal of sound cognitive-behavioral therapy, seems generally to be consistent with the idea of developing and maintaining a strong working relationship, although empiricism is added to the concept (for a review, see Keijsers et al., 2000).

It also appears that the ability to develop and work toward common goals assists with treatment success. This idea certainly is consistent with the tenets of cognitive-behavioral therapy, because an important part of the early work in this approach is the development of explicit and agreed-

TABLE 11.2. Relationship Factors Related to Treatment Outcome in Cognitive-Behavioral Therapy

Therapist-based factors	Relational factor
• Empathy	• Therapeutic collaboration or alliance
• Positive regard, authenticity, caring, and warmth	• Goal consensus and pursuit
• Secure attachment style	• Congruence
• Self-disclosure	• Feedback
	• Managing relationship disruptions
	• Recognition of and response to affect about the relationship ("transference" and "countertransference")

upon treatment goals, ideally arrived at through a consensual process. Evidence suggests that therapists who can reflect clients' distress and emotionality, or show congruence, also tend to have better outcomes, as do those who provide feedback to their clients.

There is also evidence that to maximize treatment success, it is important to attend to and manage relationship disruptions. Although it might be argued that there are no such events in an ideal therapy relationship, the therapist needs to be mindful of this possibility, and to address these events, if they occur (Leahy, 2003). Finally, the evidence suggests that effective therapists generally recognize and respond to affect about and within the relationship (traditionally referred to as *transference* and *countertransference* in the context of psychoanalytic theory; Gelso & Hayes, 2002). Although, to our knowledge, no research literature examines such issues directly, interpersonal process issues, such as resistance, have been addressed in the context of cognitive-behavioral therapy (Leahy, 2001). These types of challenges have been addressed clinically from a cognitive perspective (J. S. Beck, 2005; Chapter 10, this volume).

In addition to the general literature, several issues relevant to the cognitive-behavioral therapies have been explored in the research. These include the use of homework, the role of general and specific techniques, and the issue of "sudden change." Each of these issues is briefly discussed here.

Homework

A key tenet of cognitive-behavioral therapy is the need for a translation of the discussion that occurs during the therapy hour into assignments, or homework, between sessions. This homework may involve further assessment of problems or issues that arise in therapy, or change-oriented assignments, but the transformative part of this treatment is viewed as occurring as much (or more) between sessions as within them. Research supports the importance of homework completion, particularly early in therapy, as a positive predictor of treatment outcome (Burns & Nolen-Hoeksema, 1991; Kazantsis, Deane, & Ronan, 2000; Whisman, 1993). It stands to reason, therefore, that a key aspect of the therapy process is determining how to help the client make this translation of talk into action, and that there is a need for theory and research in this area of therapy process (Kazantsis & L'Abate, 2007).

General and Specific Techniques

Given the emphasis in the literature on the relative importance of non-specific or general techniques in psychotherapy, as opposed to theory-specific interventions, it is perhaps not surprising that this issue has been addressed in cognitive-behavioral therapy. For example, Castonguay, Goldfried, Wiser, Raue, and Hayes (1996) examined both unique and common factors that predicted outcome in a sample of 30 depressed clients. Although the general techniques in their study (therapeutic alliance and client's emotional experiencing) did predict outcome, the specific cognitive-behavioral technique of focusing on distorted cognitions actually correlated negatively with outcome. Their interpretation of this result was that some therapists may have relied inappropriately on the specific technique, instead of focusing on problems in the therapy alliance.

In contrast to the Castonguay et al. (1996) study, two Feeley and DeRubeis studies have examined general and specific techniques in cognitive therapy for depression. In both studies (DeRubeis & Feeley, 1990; Feeley, DeRubeis, & Gelfand, 1999), the specific techniques predicted more of the outcome than did the general therapist conditions. Furthermore, they also examined a measure of therapeutic alliance, and found that rather than predicting change in therapy, therapeutic alliance tended to improve only after improvement in symptomatology. As a consequence of these results, they suggested that it may be the specific interventions employed in cognitive-behavioral therapy that most lead to change in symptoms and, in turn, it is the symptom change that leads to better therapeutic alliance. These ideas need further study, particularly in disorders other than depression.

Sudden Change

A recent and somewhat serendipitous finding about the process of cognitive-behavioral therapy is that some clients do not have a smooth and gradual remission from symptoms; rather, they experience a "sudden gain." Clients who are able to have a sudden gain, then sustain it, appear to have a more stable pattern of change, as evidenced by lower likelihood of relapse following treatment (Tang & DeRubeis, 1999; Tang, DeRubeis, Beberman, & Pham, 2005; Tang, DeRubeis, Hollon, Amsterdam, & Shelton, 2007). These results hold even if these clients do not ultimately achieve greater overall change compared to other clients. This finding needs further examination, particularly in a broader range of disorders than those studied to date. However, if this pattern is found to be reliable among various disorders, it does suggest a particular process in cognitive-behavioral therapy.

TREATMENTS THAT WORK

Although it is easy to say that cognitive-behavioral therapy works, the details, of course, are much more complicated than this simple conclusion implies. Questions that should be asked include the following: For what kinds of problems does it work? Are there particular subgroups of clients for whom the treatment works? Does the therapy works equally as well or better than other therapies? What type of evidence is used to draw these conclusions, among others? The field of psychotherapy research has become a highly specialized area of science. Our goal here is not to discuss the details of that literature, but to give you at least enough information to be mindful of the issues when you consider the research. As such, we discuss the methods used to evaluate treatments, the issue of empirically supported treatments, and what we call "the evidence debate," before we review the actual evidence for various disorders.

Methods to Evaluate Treatments

As noted earlier, the field of psychotherapy research has evolved considerably since the earliest days of this treatment approach. With the advent of psychotherapy, Freud and the other early psychoanalysts primarily provided extended case studies to develop models of psychopathology and treatment. Breuer and Freud's *Studies on Hysteria*, first published in 1895 (Strachey, 1957), stands as a classic use of cases to develop broader models of both the content and process of psychological disorders. Behavioral models that first developed also employed single-case designs, and what became $N = 1$ research methods.

Over time, though, and with the development of more general models of treatment for different disorders, it was perhaps natural to see open trials of the outcomes for various treatments, in the context of various disorders. By the 1960s, comparisons between psychological therapies and control groups began to emerge in the literature, and these developed to the point that it became possible to summarize the scientific state of the literature using a method called *meta-analysis*, which collapses results across different studies and outcome measures (Smith & Glass, 1977). These early results generally supported the general efficacy of psychological treatments, but with some caveats (some therapies had better results than others, and some disorders were associated with stronger outcomes than others).

By the late 1970s, two developments occurred that have changed the field irrevocably. The first was the publication of DSM-III (American Psychiatric Association, 1980). This DSM version provided a more descriptive model of psychopathology than did previous editions, and a symptom-based model of diagnosis. With this emphasis, it became possible to evaluate treatment more clearly with respect to specific disorders. The second development was treatment manuals, which provide more standardized treatments and allow for more precision in the study of psychotherapies (Luborsky & DeRubeis, 1984). Treatment manuals also emphasize the techniques of specific therapies; whereas largely support the importance of a good therapeutic relationship, they emphasized more what the therapist is expected to do within that relationship context rather than the relationship itself.

With the establishment and acceptance of both a way to conceptualize outcome, in terms of symptoms, and the use of treatment manuals, the strategy of using randomized clinical trials to compare psychological treatments to either no-treatment comparisons or other active therapies perhaps became inevitable. This period of time was also the beginning of the "cognitive revolution" in psychology and psychotherapy, and it is not surprising that cognitive-behavioral therapies garnered a lot of the research funds. In particular, because the early results for this treatment were promising, this movement quickly gathered steam and moved the treatment to its current dominant position in the field across disciplines (Weissman et al., 2006).

The other phenomenon that helped to reify the position of cognitive behavioral therapy was the movement toward empirically supported therapies (Chambless & Ollendick, 2001). This approach used criteria similar to those employed generally in clinical trials in medicine, and allowed use of evidence from research trials to define treatments that met these criteria as "empirically supported." This approach to examining the evidence for psychological treatments has acknowledged limitations (Chambless & Ollendick, 2001; Dobson & Dobson, 2006). First, because clients are randomly assigned to treatments, emphasis in these studies is on the independent variable, which is the therapy(ies) under investigation. Consequently, client variables are considered relatively unimportant in such research. Second, because these studies use manuals, therapist flexibility in these studies is constrained. Manualized practice is not likely to reflect accurately what happens in clinical practice. Third, and, again, because of the focus on the intervention in these studies, the guidelines for inclusion or exclusion of clients in these studies are quite precise. Inclusion and exclusion rules often lead to quite homogenous samples that, again, may limit the generalizability of the results to actual clinical practice, in which clients often present with complicated or multiple problems, Despite these limitations, the randomized clinical trial has generally been recognized as an important strategy, as has the use of criteria for empirically supported therapies to review the literature and declare which therapies "work" for which problems.

Yet another force in the field that has helped to shape the current state of the evidence is the development of statistical tools to summarize data. In part because of the widespread adoption of the randomized clinical trial method, it is possible to use the statistical tool called *meta-analysis* to summarize the results of various studies in a single number. To do so, however, one must assume that client groups in each of the various studies did not significantly differ from each other at the beginning of the study, when they were randomly assigned to groups. By doing so, the results of the treatments can be directly compared (usually at the end of the acute stage of therapy), and these numbers can be averaged across studies. As summarized below, there are now many meta-analyses in various areas of cognitive-behavioral therapy, and even a review of meta-analyses (Butler et al., 2006).

One other aspect of the outcome literature that warrants brief attention is statistical and clinical significance testing. Most research literature uses traditional models of statistical significance testing to determine whether intervention is more effective on one dimension than on another. Such tests are very useful, if the assumption can be made that study groups are roughly comparable at the beginning of the study, because significant differences at the end of the study can reasonably be related to the effects of one intervention compared to another. As has been pointed out, however, it is possible to obtain a statistically significant effect in a comparative treatment study that has little practical significance. For example, if a treatment difference can be measured precisely, or if a sufficient number of research participants is used, minor differences can attain statistical significance.

Given the concerns about statistical significance, another method of evaluating research trials, referred to as *clinical significance testing*, has evolved (Jacobson & Truax, 1991). This method usually evaluates the proportion of clients given a particular treatment who start and end the study with scores on a given measure in the range of a clinically distressed population. For example, the rates of a given diagnosis at the beginning and end of treatment can be contrasted, if this comparison is of clinical importance. Alternatively, if a cutoff score on a given measure can be established to differentiate better from worse outcomes, then the percentage of people who obtain scores below that cutoff can be examined.

Although tests of clinical significance are a potential strategy to duplicate in the outcome literature clinicians' kinds of considerations, and although there are many examples of such studies, the research literature continues to focus on statistical significance testing. Also, the meta-analytic method relies on statistical results rather than the evaluation of clinical significance of results. We hope this situation will shift over time.

A REVIEW OF THE LITERATURE

So, what does the literature say? We have tried here to summarize the evidence in a way that is useful to the practitioner. Thus, rather than review specific studies in great detail, we have provided in Appendix B a list of recent review articles for various domains of cognitive-behavioral therapy. You are invited to obtain and read these articles, or the studies on which they are based, depending on your area of practice. Remember that each study has its own peculiarities that sometimes affect the results of each study, or the likelihood that the results would be achieved again, if the study were repeated.

We have also summarized the results of the studies listed in Appendix B in Table 11.3. This table lists the different specific DSM-related diagnoses treated with cognitive-behavioral therapy, and summarizes three different ways to conceptualize the success of the treatment. "Absolute efficacy" is the extent to which cognitive-behavioral therapy has better outcomes than no treatment, a waiting list, or treatment as usual. It is important to note that absolute efficacy, in this sense, actually represents different types of comparisons. The comparison of a given treatment to a waiting list or to no treatment is in some respects not a very demanding comparison, because positive outcomes are fairly easy to attain. But positive results in this type of study might be the effect of simply providing any type of care, assistance, or support to someone with a set of problems, so the results are not very telling. Comparison with treatment as usual is more demanding, because such comparisons actually involve a contrast between usual care and the additional benefit of cognitive-behavioral therapy, in contrast to usual attention and treatment. It is also worth noting that whereas earlier psychotherapy studies used no-treatment or waiting-list conditions fairly often, treatment as usual is an increasingly common comparison in more recent treatment studies, primarily due to ethical and legal concerns related to not providing any treatment during a research trial.

The next two columns represent the outcomes or efficacy of cognitive-behavioral therapy relative to two other comparisons. One of these, medication, is commonly employed in the treatment of many disorders. The other column, comparison to other psychotherapies, or to a set of psychotherapies, if the data are available (in the interest of space we do not list which ones, but the information can be found in the review articles). Bear in mind, though, that this column actually involves a number of comparisons that may become clearer as further data are gathered. For example, whereas many studies that compare cognitive-behavioral therapy to another type of psychotherapy find no significant difference, and we have concluded that there is rough equivalence in many areas, specific differences may emerge as more studies are conducted.

As seen in Table 11.3, cognitive-behavioral therapy has generated a considerable amount of supportive evidence, particularly in reference to treatment-as-usual, waiting-list, or no-treatment comparisons. In some cases, evidence is strong enough to argue that cognitive-behavioral ther-

TABLE 11.3. A Summary of Evidence for Cognitive-Behavioral Therapies

Disorder	Treatment	Type of efficacy data		
		Absolute efficacy	Efficacy relative to medications	Efficacy relative to other psychotherapies
Specific phobia	Exposure and cognitive restructuring	++	+	
Social phobia	Exposure and cognitive restructuring	++	=	=
Obsessive–compulsive disorder	Exposure and response prevention	+		+
Panic disorder	Exposure and cognitive restructuring	+	=	+
Posttraumatic stress disorder	Exposure and cognitive restructuring	++		=
Generalized anxiety disorder	Exposure and cognitive restructuring	+	=	+
Major depression	Activity, cognitive restructuring, and schema change	+	+	=
Bipolar disorder[a]	Affect regulation and cognitive restructuring	+		+
Anorexia nervosa	Eating regulation and cognitive restructuring	+	=	+
Bulimia nervosa	Eating regulation and cognitive restructuring	++	+	+
Sleep disorders	Behavioral control and cognitive restructuring	+		+
Psychosis[a]	Affect regulation and cognitive restructuring	+		+
Substance use disorders	Affect regulation, behavioral control, and cognitive restructuring	+		=

(continued)

TABLE 11.3. (*continued*)

Somatization disorder	Behavioral control and cognitive restructuring	+

Note. A blank space indicates no evidence; + indicates positive evidence; = indicates approximate equivalence; ++ indicates treatment of choice.

[a]Cognitive-behavioral therapy is used typically as an adjunct to medication in these disorders.

apy is the treatment of choice (e.g., for specific and social phobias, post-traumatic stress disorder, and bulimia nervosa). Comparative trials with medications generally show cognitive-behavioral therapies to be at least as efficacious as medications, but comparisons are absent in some areas (notably, for bipolar disorder and for psychosis, in which psychological therapies are typically used only as adjuncts to medication) and should be a focus of future research. Cognitive-behavioral therapy has been shown to have greater effects than other treatments for some disorders but to be approximately comparable to other treatments for other disorders. This aspect of the literature is perhaps the most difficult to summarize, because the comparison treatments that have been studied vary widely, from behavioral therapies without a cognitive element to short-term psychodynamically based psychotherapies, to components of the overall cognitive-behavioral treatment. If you are interested in the relative efficacy of cognitive-behavioral therapy compared to other psychosocial treatments, read the review articles for more details about these results.

Most of the comparisons in Table 11.3 represent the effects of manualized cognitive-behavioral therapies. Although manuals vary in length and in detail, most manuals do not include a single intervention but, in fact, weave together a series of interventions in a sequenced and conceptually based order. Furthermore, although there are some instances in which relatively complex manualized treatments have been taken apart into their constituent components to see which aspects of the treatment are most associated with change, such studies are relatively few compared to those that adopt the entire treatment package. As such, although we can say that cognitive-behavioral therapy "works" for a number of disorders, we are largely just beginning the research that reveals precisely why these therapies have their positive effects.

It is also important to note that the results presented in Table 11.3 are largely limited to immediate treatment effects. Although some areas have indicated that the long-term effects of cognitive-behavioral therapy are equally strong, or even stronger than the short-term results (e.g., Paykel, 2007), it is relatively difficult to conduct meta-analyses for long-term therapy results. It is also worth noting that in many of the studies to date, the appropriate focus of attention is on helping clients either to achieve fewer symptoms or not meet diagnostic criteria for a certain disorder. Therapies have other effects, though, that are less often studied. These include improvements in self-esteem and other psychological characteristics, enhanced social and work adjustment, better social and environmental supports, better health in general, or enhanced of quality of life. How much these other benefits are ancillary results of direct treatment effects, or how much they also contribute to lower symptoms remains an open question.

Treatments That Do Not Work

With the development of the outcome treatment literature, the field is increasingly able to identify treatments that do not work, or that have limited clinical outcome. Norcross, Koocher, and Garofalo (2006) surveyed a number of psychologists about discredited treatments and assessment tools, and were able to discern a number of psychological interventions that are commonly viewed as ineffective and inappropriate, or as involving unsubstantiated risk. This list includes many "New Age" therapies (e.g., "angel therapy," pyramids, orgone therapy) inappropriate extensions of models based on psychodynamic therapy (e.g., rebirthing, primal scream therapy), and miscellaneous others. Although there are one or two cognitive-behavioral therapies on the list (e.g., thought stopping for obsessional rumination), they are exceptions and are well down the list in terms of average rating of discredit.

Another perspective on the issue of treatments that do not work relates to those that actually cause harm. Lilienfeld (2007) has provided criteria for considering treatments to be harmful. These include treatments that (1) increase the variability of functioning, (2) increase some symptoms while decreasing others, (3) increase to harm friends or relatives, (4) increase deterioration, and (5) increased dropout from therapy. From this perspective, he has identified two cognitive-behavioral therapies as potentially harmful. The first potentially harmful cognitive-behavioral therapy is the immediate and universal use of critical incident stress debriefing, because, in some cases, such unneeded and rapid interventions can actually *increase* the risk of traumatic symptoms in some clients. The second is relaxation treatment for panic-prone patients, because this approach can actually *increase* the likelihood of panic.

Our point here is not to suggest that cognitive-behavioral therapies have inherent risk. Indeed, the research literature cited earlier is generally supportive of positive effects from these therapies. But any treatment, particularly if inappropriately used, can have associated risk. As a result, our suggestion is always to consider whether the treatment you are planning has an evidence base to support it. Evidence-based practice also is associated with evidence-based assessment, so that untoward or unexpected negative effects of treatment can be measured, and the treatment can be reevaluated, if necessary.

Common Principles of Therapy

A recent, considerably attractive idea is that basic principles that cut across effective forms of cognitive-behavioral therapy explain a good deal of the variance associated with the positive effects of these treatments. Barlow, Allen, and Choate (2004) have suggested that three such principles operating within cognitive-behavioral therapy explain much of the benefit of these treatments for the emotional disorders. These include (1) altering the cognitive appraisals that precede emotional disturbance, (2) preventing the avoidance of negative emotional experience, and (3) encouraging actions not associated with the dysfunctional emotion. In this regard, widespread use of methods related to cognitive reappraisal, in conjunction with exposure to emotionally disturbing stimuli, appears to be a common strategy for both the anxiety- and depression-related disorders, as well as other problems, such as eating disorders.

Barlow et al. (2004) generated the three general principles in partial response to the burgeoning number of treatment manuals in the field. Their argument was that these three principles can flexibly generate appropriate interventions for different clients who present with emotional disorders. It is not clear whether this metamodel approach to understanding the principles of therapy actually simplifies the clinician's job relative to using treatment manuals, and research that examines this issue would be welcome. The notion of an internalized model of treatment, however, is something to which we subscribe. Our hope is that by reading this book, you will see how basic principles of change have been incorporated into cognitive-behavioral practice. We also hope that you will be able to move beyond manualized practice, to a case-conceptualized and flexible use of the cognitive-behavioral approach to treatment.

Toward a Model of Evidence-Based Practice

Can we state with confidence that cognitive-behavioral therapy offers the optimal pathway to evidence-based practice? The evidence is still inconclusive. Certainly, compared to even a decade ago, the field has advanced considerably in this direction. We now have examined a number of manuals in clinical trials and have found them to be superior in outcome to a variety of comparison conditions and therapies. In some cases, however, the data that make definitive statements about absolute or even relative efficacy are wanting. There are also a number of areas in which comparative data between cognitive-behavioral therapy and other treatments suggest roughly equivalent outcomes. Thus, although this approach has accumulated some of the strongest evidence, considerable research is still needed.

Furthermore, most of the data about cognitive-behavioral therapy are based on short-term therapy outcomes, mostly in the context of efficacy research as opposed to effectiveness trials. Effectiveness trials are closer to actual clinical practice, in that such studies typically use less-controlled samples of participants, a broader range of experience in therapists providing the treatment, and are often conducted in clinical settings (Barlow, 2004). Although there is some effectiveness research on cognitive-behavioral therapy, the amount is limited. Clinicians who work in practice settings have a wonderful opportunity to conduct such work (see Wade, Treat, & Stuart, 1998, for an excellent example).

If we accept that cognitive-behavioral therapies have general research support, what are the next steps for development? We need more research, with a broader set of outcomes, so that we can fully evaluate the effects of treatment. We need more studies that evaluate both statistical and clinical significance. We need more long-term studies to be able to understand not only immediate but also long-term effects of treatment. We need cost–benefit and cost-effectiveness research, to be able to build an economic argument about the potential advantages of treatment in absolute terms or in comparison to alternative therapies. Consistent with the APA Presidential Task Force on Evidence-Based Practice (2006), we also agree that research is needed to examine client characteristics that might potentially interact with treatments, leading to better or worse outcomes. If such "aptitude × treatment interactions," as they are called, can be established, these results will help to determine whether certain therapies are preferred for specific client groups. We also need effectiveness research, as we argued earlier, to determine how well these treatments work in clinical settings.

More broadly, we also think the field has to accept that the techniques of both cognitive-behavioral therapy and the therapeutic relationship should be based on evidence. As the field moves toward evidence-based practice and the development of practice guidelines (as opposed to lists of empirically supported therapies), both the context and content of therapy will be recognized as important factors contributing to clinical outcome. As the field moves into a more mature position, we believe that integrating both aspects of evidence into practice will become easier. We have tried to provide such a beginning template in this book.

Chapter 12

❧

Myths about Cognitive-Behavioral Therapy

Client: "I didn't hear about cognitive-behavioral therapy until just recently. I have been on antidepressant medications for 20 years—why wasn't I referred years ago?"

Physician: "I don't think that my patient is appropriate for cognitive-behavioral therapy. She is severely depressed and requires medications. Cognitive-behavioral therapy is primarily an adjunctive therapy for mild to moderately depressed people. I don't think I'll make a referral."

Psychologist: "My client wasn't insightful enough for psychodynamic therapy. He couldn't handle the emotional expression and feedback in interpersonal group therapy. Perhaps he will have more success with cognitive-behavioral therapy, because it is more concrete and intellectual."

These are the types of statements we have heard about cognitive-behavioral therapy. But are they valid? In this chapter we identify common beliefs about cognitive-behavioral therapy, including those that may be held within the field. In doing so, we try to disentangle the myths from the evidence-based ideas.

Our general assumption is that clients want the most effective and efficient treatment for their problems. Clinicians want the same thing for their clients; however, as human beings, we are all prone to various ideas and beliefs—realistic or not—about many different matters. Commonly held distorted thoughts about therapy may be termed *clinical myths*. There are many different kinds of common clinical myths with regard to not only cognitive-behavioral therapy but also other treatments. Cognitive-behavioral therapists, who work in different treatment settings, typically encounter misconceptions about this type of therapy. Clinicians who have been misinformed about cognitive-behavioral therapy may not make referrals, which could create artificial barriers for clients. Distorted beliefs may also color our perceptions of the client's response to treatment. We can interpret lack of progress positively (e.g., "Clients must feel worse before they improve"; "I need to use other methods to help this particular client") or otherwise (e.g., "Cognitive-behavioral therapy doesn't work").

Within our practices, we may spend time educating, other professionals from different backgrounds and students. These educational activities likely include identifying, challenging, and correcting misconceptions about cognitive-behavioral therapy. These cognitive distortions have arisen for a variety of reasons, including the following:

- Lack of information or experience.
- Cognitive biases.
- Misunderstandings based upon misinterpretation of the literature or from training.
- Experience using other types of theoretical approaches.

There has been considerable media coverage of recent cognitive-behavioral treatment. For example, *Time* magazine (January 20, 2003) described cognitive therapy as "quick, practical and goal oriented." There was also a feature article in *Newsweek* called "Think Thin to Get Thin" (March 19, 2007) and an interview in *USA Today* with Robert Leahy (January 1, 2007) on overcoming worries. Although much of the coverage has been very positive, it has not always been comprehensive or balanced. The tendency of the popular media to provide simplified information can lead to a lack of accurate information and add to the potential for clinical myths about cognitive-behavioral therapy.

The professional and scientific communities have also contributed to the development of clinical myths. Most cognitive-behavioral researchers tend to focus on strengths of the treatments rather than limitations. Research scientists may be reluctant to share findings with the press until they achieve certainty, which is obviously a rare and unlikely event. This reluctance makes it difficult for the media to obtain balanced information. For many years there has also been debate regarding empirically supported therapies, including critical commentary (e.g., Bryceland & Stam, 2005). Because the majority of empirically supported therapies are cognitive-behavioral, there is potential for backlash by practitioners of other approaches, leading to further misunderstanding.

One of the central features of cognitive-behavioral therapy is its reliance on empirical data. Consequently, we turn to the current literature to find out what is known about these potentially distorted beliefs, and to provide evidence to challenge them. We have reviewed some of the outcome research in Chapter 11, this volume. We discuss research support for and against these beliefs, debunking some but supporting others that have provide evidence. By necessity, we briefly cover the research and, where possible, refer to other chapters in this book. You may already be prepared to challenge some of the statements that follow. After you read this chapter, we hope you will have sufficient information to counter some of the arguments and statements you may hear in clinical case conferences, meetings, or other discussions. A comprehensive review of all of the literature is beyond the scope of this chapter (see Chapter 11, this volume).

All humans are prone to holding cognitive distortions. On average, cognitive-behavioral therapists may be more likely to overestimate the efficacy of this therapy, whereas those who practice from another orientation may underestimate its efficacy. Given the different types of possible distortions, this first section of this chapter examines the more "negative" distorted beliefs likely to be held by noncognitive-behavioral practitioners, whereas the second section looks at the more "positive" beliefs of practitioners within the field. In both sections we discuss different categories of distorted beliefs, including the therapy itself, the therapy process, and appropriate clients for cognitive-behavioral treatment and training. We also include beliefs about the therapist, where possible, as well as some commonly held beliefs about the empirical findings.

NEGATIVE BELIEFS

A Sampling of Negative Beliefs about Cognitive-Behavioral Therapy

- "Because cognitive-behavioral therapy is 'manualized,' it is rigid, overly structured, and does not take the needs of individual clients into account."
- "Because cognitive-behavioral therapy is primarily a set of tools or strategies for change, these tools can be incorporated into any therapeutic framework."
- "Cognitive-behavioral therapy typically lasts between 6 and 20 sessions."
- "Cognitive-behavioral therapy does not focus on emotions. It is an 'intellectual' therapy, which does not foster 'emotional insight'."

- "Cognitive-behavioral therapy is the same thing as psychoeducation. Consequently, it may be a starting point for therapy, but it does not suffice on its' own."
- "Cognitive-behavioral therapy addresses the symptoms of the problem, but not the problem itself. As such, it does not lead to true change and 'symptom substitution' occurs."
- "Cognitive-behavioral therapy is 'antifeminist,' because it encourages logical thinking, and makes women believe that they are irrational."
- "Cognitive-behavioral therapy rests on a rational and intellectual theory that ignores the social context of problems."

These are only some of the criticisms that have been leveled at cognitive-behavioral therapy. We have heard all of these assertions in interdisciplinary clinical settings, and most of them represent misunderstandings and are easily challenged and corrected. As with most myths, however, there may be a grain of truth in some of them.

Case-formulated cognitive-behavioral therapy (see Chapter 3, this volume) is flexible and idiographic rather than rigid and overly structured. The central feature of the treatment is a cognitive-behavioral conceptual model, from which the strategies or tools logically follow. Consequently, it is clear that if the practitioner does not use a case formulation, then he or she is not using an idiographic form of cognitive-behavioral therapy. If cognitive-behavioral strategies are adopted by clinicians whose primary orientation is another model, then they also are not using cognitive-behavioral therapy. They are likely using their original treatment model to understand the client, or they practice from an "eclectic" or mixed model. For example, practitioners of other models may utilize cognitive-behavioral strategies, such as communication skills training, and incorporate these ideas into their treatment plans. This practice is common; however, the central feature that drives cognitive-behavioral treatment is the underlying theoretical understanding of clients' problems. If therapists do not have a cognitive-behavioral model but use cognitive-behavioral strategies, we argue that they are not doing cognitive-behavioral treatment. This statement is not meant as a criticism, because cognitive-behavioral therapists also may use strategies from other models (e.g., a Gestalt therapy empty-chair technique), yet still remain consistent with their own models.

Whereas individual cognitive-behavioral therapy typically includes clinical case formulation, some practices are more "manualized," and have less flexibility and scope to account for clients' idiosyncracies. These may include group treatments (e.g., social skills training for schizophrenia [Liberman, DeRisi, & Mueser, 1989]) and more structured individual protocols (MAP-3 [Barlow & Craske, 2000]). Although these programs might be characterized as "rigid" by a critic, they have also been shown to have excellent outcomes. Recall as well that limited data suggest that a case-formulated approach increases treatment utility in general, or that it leads to improved outcomes compared to a manualized cognitive-behavioral approach to treatment (see Chapter 3, this volume).

Case formulation leads to planning for individualized treatment, including the amount of treatment or "dosage" required for clients' problems. Although the typical length of treatment in outcome studies is carefully controlled and tends to be between 8 and 10 sessions for most anxiety disorders, and 16 to 20 sessions for major depressive disorder, the number of sessions varies considerably in clinical practice. A number of factors influence the length of treatment in clinical settings. Clients with more severe, or more chronic, problems likely need longer treatments than those with more acute or recent onset (Hamilton & Dobson, 2002). It is also generally assumed that clients with underlying personality disorders and interpersonal problems require longer treatment (e.g., A. T. Beck et al., 2004; Castonguay & Beutler, 2006; Linehan, 1993). Individuals with multiple problems, or comorbidity, are also likely to require more help.

A general assumption is that cognitive-behavioral therapy is of shorter duration than some other models, particularly psychodynamic therapy. Certainly, this practice is common, but limited data from applied settings compare actual numbers of sessions for practitioners from different models. Westen, Novotny, and Thompson-Brenner (2004) found that cognitive-behavioral treatments in practice were substantially longer than what was recommended in treatment manuals. Although they noted that cognitive-behavioral treatments were of shorter duration than some other approaches (e.g., eclectic–integrative or psychodynamic treatments), the average cognitive-behavioral treatment lasted 69 sessions, far longer than the vast majority of treatment manuals would suggest. These results were based upon a survey of a random sample of clinicians in the United States.

There has been some research on the *dose–response* effect, which questions duration of treatment needed to achieve meaningful change for clients. On average, it appears that between 13 and 18 sessions of treatment are needed for symptom alleviation, regardless of the type of treatment or diagnosis of the client. (Hansen, Lambert, & Forman, 2002). Although this conclusion is not specific to cognitive-behavioral treatments, numerous cognitive-behavioral trials were included in this sample. The study also found that, on average, most clients did not receive an adequate "dose" of treatment, because the average number of sessions was less than five.

Many factors that are independent of the client have a determining effect on treatment duration, including the source and amount of available funding, typical practices in the setting to which the client goes for help, and the therapist's beliefs about treatment. For example, the clients who pay directly for services may be more cost-conscious compared to clients with public funding for treatment or a third-party payer. Clients in a private practice setting typically attend fewer sessions than those in a public setting. This observation is confounded, however, by the fact that they may have less severe problems. If clients have the resources to fund their own therapy, they may function better overall and have higher levels of motivation for change. Many insurance companies, employee assistance programs, and HMOs have "caps" on the numbers of sessions or amount of available funding. These limitations force both clients and practitioners to utilize the available time efficiently and effectively. Although these caps exist for practitioners of all orientations, cognitive-behavioral therapists likely find it easier to practice within these session boundaries. Consequently, in practice, cognitive-behavioral therapists must not only be flexible and responsive to clients' needs but also practice within certain parameters.

The belief that cognitive-behavioral therapy is primarily intellectual is partially correct. The initial phase of most treatment plans, either for individual or for group cognitive-behavioral therapy, includes a psychoeducational component. Psychoeducation has been identified as one of the common elements of cognitive-behavioral therapy (see Chapter 5, this volume; Barlow, Allen, & Choate, 2004). The therapist may utilize a verbal presentation, written handouts, and assessment of the client's knowledge. Some therapists include quizzes, such as the Cognitive Therapy Awareness Scale (Wright et al., 2002), to ensure that knowledge is retained. Homework is also one of the common elements in cognitive-behavioral therapy. In most instances, clients are asked to reflect on their thoughts and to collaborate in an evidence-based or empirical process. They are likely to engage in self-monitoring, and to conduct different types of behavioral experiments. Certainly, all of these activities include a focus on an intellectual understanding of clients' problems. It is easy to see how other practitioners, who are accustomed to helping their clients identify and express emotions in therapy, may come away with the notion that the process is overly intellectual.

What critics of cognitive-behavioral therapy tend to misunderstand, or may misrepresent, is that the cognitive methods are not an end in and of themselves, but are used in the *service* of emotional and behavioral change. All types of exposure therapy (see Chapter 6, this volume) require an evocation of emotions in the presence of a feared stimulus for change to occur. The feared stimulus may be intense emotion itself, and a common intervention is emotional regulation. Direct in-session work on automatic thoughts, coupled with emotion, is common (see Chapter 7, this volume). The goal of cognitive-behavioral therapy is not intellectual awareness or insight, but reduced emotional distress, greater self-efficacy, and improved coping skills and activities. Consequently, if the therapy process stops following psychoeducation, then little change is likely. No cognitive-behavioral therapist is likely to promote the use of psychoeducation as a "stand-alone" treatment.

The way that some practitioners confuse psychoeducation and cognitive-behavioral therapy is somewhat baffling. One of us (D. D.) has heard these two terms used interchangeably by many practitioners on many occasions. This misconception not only is held by individual clinicians but also by developers of psychodynamic course curricula. For example, in a local, nationally accredited group psychotherapy training program, the term *psychoeducational* is used to refer to cognitive-behavioral group therapy. Proponents of such misrepresentation need to be challenged and reeducated.

In some settings, clinicians refer to "intellectual" and "emotional" insight, and assume that these types of insight are separable. Some clinicians also assume that emotional insight is related to "true" change, whereas intellectual insight is not. *Insight* is essentially the same thing as understanding or awareness. There are numerous types of understanding and awareness in cognitive-behavioral therapy, such as awareness of behavioral patterns, triggers, emotions, and cognitions, or understanding of the functional links among these factors. All of these types of awareness are encouraged as an early step to help clients change their lives. For true change to occur, and real-life problems to be solved, clients must not only be aware but also behave differently. If clients have different types of *experiences*, either during a session or as a result of a behavioral experiment, then their negative beliefs are likely to shift gradually. Talking *about* doing something does not generally help, whereas *practicing* or *experiencing* the behavior often does. Cognitive-behavioral therapy focuses on *doing* that leads to experiential *insight* and cognitive change.

Symptom substitution is a concept from psychodynamic therapy that has permeated general therapy vernacular (Yates, 1958). Belief in symptom substitution is related to the distorted belief that cognitive-behavioral therapy is superficial and does not tackle underlying causes of the symptoms. According to an intrapsychic psychodynamic model, if the underlying causes are not addressed, then the problem has not been resolved. Consequently, for practitioners of this model, cognitive-behavioral therapy (with the possible exception of schema-focused therapy) does not lead to true change. This distortion is easy to challenge simply by presenting the outcome data (see Chapter 11, this volume). It is increasingly difficult to argue with the positive outcomes of cognitive-behavioral therapy. If symptom substitution occurs and true change does not, then why are the research outcomes so positive? Why do some studies show that relapse rates are lower compared to medications (e.g., Hollon et al., 2006)? Generally, clients have a risk of relapse (see Chapter 9, this volume); however, the same, rather than different, problems tend to recur. There is no evidence for symptom substitution and ample evidence to oppose this viewpoint. Consequently, this myth has no substance at all. Does cognitive-behavioral therapy ignore the sociological context of problems and "blame" the client for thinking incorrectly? Some feminist theorists and clinicians would say "yes," particularly with respect to depression in women (Stoppard, 1989). The feminist model argues that depression in women may be a natural response to aspects of our society that undermine and victimize women. For example, many more women than men are victims of poverty, sexual assault, and sexual harassment, and may have fewer opportunities for advancement in the workplace. A therapeutic model that focuses primarily on "what is wrong with the self" as opposed to "what is wrong with our societal structures" might strengthen a woman's view that she has a distortion in her thinking. To mistakenly help a woman change negative thinking might implicitly encourage her to accept a problem rather than change it. To quote one of these theorists who criticize cognitive-behavioral approaches:

> It becomes clear that the theories are products of, and serve to promote, a male-biased view of mental health. Such theories appear to offer little promise of guiding researchers towards an understanding of depression that has the potential for empowering women to change their situations in ways that will prevent their continuing high rates of depression. (Stoppard, 1989, p. 47)

The truth is that many of our clients live in difficult circumstances, and that more women than men experience problems such as depression, anxiety, and domestic violence (Kessler et al., 2003; Breslau, Davis, Andreski, Peterson, & Schultz 1997; Norris, 1992). More women than men request psychotherapy of all types (McAlpine & Mechanic, 2000; Leong & Zachar, 1999). There are many reasons behind these gender differences; however, it is unfair to argue that cognitive-behavioral therapists ignore extrapsychic factors in the development, maintenance, and treatment of these problems. Cognitive-behavioral therapy, by definition, takes a collaborative stance with all clients. Therapists are expected to consider problems such as poverty or domestic violence when they develop the case formulation.

On the other hand, the cognitive model, just like many other primarily "intrapsychic" models, does focus on processes within clients. By virtue of looking for distorted thoughts, cognitive-behavioral therapists are more likely than other therapists to find them. Furthermore, some clients do react to the terms *distorted, irrational,* or *dysfunctional thinking.* We have heard clients say something to the effect—"Not only do I feel bad, but now I've learned that my thoughts are all wrong." Both of us have had clients refuse to complete a Dysfunctional Thoughts Record due to the title on the form. In one case, the client agreed to use the form when it was relabeled more descriptively as a Negative Thoughts Log, and in another case, the client revised the form and monitored functional thoughts, which led to a focus on increasing functional thoughts rather than reducing dysfunctional ones. We certainly encourage all clinicians and researchers to be sensitive to clients' concerns and feedback. We also believe that it is crucial to consider the contextual development and maintenance of problems for all clients, both men and women.

A Sampling of Negative Beliefs about the Therapy Process and the Therapeutic Relationship

- "Cognitive-behavioral therapists deemphasize the therapeutic relationship."
- "It is not necessary or common to use empathy or social support in cognitive-behavioral therapy."
- "Cognitive-behavioral therapists are not likely to utilize processes such as self-disclosure, and are likely to come across as impersonal and 'technical'."
- "Cognitive-behavioral therapists tend to be distant and do not show their emotions in therapy. They ignore expression of emotions or issues outside the content of the session."
- "It doesn't really matter what kind of therapy I use. All psychotherapies have roughly equivalent results, because the primary change is due to 'nonspecific' factors."
- "The therapy relationship is necessary and sufficient for change, so the techniques do not really matter."

Common myths in this area overlap with those regarding the therapy and the characteristics of cognitive-behavioral therapists. In our clinical experience, popular vernacular suggests that cognitive-behavioral therapy does not emphasize the therapeutic relationship, and that it focuses less on common therapeutic factors such as empathy, support, unconditional positive regard, and therapist self-disclosure. The following discussion explores assumptions regarding the psychotherapeutic process within cognitive-behavioral therapy, some of the research regarding this process, and the relationship between therapy process and outcome.

Cognitive-behavioral therapy has generally attempted to reduce clients' symptoms via cognitive and/or behavior change. Consequently, it tends to focus on the outcome rather than the process of therapy. Put another way, the therapeutic process exists in service of the clinical outcome in cognitive-behavioral therapy. Furthermore, the outcome literature has downplayed the importance of "nonspecific" factors in cognitive-behavioral therapy, in favor of emphasizing the more technical or "theory-specific" factors. Theory has tended to give rise to predictions that techniques such as behavioral activation or cognitive restructuring as opposed to relationship factors lead to change in therapy (DeRubeis & Feeley, 1990; Feeley et al., 1999). This emphasis in the outcome literature has led to a strategy that sometimes encourages nonspecific factors to be controlled rather than directly studied in cognitive-behavioral therapy. These factors include relationship variables (e.g., as the therapeutic alliance, client and therapist expectations for change) and more structural variables (e.g., length and format of treatment). Some of the myths or "distorted cognitions" seen in clinical practice and the theoretical literature indicate that these factors are equivalent across different therapies, or that they are deemphasized or somehow less important in cognitive-behavioral therapy. This deemphasis has led to a myth that the therapeutic alliance and other common factors are less important in cognitive-behavioral therapy than in therapies with other theoretical orientations. A commonly related assumption is that cognitive-behavioral therapy is presented in a technical or more didactic fashion *to the client* rather than *in relationship with the client*.

Nonspecific, multifaceted, and complex factors have alternatively been called placebo, nonspecific, and common factors in the literature. The term *placebo* has been criticized (Lambert, 2005) because, in the medical literature, it means "theoretically inert." In therapies that emphasize the therapeutic relationship as the major change "ingredient," including short-term dynamic psychotherapy, process factors are obviously not "inert." In addition, Castonguay and Grosse Holtforth (2005) strongly argue against the use of the term *nonspecific factors*, because they believe it is misleading. They prefer the term *common factors* over *nonspecific factors* and roughly distinguish between technical and interpersonal factors. Although this separation may apply to cognitive-behavioral therapy, it does not apply to interpersonal therapies, because the technical factors are themselves primarily interpersonal in nature. These authors go on to state that the therapeutic alliance is one of the most clearly defined therapeutic variables, and that more than 1,000 process–outcome findings have been reported in the literature as a whole.

According to Borden (1979), therapeutic alliance has three related components: goals, tasks, and the bond between therapist and client. The stronger the alliance, the more therapist and client agree about the therapy goals and the tasks used to achieve these goals, and the better the quality of the bond between the therapist and client. Consequently, alliance may be viewed as a specific, rather than a nonspecific, variable. The therapeutic alliance is commonly measured by the Working Alliance Inventory (Horvath & Greenberg, 1986). Although the concept originated in the psychoanalytic literature, it has more recently been discussed as a transtheoretical concept (Castonguay et al., 1996).

Virtually all texts that discuss practical applications of cognitive-behavioral therapy emphasize the importance of the therapeutic relationship or alliance in outcome. These include the original text by A. T. Beck et al. (1979), who stated that characteristics such as warmth, accurate empathy, and genuineness are "necessary but not sufficient to produce an optimum therapeutic effect" (p. 45). The importance of the therapeutic collaboration has been emphasized throughout the development of cognitive therapy, and this emphasis on interpersonal process has become more sophisticated over time. Examples include descriptions of how to address problems in the therapeutic relationship with clients who have more complex problems (J. S. Beck, 2005), how to manage resistance in cognitive therapy (Leahy, 2001), as well as how to develop an interpersonal model within cognitive therapy (Safran & Segal, 1990). It is also generally assumed that the greater the degree of interpersonal problems, the greater the emphasis on the psychotherapeutic relationship (e.g., Young et al., 2003).

With the emphasis on efficacy research in cognitive-behavioral therapy, many studies have naturally attempted to control for nonspecific factors (e.g., Heimberg et al., 1990). Fewer studies attempted to define, then study nonspecific variables in the context of cognitive-behavioral therapy. One exception is a study by Castonguay et al. (1996), which used data from a trial of cognitive therapy for depression to delineate the predictive ability of both common and unique factors. The therapeutic alliance was measured by the Working Alliance Inventory (Horvath & Greenberg, 1986). The Castonguay et al. (1996) results indicated that both the alliance and the client's emotional experiencing were related to improved outcome. As noted in Chapter 11, this volume, they found that focusing on distorted cognitions was negatively correlated with outcome.

Karpiak and Smith Benjamin (2004) presented two studies, one of which investigated short-term, individual cognitive-behavioral therapy for generalized anxiety disorder, and the other, time-limited dynamic psychotherapy (TLDP) for generalized anxiety disorder. This study investigated the specific variable of therapist affirmation and its effect on clinical outcomes. The results showed that the effect of immediate reinforcement, through affirming comments by the therapist, was very strong in the cognitive-behavioral therapy group, but less so in the TLDP group. The researchers interpreted the results as a possible reflection of the more focused nature of cognitive-behavioral therapy that, consequently, may encourage the therapist to make more specific affirming comments. They also found that higher levels of affirmation of maladaptive patient content corresponded with poorer outcomes at 12-month follow-up.

Watson and Geller (2005) studied the association among client's ratings of relationship conditions, outcome, and working alliance in both cognitive-behavioral therapy and process–experiential therapy. They found that clients' ratings of relationship conditions were predictive of outcome for both therapies. Therapists who were perceived by their clients as using empathy, congruence, and acceptance were also better able to form working alliances. The authors of this study suggested that competent therapists must be perceived as empathic, accepting, nonjudgmental, and congruent to deliver effective services, regardless of the type of therapy being delivered.

Based on an extensive review of the research results on therapist and client interpersonal behavior in cognitive-behavioral therapy, Keijsers et al. (2000) concluded that cognitive-behavioral therapists utilize relationship skills at least as much as do therapists from other theoretical orientations. For example, there appears to be no significant difference in the frequency of therapist self-disclosure between insight-oriented therapy and cognitive-behavioral therapy, as well as no association between self-disclosure and outcome (Keijsers et al., 2000). Furthermore, "the therapeutic relationship in CBT [cognitive-behavioral therapy] is characterized by a more active and directive stance on the part of therapists and higher levels of emotional support than are found in insight-oriented psychotherapies" (p. 285). They also concluded that therapeutic alliance is reliably associated with outcome across a number of studies. There appears to be a bias in the literature, however. Clients who are clearly dissatisfied with their therapists and have poor working alliances do not necessarily respond poorly, but they terminate early, dropping out of therapy. Therefore, the authors suggest that (negative) relationship factors may be a better predictor of dropout than of outcome. Most clients who complete therapy and consequent outcome data are satisfied with their therapists and have reasonably good therapeutic alliances.

Lohr, Olatumji, Parker, and DeMaio (2005) also argue against the long-held notion of nonspecific factors and define *intentional specific treatment* as characteristic features of the therapy that are both necessary and sufficient for change. They also suggest that therapies may work for reasons other than the hypothesized ones. They describe an *intentional treatment* as both one that works and works for the reasons predicted, according to the underlying theory. Many treatments may be effective, but because they may be used and described based on erroneous beliefs and intentions, they risk achieving the status of myth rather than that of evidence-based treatment. The authors provide the example of eye movement desensitization and reprocessing, which may be effective because of its use of exposure rather than use of eye movements or information reprocessing. They argue that this argument can also be applied to cognitive therapy for depression, because the behavioral activation component may be the active ingredient, contrary to the typical belief that it is the cognitive interventions that lead to change (Jacobson et al., 1996).

DeRubeis, Brotman, et al. (2005) argue for examination of the non-equivalence of different types of psychotherapies. It has been assumed that when two different treatments have equivalent outcomes, the difference is the result of "nonspecific" factors. They argue, in contrast, that the change may be the result of *different* specific factors. They discuss the outcome results of therapeutic alliance and argue that the role of the therapeutic alliance has been inconsistent, particularly in cognitive-behavioral therapy. They cite Tang and DeRubeis's (1999) work on "sudden gains," which implies that the therapeutic relationship is improved *after* good clinical outcome, rather than before. In that research, Tang and DeRubeis found that the alliance quality was reliably higher in the session following, rather than the preceding one, a sudden therapy gain.

Two studies have shown that specific, theory-guided techniques measured early in treatment predict subsequently reduction in depressive symptoms (DeRubeis & Feeley, 1990; Feeley et al., 1999). These studies imply that improved relationship quality is a consequence of positive outcomes in treatment, so it is likely to be found in cognitive-behavioral therapy but may not be predictive of outcome. Relatedly, Klein et al. (2003) found a small, but significant alliance–outcome relationship. Early alliance predicted improvement over the course of treatment, but early improvement did not predict subsequent alliance. Regardless, they state that correlation between outcome and alliance does not imply causation. DeRubeis et al.'s main point is that it is "a mistake for the field to elevate the nonspecific factors of psychotherapies at the expense of specific therapeutic techniques" (2005, p. 180).

In a commentary on the preceding article, Craighead, Sheets, Bjornsson, and Arnarson (2005) stated that the argument of specific versus nonspecific, as demonstrated in the case of therapeutic alliance, is a good example of A. T. Beck's notion of dichotomous thinking. "Establishing superiority is not the same as establishing specificity" (p. 190). They pointed out that a strong therapeutic alliance is an essential ingredient in all psychotherapies, including cognitive-behavioral therapy, and that what are labeled as nonspecific and specific variables are inextricably linked. For example, scales measuring competence typically assess non-specific factors. The Cognitive Therapy Scale (see Appendix A), which has been used in many treatment outcome studies, has six items on general therapeutic skills and five items on more theory-specific skills (Young & Beck, 1980). Consequently, to be considered competent in cognitive therapy, the therapist, by definition, must be rated as having good general therapy skills include understanding and empathy, warmth, genuineness, and responsiveness to the client's verbal and nonverbal feedback.

Goldfried et al. (2003) argued that self-disclosure is an effective tool for strengthening the alliance and facilitating change in cognitive-behavioral therapy. There appears to be no significant difference in the frequency of therapist self-disclosure between insight-oriented and cognitive-behavioral therapy. They also noted, importantly, that there is no strong association between self-disclosure and outcome. Contrary to some myths, there do not appear to be strong data suggesting that cognitive-behavioral therapists are cold or perfunctory in the way they conduct therapy (Keijsers et al., 2000).

Consequently, it seem clear from these reviews and studies, as well as many clinical texts, that cognitive-behavioral therapists are support-ive and empathic, and focus on developing a positive therapeutic alli-ance, similar to therapists from other theoretical orientations. What is less clear is the proportion of outcome that can be attributed to these variables. It is extremely difficult, if not impossible, to separate these variables from each other and from more technical aspects of treat-ment. It may be that, as some of these studies suggest, the positive clinical outcomes in cognitive-behavioral therapy enhance the positive treatment relationships that are observed. To assert that cognitive-behavioral therapy deemphasizes or disregards the therapeutic rela-tionship is clearly incorrect.

A Sampling of Negative Beliefs Regarding the Client and Predictors of Outcome

- "Cognitive-behavioral therapy is most appropriate for clients who are not 'psychologically minded' or insightful."
- "Clients who benefit the most from cognitive-behavioral therapy are those who require structure, teaching, and direct guidance."
- "Cognitive-behavioral therapy is most appropriate for clients who are quite bright and intellectual, because these clients are used to

reading materials and are able to reflect on their own thought processes."
- "Cognitive-behavioral therapy is most appropriate for clients with mild problems. Clients with serious problems require medication to control their symptoms."
- "Cognitive-behavioral therapy may be useful for mild problems, but only as an adjunctive therapy for 'real' clinical problems."
- "Cognitive-behavioral therapy works best with motivated clients who are willing to do homework outside of the sessions."
- "Most research findings do not apply to my clients. My clients are more complex, more distressed, or more acutely disordered than most clients."

If referral sources have inaccurate information about the types of clients who may benefit from cognitive-behavioral therapy, then it is quite likely that they will make inappropriate referrals. Clients who might benefit may not be referred or, conversely, clients who are not likely to benefit may be referred. It is common for referral sources to make assumptions about the types of clients who may be appropriate for this type of treatment. Unfortunately, these assumptions can have an impact on clients' ability to access needed treatments. For example, as a beginning practitioner in a psychiatric day program setting, one of us (D. D.) frequently received referrals of clients who had numerous past treatment failures. At other times, clients who were perceived by their physicians as not being psychologically minded were referred for treatment, because they were deemed "incapable" of benefiting from insight-oriented therapies. The belief in the suitability of cognitive-behavioral therapy for clients judged to be less insight-focused, more concrete in their thinking, and possibly less intelligent comes from the notion that the demands on the client are less than those for other treatments, because cognitive-behavioral therapy tends to be more structured and directive than some other types of therapy. It is likely that the former belief may affect the decision to refer a client to insight-oriented therapy instead of cognitive-behavioral therapy, whereas the latter belief may affect a decision to utilize cognitive-behavioral therapy or medication treatment, because these models are thought to place lower demands upon the client.

Ironically, we have also seen evidence for the opposite belief— that cognitive-behavioral therapy is most appropriate for bright and psychologically minded clients, because they may be accustomed to educational materials, homework, and reflecting on their own thought processes.

Given these opposing, and possibly dysfunctional, beliefs about cognitive-behavioral therapy on the part of referral sources, what does the evidence indicate about non-symptom-based predictors of outcome? Predictors may include demographic factors (gender, age, socioeconomic status, ethnicity), psychological factors (intelligence, "psychological mindedness," motivation to change), communication factors (ability to form a relationship with the therapist, openness), and therapy-related factors (compliance, expectations, "readiness" for change).

Keijsers et al. (2000) completed an extensive review of the research literature exploring the effect of interpersonal behaviors of the client, as well as the therapist, on the outcome in cognitive-behavioral therapy. They found that clients tend to communicate similarly across different types of therapy, and that there is a positive relationship between clients' degree of openness and therapy outcome. No data were available on the effect of self-exploration and insight on outcomes, possibly because these factors tend not to be emphasized as common variables in cognitive-behavioral therapy. Somewhat surprisingly, empirical findings related to the importance of client motivation and participation in homework were disappointing.

A client's attitude toward therapy is an important variable when considering therapy dropout and outcome. Therapy attitudes include the degree of client motivation, as well as expectations about changes in therapy. These attitudes may have a greater impact in short-term, goal-oriented psychotherapies such as cognitive-behavioral therapy, because the time constraints require that therapy proceed quickly and in a goal-oriented fashion (Koss & Shiang, 1994). One of the clearest results from the Keijsers et al. (2000) study was the strong relationship between low motivation and dropout. Simply put, clients who are less motivated stop coming to treatment. Thus, attitude and relationship factors may be better predictors of early treatment termination than of outcome. As noted earlier (Tang & DeRubeis, 1999), early improvement may lead to better alliance, which may in turn lead to higher motivation and adherence to treatment.

Furthermore, a number of studies have found that clients who agree with the cognitive-behavioral treatment rationale are more likely to have successful outcomes compared to clients who do not "buy into" the rationale (Addis & Jacobson, 2000). For example, Fennell and Teasdale (1987) provided to clients at the intake for therapy an explanatory pamphlet about cognitive-behavioral therapy for depression. Their results showed that clients who accepted this pamphlet changed more rapidly during the first four sessions of treatment compared to clients who did not accept the pamphlet. In addition, the same clients had better outcomes at the treatment follow-up. Addis and Jacobson (1996) provided their clients with a rationale for the causes and treatment of depression, using the same pamphlet used by Fennell and Teasdale (1987). The results again indicated that clients who perceived the treatment to be helpful had better outcomes. Using a measure of "patient willingness" to use positive coping strategies, Burns and Nolen-Hoeksema (1991) found that willingness was related to better outcomes in cognitive-behavioral therapy for depression. Finally, Keijsers, Hoogduin, and Schaap (1994) found that motivation was significantly related to outcome in the behavioral treatment of obsessive–compulsive disorder.

In a review of pretreatment patient predictors of outcome for cognitive therapy of depression, Hamilton and Dobson (2002) found that a number of symptom variables (e.g., severity and chronicity of symptoms) were associated with poorer outcomes. There has been limited research, however, assessing the effects of demographic factors on outcome in cognitive-behavioral therapy. Hamilton and Dobson were only able to demonstrate that married clients have better outcomes than unmarried individuals, which may well be related to better social skills, or increased social support for clients in marital relationships, rather than an effect of marriage per se.

Castonguay and Beutler (2006) have identified empirically based principles of therapeutic change that cut across different psychotherapy models. These principles identify both client and therapist characteristics, relational conditions, therapist behaviors, and the types of interventions that best lead to change. These authors state that principles are more general than theory driven techniques, and more specific than theoretical formulations. They note in their extensive review of the current psychotherapy literature across the more common clinical problems (dysphoric disorders, anxiety disorders, personality disorders, and substance use disorders) that some general conclusions regarding client characteristics and therapy outcomes may be drawn. Clients with high levels of impairment, as well as Axis II diagnoses, benefit less from all types of psychotherapy than do clients without these characteristics. Clients with these characteristics are also likely to require longer treatment. Furthermore, clients with financial and/or occupational problems may benefit less than people without these concerns. Increased age is also a negative predictor of response. Matching client–therapist backgrounds (e.g., ethnicity) improves treatment outcome somewhat; however, clients from underserved ethnic or racial backgrounds do not improve as much from typical psychotherapeutic interventions as do clients from the majority population.

A Sampling of Negative Beliefs about Training and Cognitive-Behavioral Therapy

- "Cognitive-behavioral therapy is a straightforward approach that can be learned by anybody with a minimal amount of training and supervision. Going to a few workshops or reading several books should suffice."
- "Paraprofessionals trained to use cognitive-behavioral therapy are just as effective as highly trained therapists."

Most therapists believe that their form of therapy requires considerable skill, training, and experience to achieve positive outcomes. Graduate and residency programs in mental health often requires years of background and focused training experience, often under intensive supervision. There are, however, relatively few solid data that directly addresses the debate over whether experience and professional training make a difference in client outcome. Furthermore, what research does exist often fails to favor more highly trained therapists. Therapists with and without training in specific therapeutic techniques achieve positive client outcomes (Lambert, 2005).

There is some evidence that is worthy of attention. Bright et al. (1999) investigated the efficacy of professional versus paraprofessional therapists' provision of group cognitive-behavioral therapy and mutual support for clients with depression. Therapists were classified according to their level of education. Of note, the professional therapists were actually students in doctoral clinical and counseling psychology, with an average of 4 years' postsecondary supervised psychotherapy training. The paraprofessional therapists were not students, nor did they have advanced training in psychology. In this trial, clients in the cognitive-behavioral therapy group led by the professionally trained therapists were less depressed at posttreatment than clients in the group led by the para-professionals. The results indicated that a comparable number of clients were classified as nondepressed following treatment within the mutual support groups. Consequently, professional and educational training was related to outcome, but only in the cognitive-behavioral therapy condition. These results may be confounded, however, because about half of the paraprofessionals had previous experience in leading groups, whereas the students did not. The paraprofessionals may have been more effective than the professionals at leading mutual support groups, due to their prior experience. Successful delivery of cognitive-behavioral therapy with groups may require more skill and experience than therapy with individuals.

Huppert et al. (2001) found that clients treated by therapists with more general psychotherapy experience showed greater improvement in cognitive-behavioral therapy for panic disorder than clients treated by therapists without such experience. However, *experience* was related more to treatment outcome when it was defined as years of experience practicing psychotherapy in general, rather than specific years of practicing cognitive-behavioral therapy. Haby et al. (2006) found that cognitive-behavioral therapy provided by psychologists had better outcomes than that provided by therapists. Further details about training were not provided.

Burns and Nolen-Hoeksema (1992) examined the relationship between therapists' years of experience and outcome in cognitive-behavioral therapy for depression. They provided controls for nonspecific factors, including therapeutic alliance and therapist empathy, compliance with homework, and client income. Similar to the Bright et al. (1999) trial, this study supported the need for experienced therapists in the delivery of cognitive-behavioral therapy. Results indicated that the clients of novice therapists improved significantly less than did clients of more experienced therapists. Specifically, scores on the BDI at posttreatment for clients treated by more senior therapists were significantly lower than scores of clients treated by the novice therapists.

POSITIVE (BUT DISTORTED) BELIEFS

We hope that some of the negative beliefs listed at the beginning of this chapter about cognitive-behavioral therapy have been challenged by our discussion and literature review. Our goal is to provide accurate information, as opposed to an unrealistic promotion of cognitive-behavioral therapy. By doing so, we likely have already challenged some of the more likely myths about cognitive-behavioral therapists. Any type of approach that is unquestioned or zealously advocated for use across most problems runs the risk of either being, or being seen to be, a "snake oil" cure or a "one-size-fits-all" solution that does few clients much good! Although there is much to promote about cognitive-behavioral therapy, there are also reasons to be humble and to appreciate other types of effective interventions.

A Sampling of Positive Beliefs about Cognitive-Behavioral Therapy, Its Empirical Support, and Training

- "Cognitive-behavioral therapy is applicable to almost any problem."
- "Most problems are resolved within 12–20 sessions."

- "All aspects of cognitive-behavioral therapy are supported by empirical data. Because I practice cognitive-behavioral therapy, my work is empirically supported."
- "Because cognitive-behavioral therapy works, it is the client's fault if he or she does not improve."
- "Cognitive-behavioral therapy is difficult to learn for people without extensive training and supervision. The field should control its use."

These and other statements we have made in this chapter will continue to be subjected to healthy debate. Although the results of many outcome trials demonstrate the efficacy of cognitive behavioral therapy (see Chapter 11, this volume), outcome differences among the different types of psychological treatments are typically much less than when the treatment is compared to placebo or to waiting-list control. Generally, we may know that "packages" of treatment are effective. We also may know some of the components of the treatments that are relatively effective; however, much less is known about the effectiveness of typical clinical practice and applications. For more information regarding these arguments, see Chapter 11, this volume.

According to Castonguay and Beutler (2006), estimates of the differences among treatments account for no more than 10% of the variability in client change. Many critics of technique-focused therapies argue that the therapeutic relationship is the key ingredient of change; however, Castonguay and Beutler (2006) state that the therapeutic alliance accounts for a similar amount of change. Other therapist and relationship factors separately likely account for even less than 10% of the change. Obviously, we do not fully understand a great deal about the change process and the interaction between the differing variables.

According to our arguments in this and other chapters in this text, many problems cannot be resolved in a short period of time. Although symptom reduction may occur and new skills may be learned, chronic problems, interpersonal issues, and multiple concerns are likely to take longer to resolve when they exist, and longer therapy is recommended for clients with such problems. If the treatment does not work, other treatment options, or a new conceptualization, likely should be considered. Cognitive-behavioral therapy is not suitable for all problems, and nonpsychotherapy options should be kept in mind as part of the treatment options that are considered, including occupational therapy for work-related problems), pastoral counseling for existential or spiritual problems, grief counseling for loss, and community support or self-help groups. As therapists, we may lose sight of basic problems, such as lack of adequate housing or financial resources. If a client requires

basic assistance, then resources such as housing, financial aid, or transportation services are necessary prior to any type of psychotherapy. As
cognitive-behavioral therapists, it is crucial that we continue to question
the work we do, with respect both to individual clients and to the field
as a whole.

Chapter 13

Starting and Maintaining a Cognitive-Behavioral Practice

"I have completed training and am eager to have a primarily cognitive-behavioral practice, as well as to work within a scientist-practitioner model. I have learned how to complete assessments and provide therapy, but how do I start? What do I do next? How can I promote my practice?" In this final chapter, we review the practical aspects for starting a cognitive-behavioral practice, whether in a health care or hospital setting or in private practice. Many different types of settings exist. However, many of the practical aspects are the same or may be easily modified for different systems. Because of you may many desire further training and supervision, we also review ways to further your skills.

In this chapter, we raise a series of questions to consider when obtaining and accepting referrals for your practice. We assume that you have been trained in the basic elements of professional practice and are aware of your jurisdiction's requirements for licensing, advertising, professional ethics, and behavior. We review issues that are unique to cognitive-behavioral therapy and take the viewpoint that some existing systems can be modified to enhance your cognitive-behavioral practice. We do not review all of the practical matters in arranging for an assessment or beginning treatment, such as initial contacts with potential clients, preparations for the visit, fee setting, introductions, or professional and ethical behavior. These issues are not unique to cognitive-behavioral therapy, but are part of any good professional clinical practice. This chapter begins with a discussion of some methods to obtain and accept referrals, moves on to review tips for communicating what you do, then on to services that may increase your referral base. Finally, we discuss ways to assess your competence, as well as methods to obtain further training and supervision.

OBTAINING AND ACCEPTING REFERRALS

Where do referrals come from, and how can you increase the referral base for your practice? To obtain and accept referrals, it is important to keep in mind the setting in which you work, the training you have received, the clientele and types of problems you work with competently, and any limitations you need to place upon your practice. Asking yourself some key questions will help to focus your efforts on building a manageable practice that fits your skills and needs.

What Is Your Practice Setting, and What Is Your Role in It?

There are often practical limits to services that clinicians can provide, depending on the setting within which they practice. Some of the common settings include individual private practice, group practices, and health care settings, such as a mental health clinic or hospital, or HMOs. Other settings include college- or university-based clinics, or specialized research facilities. The sources of payment include direct fee for service and third-party payments (e.g., insurance or employee assistance plans or salaries). The payment schemes and proportions for public versus private payments vary tremendously from country to country; consequently, they are not be reviewed in this chapter.

The greatest flexibility for practitioners exists within direct fee-for-service settings, because clinicians can generally dictate their own terms of work. There are some downsides of private practice. Because earnings are based on billable time, which depends directly on seeing clients, you might feel the push to see as many clients as possible. This understandable push to earn an income, and the market forces related to service demand, may make it difficult to establish particular areas of expertise. Some of the techniques that have excellent empirical support, such as *in vivo* exposure therapy, may not be cost-effective for the clinician due to the large amounts of time involved or the high cost to the client for the time expenditure required. Some types of interventions, such as cognitive-behavioral group therapy, tend to be more difficult to establish in private practice because of the large numbers of referrals required to begin a group. Developing an exclusively cognitive-behavioral practice may be possible in some larger settings but impractical in others, where there may be demands for diagnostic or other types of assessments, or a broader range of interventions.

If you are an employee within a private practice or for-profit agency, you may have limited options to set your own agenda or choose your own clientele. Rather, clients may be directly assigned to you by a program manager, or you may be expected to take clients on a "first come, first served" basis. If you work within a specialty clinic, you may have limited options in terms of the problem areas you treat but greater options for innovation and research. If you work in a publicly funded program, you may also have few options other than to see clients as they are referred to you. Furthermore, some settings do not provide cognitive-behavioral therapy as a specialty service, but offer this type of therapy as part of an array of services to clients. Your role may be to provide cognitive-behavioral therapy only, or to provide it as only part of what you do.

Although practice settings are often part of a greater system, such as hospitals, managed care companies, or larger regional health care systems, there typically is room for innovation with respect your role within that setting. Consider how you may influence and expand your role as a cognitive-behavioral therapist. Often these influences include building upon your areas of expertise, special interests, and competence. In our experience, the increasing public demand for cognitive-behavioral therapies and the evidence base for the efficacy of these treatments can be used to expand these activities in a range of health service and other practice settings. The possibility for marketing your work exists in all settings, despite differences in the way services are funded.

What Are Your Areas of Expertise and Interest?

Consider the possibilities and limitations of your clinical practice, and your areas of expertise and interest. Are your interests and areas of expertise related to a diagnostic problem, a type of intervention, or a variation on current practices? How do you want to grow and develop in the future? Areas of expertise typically begin with your academic research and supervised training. But, as you look to the future, do you plan to be a "generalist" or a "specialist"? Is a range of choices possible within your setting? Making decisions about your areas of expertise, then working within those limits, helps to focus the work you do. This focus helps you to define your expertise further and cultivate certain referrals to your practice, allowing you to be more in charge of your own work. Defining your work yourself, as opposed to being reactive to forces outside of your control, no doubt lead to increased work satisfaction. Almost all work settings have some flexibility, even though it may not be immediately obvious to you. See discussions with your supervisor or manager, or speaking up in case consultation meetings, as opportunities to practice assertive communication skills.

What Are Your Limits of Competence?

In addition to your specialty area, you may be more or less competent in other areas. It is important to be clear in your own mind regarding your limits of competence. Indeed, it is likely that your professional code of ethics dictates self-knowledge of competence, then working within that level of expertise. Limits of competence may be related to providing services for specific populations and certain problems (e.g., adolescents with eating disorders, adults with comorbid Axis I disorders and medical problems, distressed couples), or they may relate to specific interventions (dialectical behavior therapy, interoceptive exposure). Likewise, it is important to be clear about your limits of competence and not accept referrals of members of populations or problems for which you have not had appropriate training or supervision. For new practitioners, it may be tempting to accept a wide array of referrals. However, this practice is not wise and may in the worst case lead to incompetent and irresponsible practice.

There is a growing literature on the assessment of competence in cognitive-behavioral therapy (McGlinchey & Dobson, 2003). Although many therapists see competence as a learned skill or proficiency that becomes a more or less enduring feature of their work, it is also important to realize that competence may vary over time. It is only responsible practice to place temporary limits on your practice for personal reasons, such as your own mental health, addictions, and family or medical problems. Obtain further training, supervision, or treatment, as appropriate, if you need to change your practice or reduce the limits of your competence. If you have been trained in psychotherapy, but not specifically cognitive-behavioral interventions, we encourage you to obtain supervised training, in addition to reading and attending workshops.

What Are the Exclusion Criteria for Your Setting?

Many clinics, practices, and clinicians have preferred types of clients, whom they often advertised for in the media and other outlets. Some practices and clinics also have exclusion criteria for referrals. These are most common in specialty clinics or research settings in which it is important to reduce variability in research samples to test certain hypotheses. Most psychotherapy research that involves randomized clinical trials has employed numerous exclusion criteria. For example, Table 13.1 lists

TABLE 13.1. Exclusion Criteria in Psychotherapy Outcome Trials for Major Depressive Disorder

Example 1: DeRubeis, Hollon, et al. (2005)

1. History of bipolar disorder.
2. Substance abuse or dependence judged to require treatment.
3. Current or past psychosis.
4. Another DSM-IV Axis I disorder judged to require treatment in preference to depression.
5. Axis II diagnosis of antisocial, borderline, or schizotypal personality disorder.
6. Suicide risk requiring immediate hospitalization.
7. Medical condition that contraindicates study medications.
8. Nonresponse to an adequate trial of antidepressant in the preceding year.

Example 2: Dimidjian et al. (2006)

1. Lifetime diagnosis of psychosis or bipolar disorder, organic brain syndrome, or mental retardation.
2. Substantial and imminent suicide risk.
3. Current or primary diagnosis of alcohol or drug abuse or dependence, or a positive toxicology screen.
4. Primary diagnosis of panic disorder, obsessive–compulsive disorder, psychogenic pain disorder, anorexia, or bulimia.
5. Presence of antisocial, borderline, or schizotypal personality disorder.
6. Nonresponse to an adequate trial of either cognitive therapy or antidepressant within preceding year.

exclusion criteria for two recent studies comparing psychological and medical therapies for major depressive disorder.

In many settings, it is not practical or reasonable to exclude from therapy the clients who present with many of the exclusion criteria in Table 13.1. It is important to note that if you are using these types of research studies to justify certain treatment practices, but are not using the same inclusion and exclusion criteria that existed in the original research, then your research results may or may not translate into your practice. For example, you may find that if you do not exclude certain types of clients who were excluded in the research, then you may need to modify your interventions when clients present with multiple problems.

On the other hand, exclusion criteria can potentially be used to advantage in some practice settings. The criteria might include not accepting referrals when substance abuse or dependence is a primary problem, when an Axis II diagnosis has been documented, or when communication is likely to be an issue (e.g., literacy problems, or when the client's English is not sufficiently developed to conduct therapy). In addition, cognitive-behavioral interventions are likely to have lower success rates when applied to clients with multiple problems. At best, the outcomes are much more difficult to predict. If other interventions are available and have known empirical support, such clients can be referred to another service. Possible exclusion criteria in an outpatient mental health clinic may include a primary problem of substance abuse, suicide risk or another crisis sufficient to warrant admission to hospital, a primary medical problem that would be likely to interfere with the ability to attend sessions, and/or inability to communicate in the languages offered in the clinic (unless translation services exist). Other services that exist in your community may be more appropriate for these clients (e.g., inpatient psychiatric services, addiction programs). It is generally good practice to keep lists of other resources available, so that you are able to offer suggestions to those who contact you or the clinic looking for services but do not meet criteria for the program. It can be tempting to offer services to clients with the highest needs or the most problems, but to do so likely ensures more treatment failures for a new practitioner. Although it may be difficult for clients with multiple problems to find help, solving this problem is beyond the scope of your practice. There are likely to be referrals of clients with multiple problems, for whom no available option is preferable to cognitive-behavioral therapy. This treatment may be helpful for these clients. However, referral to an experienced provider may be the best choice.

COMMUNICATING SPECIALTIES, LIMITS, AND EXCLUSION CRITERIA TO POTENTIAL CLIENTS

Once you have identified your own areas of expertise, any limits to competence, and your role within your practice setting, it is important to communicate this self-knowledge to your "marketplace." It is vital that you communicate your abilities, as well as your personal restrictions of practice, confidently to your clientele. Communication may include written documentation (e.g., clinic pamphlets, websites), providing such information during initial telephone contact, or informing clients what you can and cannot do at the time of the first visit.

Communicate your competencies to referral sources (e.g., physicians, insurance companies, other practitioners and clinics). Building a sound cognitive-behavioral practice includes developing excellent communication skills and clearly discussing the services you do and do not provide to your clients. Our perspective is that your practice will grow more, and in a more positive direction, if you focus efforts on your areas of success rather than trying to be all things to all people, and likely having more treatment failures.

Selecting Initial Clients

If possible, select some early clients with whom you are likely to demonstrate efficacy and the clinical utility of your services. The acceptance of referrals of clients with clear problems, and for whom you will be able to provide effective services, is one of the best ways to communicate expertise to your referral sources or the team within which you work. Your job role may or may not make this selection feasible, because some clinics assign clients in the order within which they are referred or have other practices that give minimal control to the clinician. It is often possible, however, to have an influence or to be assertive in stating your preference or communicating your clinical expertise to those with decision-making power. Do not hesitate to use the behavioral communication skills you have learned (see Chapter 6, this volume)!

New practitioners in agencies often receive difficult referrals, because the referral source may hope that new and improved options exist for complex issues and/or long-term problems. These referrals often indicate past treatment failures, and it can be flattering to receive such referrals expressing confidence in your abilities. You may even have an automatic thought, such as "Cognitive-behavioral therapy is likely to help this client's problem(s) where past treatments have not." Be aware that this thought is not necessarily accurate. Indeed, past treatment failure is likely a good predictor of future treatment failure. It can be very helpful for you and your beginning practice to be strict about following inclusion and exclusion criteria in the initial part of setting up a practice and developing your caseload. As the practice builds, you may be more able to be liberal and flexible in your selection criteria. This is not to say that these clients do not have important needs, or that services to help them do not exist. As you learn about services offered within your community, you can provide referral options for those clients you do not accept into your practice.

Establishing a Caseload

How many clients should you see in an average week? What proportion of direct service compared to indirect service should you establish? It is extremely important to have a balanced work week with a variety of different types of activities: individual cognitive-behavioral sessions, group treatments, outside office exposure sessions, giving or receiving supervision and consultation, meetings, reading, and research projects. Leave yourself time for planning, completing clinical records, and writing reports. Most new practitioners require considerable time for reporting requirements. Many services have databases or billing systems that the therapist needs to complete. Administrative work also takes time, depending on your role. Checking e-mail messages, returning telephone calls, and dealing with client emergencies are also ways in which clinicians use their time. Last, but certainly not less important, are personal needs, such as peer support, engaging with your colleagues, and taking breaks. When determining the number of clients you should see on average, include all of these time expenditures in the equation. Most practitioners need to leave 30–60% of their time available for indirect service, depending on other responsibilities and roles. Of course, in a direct fee-for-service setting, the therapist is not paid for indirect service time, so income is significantly affected. When you calculate your hourly rate, be sure to include all of these factors. If the hours in the week seem to disappear quickly, be sure to spend a week or two using a self-monitoring record to keep track of the ways you spend your time. You can then modify your schedule as needed.

Just as important as the number of clients you see per week is the balance of your caseload. Some services are likely to have high rates of "no shows" or cancellations. For example, clients seen in outpatient addictions programs may be less prone to follow through with treatment. Clients who have high anxiety about leaving their homes or who lack resources, such as transportation, may struggle to attend sessions. Ask your colleagues about attendance rates in your workplace, if you are new to the service. Some clinicians overbook their weekly sessions, somewhat like the airlines. Cautiously used, this approach can prevent down time, but can also lead to harried schedules if all clients attend. You can also take steps to increase attendance and improve adherence (see Chapter 10, this volume), sometimes simply through confirmation calls to your clients.

Another aspect of caseload balance includes the proportion of challenging clients you have, or those who are prone to crises. Some clients require more therapist time than others, not only because of direct needs, such as more sessions, telephone calls, and consultation, but also because of preparation, reporting, and sometimes worry. Although it is ideal to leave your thoughts about a client at work, this degree of personal control is difficult in practice. Maintain self-awareness and be realistic about how many challenging clients you can manage. In addition, the type of problem that is difficult for one clinician may not be for another. Keeping your own Thought Records can help you to determine the kinds of predictions or thoughts you have about clients. These thoughts can guide you to establish your caseload. One of us (D. D.) has also learned not to schedule challenging clients (e.g., those who might require hospital admission or other services) late in the day or on Friday afternoon, when colleagues have gone or it is difficult to find support. If you leave work with the problem unresolved, you are also more likely to think about it over the weekend. Similarly, in scheduling clients, consider your own needs for balance and variety, as well as your client's scheduling requirements.

COMMUNICATING TO YOUR "MARKETPLACE"

Once you have clarified your areas of expertise, and that your areas of practice are within the scope of the setting in which you work, who comprises your "market", or to whom you should be communicating about your services, will become clear. The market may vary—from the community as a whole to smaller segments of that community. If your workplace requires physician referrals, then the "market" is the group of physicians that is likely to request cognitive-behavioral therapy for their patients. If direct referrals from potential clients are typical, then your challenge is to get your message out, so that potential "buyers" know that your practice exists and is a good option for them. Your services have a "market" in all settings, whether private or publicly funded.

Being clear about your potential "buyers" helps you to clarify the message you develop to advertise your services. If you work in a hospital or mental health clinic setting, where marketing and "advertising" is not an issue, then communication about your services is still important. This communication might include a range of activities, including the development of informational handouts or brochures, doing inservice training for staff, or presenting at local or other types of conferences. Other communication activities may include placing an advertisement in the Yellow Pages of the telephone book, putting notices in local newsletters, or releasing public service announcements. All these activities help to establish not only your specific services but also the relevance of cognitive-behavioral therapy in general. There is likely to be regional variation in the effectiveness of different strategies. Be sure to talk to your colleagues to obtain suggestions about what has worked best for them. Next we describe effective strategies for increasing the scope and size of your cognitive-behavioral practice.

WAYS TO INCREASE YOUR
COGNITIVE-BEHAVIORAL PRACTICE

Doing effective work is the most best way to increase your practice in the long run; however, beginning cognitive-behavioral therapists do not have past client successes on which to depend. A common way to promote any clinical practice is to advertise in the Yellow Pages, or to place notices in newsletters or community newspapers. These strategies will no doubt increase the exposure of your services and, we hope, lead to referrals. You need to be clear about what you do and do not do, when referrals from these sources contact you. Some members of the public have difficulty discriminating among different types of mental health professionals, let alone differentiating between cognitive-behavioral therapy and other treatment models, so referrals from these sources will likely need a moderate amount of education and assessment to ensure that you are the appropriate therapist for them.

Conduct a local workshop, or a continuing education course, for the general public. These educational activities can be offered in a number of different venues, including continuing education programs through colleges, universities, or boards of education. These types of institutions typically offer programs several times per year, which can be an excellent way to create some recognition locally, as well as to highlight cognitive-behavioral therapy in general. In our community, two psychologists offer a mindfulness-based stress reduction course through the continuing education program at the local university twice per year. The course has become so popular that a waiting list is established virtually every time it is offered. It is common to receive requests and referrals following such a public education activity.

Offer a presentation to the public. Potential venues include consumer groups, local branches of self-help groups, mental health associations, and college-, university-, or association-sponsored career days. While it is common to receive either no stipend or a small honorarium for your services, you frequently reap the benefits later on, when potential clients call your practice. Pubic presentations are a positive way to give local recognition to both your practice and cognitive-behavioral therapy.

Write and talk about what you do. Writing may include brochures, web-based materials, or articles in local newspapers, magazines, and media outlets. Talking about your work might include media interviews, such as radio and television. Media sources are often looking for news items, and the development of an innovative, effective cognitive-behavioral therapy may be of interest to such agencies. Mention cognitive-behavioral therapy by name in your written and oral work.

Become active in your professional and cognitive-behavioral therapy associations. Many of these associations have referral services that are useful sources of new clients. For example, the Academy of Cognitive Therapy (*www.academyofct.org*) lists members by geographic area. This listing can prove to be an effective way to develop your practice, because potential clients increasingly search the world wide web for services.

It is easier to become known when your name is associated with a specialty service, than when you offer either generic services or claim expertise in a broad range of areas. For example, it is more credible and easier to remember that "Dr. Jones provides cognitive-behavioral therapy for anxiety disorders," compared to "Dr. Jones provides psychotherapy for adults." The latter service is general and not a unique service. If possible, consider what other specialty services practitioners offer in your community and work toward providing a unique element or new component to what is available. Consider gaps or areas not currently being served. For example, one of us (D. D.) realized that there were a large number of local services for people with severe and persistent mental illness (e.g., schizophrenia) early in her practice. There was, however, no organized service for individuals with social anxiety disorder, despite the considerable research data that demonstrate the efficacy of both individual and group cognitive-behavioral treatment for social anxiety. Her decision to shift her work and obtain new training in this area led to a shift in her career direction.

If the referral is from someone other than the client, send thank-you notes, as well as assessment and treatment information to the referral source (with the client's consent). The referral source (typically, your client's family physician) may see the client on an ongoing basis, long after your cognitive-behavioral therapy has been completed. The information you send serves as not only a progress note but also a reminder that you appreciate the referral and might be willing to accept other referrals in the future. Send updates to referral sources, if there has been any change in your practice, such as a new location, a new area of expertise, new partners, or any new services. If you require additional exposure, consider activities such as a newsletter or update sheet about your practice. Having your name or your clinic's name noted frequently is one of the best ways to keep the practice viable and healthy.

The most important way to promote your cognitive-behavioral practice is to work effectively with your clients. Providing evidence-based treatment and helping to reduce clients' distress and to solve their problems leads to more referrals. Clients can appreciate that cognitive-behavioral therapy will not be 100% effective for all problems. However, if they feel that they have been respected, that their needs were considered, and that some positive results occurred, they are likely to return in the future if needed, and they will often refer other people. Word of mouth is usually the best source of referrals. If clients return in the future, it is important to see this return as a vote of confidence in your treatment, not as a treatment failure. If you do a good job, you, fortunately, may have the problem of looking for ways to limit the number of your referrals!

FURTHER TRAINING AND SUPERVISION
IN COGNITIVE-BEHAVIORAL THERAPY

Cognitive-behavioral therapy has a number of evidence-based applications with broad applicability across a range of clinical problems. Having reached this point in the book, you may wonder where to obtain further training to increase your expertise in cognitive-behavioral therapy. We now turn our attention to issues related to training and supervision. How can you decide whether you are a competent cognitive-behavioral therapist? What level of competence is needed before a practitioner can be identified as "expert"? There is surprisingly little research on these topics. What follows here is our clinical wisdom regarding evidence-based training methods.

Thinking about Competence

Most beginning therapists want to reassure themselves that they are competent in the work that they do. The "impostor syndrome" is common in graduate and residency programs, in which the students think that perhaps they should not be there, that they are really "fooling" the supervisors into thinking they are more knowledgeable or competent than they really are. Some professionals harbor this set of negative cognitions well into their practice.

We all seek to provide optimal care to our clients. An important distinction is made between treatment adherence and competence, both of which are seen as aspects of overall treatment integrity (McGlinchey & Dobson, 2003; Perepletchikova & Kazdin, 2005). *Treatment adherence* occurs when a therapist adheres or sticks to a particular therapy. Adherence has both a positive and negative element; thus, *adherence* means doing the things that are included in a given treatment and *not* doing things that are not included in the treatment. For example, a positive element of most cognitive-behavioral therapy treatments is exposure; a negative element would be dream interpretation.

What aspects are associated with good adherence in cognitive-behavioral therapy? These aspects depend on the particular problems being treated and the particular model being applied. For example, schema-related interventions are not incorporated into Barlow and Craske's (2000) MAP-3 therapy, but they are a regular feature of cognitive therapy for depression (A. T. Beck et al., 1979). Thus, the specific details of the treatment plan dictate what the therapist should do. Practically speaking, adherence is maximized when the therapist does only what is in a given treatment manual. If the treatment is not based on a manual, then cognitive-behavioral therapy adherence is maximized when the therapist uses only interventions found in books on cognitive-behavioral therapy.

Adherence to cognitive-behavioral therapy does not ensure competence. It is easy to imagine the use of any intervention at the wrong phase of treatment, or in an inappropriate manner for a specific client. For example, doing schema work in a first treatment session is often not reflective of competent practice, just as waiting until the final session to do exposure with a person with social phobia would be considered incompetent treatment. Consequently, it is possible to be adherent but not competent. In contrast, you cannot be a competent cognitive-behavioral therapist if you do not adhere to the model. Competence builds on, but is distinct from, adherence.

Of the scales developed to measure both adherence and competence in cognitive-behavioral therapy, one of the best is the Cognitive Therapy Adherence and Competence Scale (CTACS; Barber, Liese, & Abrams, 2003). The CTACS includes 21 items, each of which is rated for both adherence and competence. Raters can be either experts or trained nonspecialists. The items include typical cognitive-behavioral activities, such as setting an agenda, assigning homework, and doing cognitive restructuring. CTACS, developed for use in a trial of cognitive-behavioral therapy for substance abuse, has now been modified for use in general practice. It has demonstrated good reliability (McGlinchey & Dobson, 2003).

The most commonly used scale of adherence or competence is the Cognitive Therapy Scale (CTS; Young & Beck, 1980; see Appendix A in this volume). The CTS was developed rationally to be an index of the quality of cognitive therapy. Each of its 11 items is scored from 0 to 6, for a range of 0 to 66. The items can be roughly divided into general skills (e.g., setting an agenda, collaborative empiricism) and specific cognitive-behavioral therapy items (e.g., using appropriate interventions, doing the interventions with skill, homework). It should be noted that the general skills category also includes items related to the therapeutic relationship, and not all items are specific to cognitive therapy. The CTS is intended to be completed by an "expert" in cognitive therapy, and the ratings are completed after listening or viewing an entire session. Interrater reliability estimates of the CTS are good for the overall scale (Vallis, Shaw, & Dobson, 1986; Dobson, Shaw, & Vallis, 1987).

Part of the reason for its widespread is that the CTS has been adopted by the Academy of Cognitive Therapy (*www.academyofct.org*) as the measure of competent treatment, as part of the criteria for Academy membership. More specifically, the Academy of Cognitive Therapy has adopted a pass score of 40 (out of 66) as one of the measures of competent cognitive therapy. Specific research trials have also adopted this same "redline" score of 40 as the index of competence (Shaw & Dobson, 1988).

Even though the CTS is meant to be rated by "experts" in cognitive therapy, and as such, the extent to which the person being rated scores well is dictated in part by the expert, there is no reason why this scale should not be used by supervisees and trainees working to improve their skills. We know that not all "experts" agree on the case conceptualization of any given client, just as there is no guarantee regarding competence ratings. Also, because there is so much variability among clients, there is really no "ideal" or "gold standard" format for cognitive-behavioral therapy. Fortunately, there is evidence that training can improve agreement about case conceptualizations and therapy ratings (Kuyken et al., 2005), which provides some evidence that use of the CTS is a reasonable standard for assessing competence. Practice using the CTS on yourself by observing videotaped sessions, or ask one of your colleagues or supervisors to provide his or her opinion.

How Can We Maximize Treatment Integrity?

Treatment integrity is a consideration when both adherence and competence matter. Settings in which both issues are important include training settings, such as graduate school, and research trials in which a fairly pure test of the treatment is required. Although we have no data to support this contention, our experience and the wisdom we hear from other trainers indicate that high treatment integrity occurs most easily with trainees who have not been trained in a prior theoretical model. Prior training and experience with other treatments seem to lead to "proactive interference," either in case conceptualization or practice. For example, earlier exposure to psychodynamic training may be associated with a trainee's search for unconscious processes, which is certainly not adherence to cognitive-behavioral therapy. One of us (K. S. D.) had a trainee, previously trained in humanistic therapy, who would revert to nondirective and supportive statements when flustered or unsure about what to do. The more active and interventionist style of cognitive-behavioral therapy was a struggle for this trainee. This is not to say that therapists trained in other models cannot be trained in cognitive-behavioral therapy, but our experience indicates that it is more of a struggle for them. In effect, they have to unlearn some of their "bad habits" from previous training.

Some therapists want to integrate the interventions of cognitive-behavioral therapy into their existing practices, particularly whether they see themselves as expert in another treatment model. Essentially, they see the possibility of being an eclectic therapist but using interventions from cognitive-behavioral therapy. Our perspective is that to be eclectic and cognitive-behavioral at the same time is not possible. Cognitive-behavioral therapy has an underlying model, a case conceptualization framework, and a set of interventions that make it a system of psychotherapy in exactly the same way that psychodynamic therapy is. From our perspective, it *may* be possible for a talented therapist to internalize different models of treatment and choose the most appropriate one for a given client, but such therapists are the exception rather than the rule.

Clients may become confused when therapists try to practice in an eclectic fashion. How do clients understand a cognitive-behavioral therapist who suddenly recommends work on "the inner child" to address early childhood experiences? Is the cognitive-behavioral therapy insufficient for their problems? Are they too difficult to treat with a single intervention? Was the cognitive-behavioral approach "wrong" for them? Both therapists and clients need to build a model for integrated practice, which in cases like this may be a challenge.

How Should Treatment Integrity Be Trained?

If we accept that the goals of training are to help the trainee become both adherent and competent, how are these goals best attained? To our knowledge, there is no real evidence about the optimal methods of training, the optimal time line for training, or the range of interventions needed. There is some evidence that important influences on self-perceived competence include education, practice, self-reflection, knowledge about standards of practice, and therapist mental health (Bennett-Levy & Beedie, 2007), but how do we incorporate these ideas into training? Table 13.2 presents some of our best ideas about how ideally to train a competent cognitive-behavioral therapist. These are offered in the spirit of suggestions, though, because we really do not have the evidence base to say with any certainty whether this is truly an optimal (or even feasible) strategy.

Who Should Provide What Services?

Even if they work in specialty clinics or limit their practices to certain age groups, most cognitive-behavioral therapists strive for a general competence in their clinical skills and abilities. However, this suggestion may not be practical, for the following reasons:

1. It is likely that not all therapists need to provide all services. For example, although a person with advanced assessment–case conceptualization–treatment planning skills needs to be involved in the beginning stages of treatment, that same person need not necessarily do all aspects of treatment. For a significant component of exposure-based

TABLE 13.2. Ways to Maximize Competence in Cognitive-Behavioral Therapy

1. Read widely in the approach before attempting to work with clients. Get a good conceptual understanding of the DSM, read about models of psychopathology, and know the prototypical case conceptualization of the common clinical problems treated with cognitive-behavioral therapy.
2. Develop good interpersonal skills, including reflective listening and feedback skills.
3. Optimize personal mental health through a balanced life style and practice of good cognitive-behavioral skills (i.e., practice what you preach).
4. Develop good assessment skills, including the use of interview methods and the administration, scoring, and interpretation of common psychometric tools.
5. Watch some training tapes, ideally with someone who can describe or interpret the therapist's behavior in the training sessions (if such commentary is not provided in the tapes).
6. Begin training with a highly structured, manualized treatment. Read the manual and get close supervision on the first few cases to ensure that you are able to interpret and implement the manual adequately. Aim for adherence first, and competence later.
7. Continue supervised training with problems and disorders that do not have clear manualized treatment. Develop your ability to conceptualize a variety of different clinical presentations using written case conceptualizations.
8. Develop a peer supervision team in your work setting, or with like-minded therapists, to continue to discuss cases.
9. Use audiotapes and/or videotapes to observe yourself and others on your team. Rate yourself with the CTS. Compare your own ratings with those of your colleagues or trainees.
10. Attend continuing education seminars and workshops to expand your case conceptualization and intervention skills. Try not to become tied to a few interventions; instead, become versatile in treatment styles and methods.
11. Supervise someone else in cognitive-behavioral therapy. Teach an inservice seminar or course. Write an article. Having to describe the model and work helps to clarify it in your own mind.
12. Consider a specialty credentialing, with an organization such as the Academy of Cognitive Therapy or the British Association of Behavioural and Cognitive Psychotherapy, if you live in the United Kingdom. External review sets a high standard and can help to establish your expertise in both your own mind and in the minds of those around you.

interventions, for example, if may be possible to have a behavioral technician or trainee undertake the actual administration of this component of treatment.

Davidson (1970) proposed a trilevel system of providers for behavioral therapy: (a) an advanced, doctoral-level person with program development, evaluation, and implementation responsibilities; (b) a clinician with broad training, and the ability to plan and implement treatment; and (c) behavioral technicians, whose role is to provide aspects of treatment, such as exposure, under supervision. It may be possible to integrate the use of paraprofessionals into a model of care, with registered or licensed professionals planning and organizing care, but with specially trained providers doing some of the frontline work. Although such a multilevel set of practitioners is inconsistent with the normative way that professions consider the issue of credentialing and service provision, it may be a more efficient and effective way to plan services. One of us (D. D.) has frequently incorporated others into treatment, particularly in the implementation of exposure therapy.

2. Not all clients need the services of a specialist or even a health care professional. The idea associated with a "stepped care" model of services is that clients be assessed for the severity and chronicity of their problems, and that only the necessary services should be provided. For example, for persons with a fairly mild first episode of depression, a self-help program may be entirely sufficient to help them recover functioning. Persons with more chronic courses of depression, or with severe episodes or multiple presenting problems, on the other hand, may require an experienced clinician, or even a treatment team, to conceptualize fully and treat the various aspects of clients' problems. Stepped care has achieved some support in North America, and has been integrated into some practice guidelines, such as those published by the National Institute for Health and Clinical Excellence in the United Kingdom (*www.nice.org. uk*). These types of "therapy extenders" can be of tremendous assistance for cognitive-behavioral therapists working in busy clinics with long waiting lists.

3. It is unlikely that the average therapist can be competent across the broad range of populations, problems, and interventions subsumed under the spectrum of cognitive-behavioral therapy. Except perhaps in small towns, or in centers where there are few practitioners, our general view is that therapists should try to specialize to some extent, and to become known for excellence of care in these specialty areas.

It is worth noting, too, that most therapists do not work in specialty clinics. Nonspecialty mental health services often encourage therapists to take clients who present with a broad range of problems. In some cases, therapists also work across a range of age groups and treatment formats. Within private practice, there is a tendency to accept a broad range of clients to maximize earning potential. These types of issues are particularly acute in smaller centers or remote areas, where the possibility of specialization in services is more difficult. Although we accept that these issues may challenge optimal provision of services, we also believe that it is incumbent on therapists to be cognizant of these pressures to practice outside of their range of competence, and to resist them. As noted earlier, we do not endorse a generic idea of therapeutic competence, and although we do accept the idea that a given therapist may be competent in different models, we suspect that it is the rare clinician who can attain this state.

Specialty Credentialing

Models for specialty credentialing in cognitive-behavioral therapy have emerged in recent years, and further development in this area is likely in the years to come. These models have emerged for several good reasons, including a desire to identify appropriately trained service providers, a desire for people with a shared identity to belong to a "home" organization, and the potential for improving marketing and income by possessing an additional credential (Dobson, Beck, & Beck, 2005). As noted above, some credentialing organizations are even having a broader influence on the training methods and standards in the field.

An issue associated with any credentialing process is the extent to which it improves the quality of service and protects the clients who receive that service, as opposed to the guild or financial issues of the people who create and maintain the credential. The process of credentialing tends to be more credible if there are real concerns about the quality of providers who do not possess that certain credential. The credibility of a credential is also enhanced as the difficulty of obtaining that credential increases (although the potential number of people who can attain the credential goes down). In contrast, credentialing is more difficult to substantiate if the credential is simply a barrier that allows only some people to practice, and if the credential serves largely to protect the interests of those with that credential. Although as yet there is no requirement for membership in the Academy of Cognitive Therapy, we both joined this organization because we believe it meets the test of providing a credible credential. It also provides an international community of therapists with a common framework. Will specialty credentialing in cognitive-behavioral therapy be defensible over time? We shall see.

COMING FULL CIRCLE: THE CONTEXT MATTERS

We began this book with a discussion of some of the contextual factors associated with the development and promotion of cognitive-behavioral therapy. As clinicians, we tend to focus on our individual clients and their needs, and sometimes we do not have much time to think about contextual factors. But the context within which these clients' needs have developed matters! Many variables are at play and affect service delivery. We have tried to address this concern in Table 13.3, which is our effort to offer practical suggestions for how you can promote cognitive-behavioral

TABLE 13.3. Practical Ideas to Disseminate Cognitive-Behavioral Therapy

1. Develop good treatment integrity, with both adherence and competence, in the services you provide.
2. Obtain peer or other supervision to remain current and to practice at a high level of quality.
3. Use treatment "extenders," such as the telephone or other methods, to reach out to your clients, if necessary or appropriate.
4. Participate in the training of the next generation of service providers.
5. Promote evidence-based practice within your practice setting. Be bold about such promotion, even in interdisciplinary settings.
6. Talk to primary care physicians, funding agencies, and other "gatekeepers" of services to ensure they are knowledgeable about the evidence base for cognitive-behavioral therapy.
7. Consider dissemination of information on cognitive-behavioral therapy to the public through talks at local agencies, schools, and libraries, or writing in local media outlets.
8. Become a member and get involved with local, national, or international associations that promote and advocate for evidence-based practice, such as cognitive-behavioral therapy. A list of national organizations can be found on the website of the International Association of Cognitive Psychotherapy (*www. cognitivetherapyassociation.org*).

---

therapy. How far you want to take these ideas, of course, is a personal matter, but we hope to have perhaps inspired you in these suggestions at some level.

The demand for cognitive-behavioral therapy far outstrips the availability of resources. We have briefly discussed some ways to extend services within your practice. Ultimately, the training and broad availability of cognitive-behavioral therapy is going to be affected most by governmental policies and practices related to health care. Dissemination will take place at different levels and in diverse ways in the far-flung parts of the world, and disseminators will need to be cognizant of local needs, cultural practices, and funding abilities (Hamilton & Dobson, 2001). National and international associations need to assume a primary role in the appropriate international dissemination of this treatment model. Ideally, organizations, such as the International Association of Cognitive Psychotherapy, can work with other international associations, such as the World Federation of Psychotherapy, and in concert with global agencies, such as the World Health Organization (WHO) and the United Nations Education, Scientific and Cultural Organization (UNESCO), to promote evidence-based practice in general therapy and in cognitive-behavioral therapy in particular.

To the extent possible, both we as individual therapists and the field as a whole need to build on past successes and anticipate future needs. Chapter 1 of this book, we reviewed some of the contextual factors that have led to the development of cognitive-behavioral therapy. There are a number of challenges ahead. Some of the challenges include the impact of globalism on local culture, the use and misuse of communication systems, the mental health implications of the "shrinking world," the adaptation and dissemination of treatments among diverse cultures, the integration of cognitive-behavioral therapy into local or indigenous mental health practices, and the daunting demands of global training. Over time, we need to continue to integrate science and practice in their "real-world" contexts. Just as in our work with individual clients, the context matters.

Appendix A

The Cognitive Therapy Scale

Therapist: _____ Client: _____ Date of Session:_____

Tape ID#: _____ Rater: _____ Date of Rating: _____

Session# _____ ( ) Videotape ( ) Audiotape ( ) Live Observation

Directions: For each item, assess the therapist on a scale from 0 to 6, and record the rating on the line next to the item number. Descriptions are provided for even-numbered scale points. *If you believe the therapist falls between two of the descriptors, select the intervening odd number (1, 3, 5).* For example, if the therapist set a very good agenda but did not establish priorities, assign a rating of 5 rather than 4 or 6.

If the descriptions for a given item occasionally do not seem to apply to the session you are rating, feel free to disregard them and use the more general scale below:

0	1	2	3	4	5	6
Poor	Barely Adequate	Mediocre	Satisfactory	Good	Very Good	Excellent

Please do not leave any item blank. For all items, focus on the skill of the therapist, taking into account how difficult the patient seems to be.

Note. For instructions on administering and interpreting the Cognitive Therapy Scale, see Chapter 13, this volume. The Cognitive Therapy Scale and Cognitive Therapy Scale manual copyright 1980 by Jeffrey E. Young and Aaron T. Beck. Reprinted with permission from the Academy of Cognitive Therapy.

Part I. General Therapeutic Skills

_____ 1. Agenda

       0 Therapist did not set agenda.

       2 Therapist set agenda that was vague or incomplete.

       4 Therapist worked with patient to set a mutually satisfactory agenda that included specific target problems (e.g., anxiety at work, dissatisfaction with marriage).

       6 Therapist worked with patient to set an appropriate agenda with target problems, suitable for the available time. Established priorities and then followed agenda.

_____ 2. Feedback

       0 Therapist did not ask for feedback to determine patient's understanding of, or response to, the session.

       2 Therapist elicited some feedback from the patient, but did not ask enough questions to be sure the patient understood the therapist's line of reasoning during the session *or* to ascertain whether the patient was satisfied with the session.

       4 Therapist asked enough questions to be sure that the patient understood the therapist's line of reasoning throughout the session and to determine the patient's reactions to the session. The therapist adjusted his or her behavior in response to the feedback, when appropriate.

       6 Therapist was especially adept at eliciting and responding to verbal and nonverbal feedback throughout the session (e.g., elicited reactions to session, regularly checked for understanding, helped summarize main points at end of session).

_____ 3. Understanding

       0 Therapist repeatedly failed to understand what the patient explicitly said, thus consistently missing the point. Poor empathic skills.

       2 Therapist was usually able to reflect or rephrase what the patient explicitly said, but repeatedly failed to respond to more subtle communication. Limited ability to listen and empathize.

       4 Therapist generally seemed to grasp the patient's "internal reality" as reflected by both what the patient explicitly said and what the patient communicated in more subtle ways. Good ability to listen and empathize.

       6 Therapist seemed to understand the patient's "internal reality" thoroughly and was adept at communicating this understanding through appropriate verbal and nonverbal responses to   the patient (e.g., the tone of the therapist's response conveyed a sympathetic understanding of   the patient's "message"). Excellent listening and empathic skills.

_____ 4. Interpersonal Effectiveness

    0 Therapist had poor interpersonal skills. Seemed hostile, demeaning, or in some other way destructive to the patient.

    2 Therapist did not seem destructive but had significant interpersonal problems. At times, therapist appeared unnecessarily impatient, aloof, insincere, *or* had difficulty conveying confidence and competence.

    4 Therapist displayed a *satisfactory* degree of warmth, concern, confidence, genuineness, and professionalism. No significant interpersonal problems.

    6 Therapist displayed *optimal* levels of warmth, concern, confidence, genuineness, and professionalism, appropriate for this particular patient in this session.

_____ 5. Collaboration

    0 Therapist did not attempt to set up a collaboration with the patient.

    2 Therapist attempted to collaborate with the patient, but had difficulty *either* defining a problem that the patient considered important *or* establishing rapport.

    4 Therapist was able to collaborate with the patient, focus on a problem that both patient and therapist considered important, and establish rapport.

    6 Collaboration seemed excellent; therapist encouraged patient as much as possible to take an active role during the session (e.g., by offering choices) so therapist and patient could function as a "team."

_____ 6. Pacing and Efficient Use of Time

    0 Therapist made no attempt to structure therapy time. Session seemed aimless.

    2 Session had some direction, but the therapist had significant problems with structuring or pacing (e.g., too little structure, inflexible about structure, too slowly paced, too rapidly paced).

    4 Therapist was reasonably successful at using time efficiently. Therapist maintained appropriate control over flow of discussion and pacing.

    6 Therapist used time efficiently by tactfully limiting peripheral and unproductive discussion, and by pacing the session as rapidly as was appropriate for the patient.

Part II. Conceptualization, Strategy, and Technique

_____ 7. Guided Discovery

    0 Therapist relied primarily on debate, persuasion, or "lecturing." Therapist seemed to be "cross-examining" the patient, putting the

patient on the defensive, or forcing his or her point of view on the patient.

2 Therapist relied too heavily on persuasion and debate rather than on guided discovery. However, the therapist's style was supportive enough that the patient did not seem to feel attacked or defensive.

4 Therapist, for the most part, helped the patient see new perspectives through guided discovery (e.g., examining evidence, considering alternatives, weighing advantages and disadvantages) rather than through debate. Used questioning appropriately.

6 Therapist was especially adept at using guided discovery during the session to explore problems and help the patient draw his or her own conclusions. Achieved an excellent balance between skillful questioning and other modes of intervention.

_____ 8. Focusing on Key Cognitions or Behaviors

0 Therapist did not attempt to elicit specific thoughts, assumptions, images, meanings, or behaviors.

2 Therapist used appropriate techniques to elicit cognitions or behaviors; however, the therapist had difficulty finding a focus *or* focused on cognitions/behaviors that were irrelevant to the patient's key problems.

4 Therapist focused on specific cognitions or behaviors relevant to the target problem. However, therapist could have focused on more central cognitions or behaviors that offered greater promise for progress.

6 Therapist very skillfully focused on key thoughts, assumptions, behaviors, etc., that were most relevant to the problem area and offered considerable promise for progress.

_____ 9. Strategy for Change (*Note.* For this item, focus on the quality of the therapist's strategy for change, not on how effectively the strategy was implemented or whether change actually occurred.)

0 Therapist did not select cognitive-behavioral techniques.

2 Therapist selected cognitive-behavioral techniques; however, the overall strategy for bringing about change either seemed vague *or* did not seem promising in helping the patient.

4 Therapist seemed to have a generally coherent strategy for change that showed reasonable promise and incorporated cognitive-behavioral techniques.

6 Therapist followed a consistent strategy for change that seemed very promising and incorporated the most appropriate cognitive-behavioral techniques.

____ 10. Application of Cognitive-Behavioral Techniques (*Note.* For this item, focus on how skillfully the techniques were applied, not on how appropriate they were for the target problem or whether change actually occurred.)

    0 Therapist did not apply any cognitive-behavioral techniques.

    2 Therapist used cognitive-behavioral techniques, but there were *significant flaws* in the way they were applied.

    4 Therapist applied cognitive-behavioral techniques *with moderate skill.*

    6 Therapist *very skillfully* and resourcefully employed cognitive-behavioral techniques.

____ 11. Homework

    0 Therapist did not attempt to incorporate homework relevant to cognitive therapy.

    2 Therapist had significant difficulties incorporating homework (e.g., did not review previous homework, did not explain homework in sufficient detail, assigned inappropriate homework).

    4 Therapist reviewed previous homework and assigned "standard" cognitive therapy homework generally relevant to issues dealt with in session. Homework was explained in sufficient detail.

    6 Therapist reviewed previous homework and carefully assigned homework drawn from cognitive therapy for the coming week. Assignment seemed "custom tailored" to help the patient incorporate new perspectives, test hypotheses, experiment with new behaviors discussed during session, etc.

____ Total Score on Part I: General Therapeutic Skills
____ Total Score on Part II: Conceptualization, Strategy, and Technique
____ Total CTS Score

Part III. Additional Considerations

1. Did any special problems arise during the session (e.g., nonadherence to homework, interpersonal issues between therapist and patient, hopelessness about continuing therapy, relapse)?

____ No   ____ Yes
____ (b) *If yes:*

    0 Therapist could not deal adequately with special problems that arose.

    2 Therapist dealt with special problems adequately but used strategies or conceptualizations inconsistent with cognitive therapy.

    4 Therapist attempted to deal with special problems using a cognitive framework and was *moderately skillful* in applying techniques.

      6 Therapist was very skillful at handling special problems using cognitive therapy framework.

2. Were there any significant unusual factors in this session that you feel justified the therapist's departure from the standard approach measured by this scale?
____ No   ____ Yes (Please explain below.)

_____

_____

_____

Part IV. Overall Ratings and Comments
1. How would you rate the clinician overall in this session, as a cognitive therapist?

0	1	2	3	4	5	6
Poor	Barely Adequate	Mediocre	Satisfactory	Good	Very Good	Excellent

2. If you were conducting an outcome study in cognitive therapy, do you think you would select this therapist to participate at this time (assuming this session is typical)?

0	1	2	3	4
Definitely Not	Probably Not	Uncertain–Borderline	Probably Yes	Definitely Yes

3. How difficult did you feel this patient was to work with?

0	1	2	3	4	5	6
Not Difficult–Very Receptive			Moderately Difficult			Extremely Difficult

4. Comments and Suggestions for Therapist's Improvement:

_____

_____

_____

_____

Review Articles Regarding the Efficacy of Cognitive-Behavioral Therapy

GENERAL

Butler, A. C., Chapman, J. E., Forman, E. M., & Beck, A. T. (2006). The empirical status of cognitive-behavioral therapy: A review of meta-analyses. *Clinical Psychology Review, 26*, 17–31.

Bandelow, B., Seidler-Brandler, U., Becker, A., Wedekind, D., & Rüther, E. (2007). Meta-analysis of randomized controlled comparisons of psychopharmacological and psychological treatments for anxiety disorders. *World Journal of Biological Psychiatry, 8*, 175–187.

Deacon, B. J., & Abramowitz, J. S. (2004). Cognitive and behavioral treatments for anxiety disorders: A review of meta-analytic findings. *Journal of Clinical Psychology, 60*, 429–441.

Norton, P. J., & Price, E. C. (2007). A meta-analytic review of adult cognitive-behavioral treatment outcome across the anxiety disorders. *Journal of Nervous and Mental Disease, 195*, 521–531.

Siev, J., & Chambless, D. L. (2007). Specificity of treatment effects: Cognitive therapy and relaxation for generalized anxiety and panic disorders. *Journal of Consulting and Clinical Psychology, 75*, 513–522.

SPECIFIC PHOBIA

Choy, Y., Fyer, A. J., & Lipsitz, J. D. (2007). Treatment of specific phobia in adults. *Clinical Psychology Review, 27*, 266–286.

SOCIAL ANXIETY DISORDER

Fedoroff, I. C., & Taylor, S. (2001). Psychological and pharmacological treatments of social phobia: A meta analysis. *Journal of Clinical Psychopharmacology, 21,* 311–324.

Gould, R. A., Buckminster, S., Pollack, M. H., Otto, M. W., & Yap, L. (1997). Cognitive-behavioral and pharmacological treatment for social phobia: A meta-analysis. *Clinical Psychology: Science and Practice, 4,* 291–306.

Heimberg, R. G. (2002). Cognitive-behavioral therapy for social anxiety disorder: Current status and future directions. *Biological Psychiatry, 51,* 101–108.

Rodebaugh, T. L., Holaway, R. M., & Heimberg, R. G. (2004). The treatment of social anxiety disorder. *Clinical Psychology Review, 24,* 883–908.

Taylor, S. (1996). Meta-analysis of cognitive-behavioral treatments for social phobia. *Journal of Behavior Therapy and Experimental Psychiatry, 27,* 1–9.

OBSESSIVE–COMPULSIVE DISORDER

Abramowitz, J. S. (1997). Effectiveness of psychological and pharmacological treatments for obsessive–compulsive disorder: A quantitative review. *Journal of Consulting and Clinical Psychology, 65,* 44–52.

Abramowitz, J. S., Taylor, S., & McKay, D. (2005) Potentials and limitations of cognitive treatments for obsessive-compulsive disorder. *Cognitive Behaviour Therapy, 34,* 140–147.

Van Balkom, A. J. L. M., van Oppen, P., Vermeulen, A. W. A., van Dyck, R., Nauta, M. C. E., & Vorst, H. C. M. (1994). A meta-analysis on the treatment of obsessive–compulsive disorder: A comparison of antidepressants, behavior, and cognitive therapy. *Clinical Psychology Review, 14,* 359–381.

PANIC DISORDER

Gould, R. A., Otto, M. W., & Pollack, M. H. (1995). A meta-analysis of treatment outcome for panic disorder. *Clinical Psychology Review, 8,* 819–844.

Landon, T. M., & Barlow, D. H. (2004). Cognitive-behavioral treatment for panic disorder: Current status. *Journal of Psychiatric Practice, 10,* 211–226.

Mitte, K. (2005). A meta-analysis of the efficacy of psycho- and pharmacotherapy in panic disorder with and without agoraphobia. *Journal of Affective Disorders, 88,* 27–45.

van Balkom, A. J. L. M., Bakker, A., Spinhoven, P., Blaauw, B. M. J. W., Smeenk, S., & Ruesink, B. (1997). A meta-analysis of the treatment of panic disorder with or without agoraphobia: A comparison of psychopharmacological, cognitive-behavioral, and combination treatments. *Journal of Nervous and Mental Disease, 185,* 510–516.

POSTTRAUMATIC STRESS DISORDER

Bisson, J., & Andrew, M. (2007). Psychological treatment of post-traumatic stress disorder. *Cochrane Database System Review, 3,* CD00338.

Harvey, A. G., Bryant, R. A., & Tarrier, N. (2003). Cognitive behaviour therapy for posttraumatic stress disorder. *Clinical Psychology Review, 23,* 501–522.

Seidler, G. H., & Wagner, F. E. (2006). Comparing the efficacy of EMDR and trauma-focused cognitive-behavioral therapy in the treatment of PTSD: A meta-analytic study. *Psychological Medicine, 36,* 1515–1522.

Van Etten, M., & Taylor, S. (1998). Comparative efficacy of treatments for posttraumatic stress disorder: A meta-analysis. *Clinical Psychology and Psychotherapy, 5,* 126–145.

GENERALIZED ANXIETY DISORDER

Gould, R. A., Otto, M. W., Pollack, M. H., & Yap, L. (1997). Cognitive behavioral and pharmacological treatment of generalized anxiety disorder: A preliminary meta-analysis. *Behavior Therapy, 28,* 285–305.

Hunot, V., Churchill, R., Teixeira, V., & Silva de Lima, M. (2007). Psychological therapies for generalised anxiety disorder. *Cochrane Database System Review,* CD001848.

Mitte, K. (2005). Meta-analysis of cognitive-behavioral treatments for generalized anxiety disorder: A comparison with pharmacotherapy. *Psychological Bulletin, 131,* 785–795.

MAJOR DEPRESSION

Bledsoe, S. E., & Grote, N. K. (2006). Treating depression during pregnancy and the postpartum: A preliminary meta-analysis. *Research on Social Work Practice, 16,* 109–120.

Feldman, G. (2007). Cognitive and behavioral therapies for depression: Overview, new directions, and practical recommendations for dissemination. *Psychiatric Clinics of North America, 30,* 39–50.

Hollon, S. D., Thase, M. E., & Markowitz, J. C. (2005). Treatment and prevention of depression. *Psychological Science in the Public Interest, 3,* 39–77.

Paykel, E. S. (2007). Cognitive therapy in relapse prevention in depression. *International Journal of Neuropsychopharmacology, 10,* 131–136.

Wampold, B. E., Minami, T., Baskin, T. W., & Tierney, S. C. (2002). A meta-(re)analysis of the effects of cognitive therapy versus "other therapies" for depression. *Journal of Affective Disorders, 68,* 159–165.

BIPOLAR DISORDER

Colom, F., & Vieta, E. (2004). A perspective on the use of psychoeducation, cognitive-behavioral therapy and interpersonal therapy for bipolar patients. *Bipolar Disorders*, *6*, 480–486.

Jones, S. (2004). Psychotherapy of bipolar disorder: A review. *Journal of Affective Disorders*, *80*, 101–114.

Miklowitz, D. J., & Otto, M. W. (2006). New psychosocial interventions for bipolar disorder: A review of literature and introduction of the systematic treatment enhancement program. *Journal of Cognitive Psychotherapy: An International Quarterly*, *20*, 215–230.

Zaretsky, A. E., Rizvi, S., & Parikh, S. V. (2007). How well do psychosocial interventions work in bipolar disorder? *Canadian Journal of Psychiatry*, *52*, 14–21.

ANOREXIA NERVOSA

Bowers, W. A., & Andersen, A. E. (2007). Cognitive-behavior therapy with eating disorders: The role of medications in treatment. *Journal of Cognitive Psychotherapy: An International Quarterly*, *21*, 16–27.

Rosenblum, J., & Forman, S. (2002). Evidence-based treatment of eating disorders. *Current Opinion in Pediatrics*, *14*, 379–383.

BULIMIA NERVOSA

Hay, P. J., Bacaltchuk, J., & Stefano, S. (2007). Psychotherapy for bulimia nervosa and binging. *Cochrane Database System Review*, *3*, CD000562.

SLEEP DISORDERS

Edinger, J. D., Melanie, T., & Means, K. (2005). Cognitive-behavioral therapy for primary insomnia. *Clinical Psychology Review*, *25*, 539–558.

Montgomery, P., & Dennis, J. (2004). A systematic review of non-pharmacological therapies for sleep problems in later life. *Sleep Medicine Reviews*, *8*, 47–62.

Wang, M.-Y., Wang, S.-Y., & Tsai, P.-S. (2005). Cognitive behavioural therapy for primary insomnia: A systematic review. *Journal of Advanced Nursing*, *50*, 553–564.

PSYCHOSIS

Lawrence, R., Bradshaw, T., & Mairs, H. (2006). Group cognitive behavioural therapy for schizophrenia: A systematic review of the literature. *Journal of Psychiatric and Mental Health Nursing*, *13*, 673–681.

Penn, D. L., Waldheter, E. J., Perkins, D. O., Mueser, K. T., & Lieberman, J. A. (2005). Psychosocial treatment for first-episode psychosis: A research update. *American Journal of Psychiatry*, *162*, 2220–2232.

Turkington, D., Dudley, R., Warman, D. M., & Beck, A. T. (2004). Cognitive-behavioral therapy for schizophrenia: A review. *Journal of Psychiatric Practice*, *10*, 5–16.

SUBSTANCE USE DISORDERS

Denis, C., Lavie, E., Fatseas, M., & Auriacombe, M. (2007). Psychotherapeutic interventions for cannabis abuse and/or dependence in outpatient settings. *Cochrane Database System Review*, *3*, CD005336.

Morgenstern, J., & McKay, J. R. (2007). Rethinking the paradigms that inform behavioral treatment research for substance use disorders. *Addiction*, *102*, 1377–1389.

SOMATIZATION AND SOMATOFORM DISORDERS

Looper, K. J., & Kirmayer, L. J. (2002). Behavioral medicine approaches to somatoform disorders. *Journal of Consulting and Clinical Psychology*, *70*, 810–827.

Mai, F. (2004). Somatization disorder: A practical review. *Canadian Journal of Psychiatry*, *49*, 562–662.

References

Abramowitz, J. S., Taylor, S., & McKay, D. (2005). Potentials and limitations of cognitive treatments for obsessive–compulsive disorder. *Cognitive Behaviour Therapy, 34*, 140–147.

Abramson, L. Y., & Alloy, L. B. (2006). Cognitive vulnerability to depression: Current status and developmental origins. In T. E. Joiner, J. S. Brown, & J. Kistner (Eds.), *The interpersonal, cognitive, and social nature of depression* (pp. 83–100). Mahwah, NJ: Erlbaum.

Achenbach, T. (2005). Advancing assessment of child and adolescent problems: Commentary on evidence based assessment of child and adolescent disorders. *Journal of Clinical Child and Adolescent Psychology, 34*, 542–547.

Addis, M. E., & Jacobson, N. S. (1996). Reasons for depression and the process and outcome in cognitive-behavioral psychotherapies. *Journal of Consulting and Clinical Psychology, 64*, 1417–1424.

Addis, M. E., & Jacobson, N. S. (2000). A closer look at the treatment rationale and homework compliance in cognitive-behavioral therapy for depression. *Cognitive Therapy and Research, 24*, 313–326.

American Psychiatric Association. (1980). *Diagnostic and statistical manual of mental disorders* (3rd ed.). Washington, DC: Author.

American Psychiatric Association. (2000). *Diagnostic and statistical manual of mental disorders* (4th ed., text rev.). Washington, DC: Author.

Antony, M., & Barlow, D. (Eds.). (2002). *Handbook of assessment and treatment planning for psychological disorders.* New York: Guilford Press.

Antony, M., Ledley, D. R., & Heimberg, R. (Eds.). (2005). *Improving outcomes and preventing relapse in cognitive-behavioral therapy.* New York: Guilford Press.

Antony, M., Orsillo, S., & Roemer, L. (Eds.). (2001). *Practitioner's guide to empirically based measures of anxiety.* New York: Springer.

Antony, M., & Swinson, R. (2000). *Phobic disorders in adults: A guide to assess-*

297

ment and treatment. Washington, DC: American Psychological Association Press.

APA Presidential Task Force on Evidence-Based Practice. (2006). Evidence-based practice in psychology. *American Psychologist, 61*, 271–285.

Bandelow, B., Seidler-Brandler, U., Becker, A., Wedekind, D., & Rüther, E. (2007). Meta-analysis of randomized controlled comparisons of psychopharmacological and psychological treatments for anxiety disorders. *World Journal of Biological Psychiatry, 8*, 175–187.

Barber, J. F., Liese, B. S., & Abrams, M. J. (2003). Development of the Cognitive Therapy Adherence and Competence Scale. *Psychotherapy Research, 13*, 205–221.

Barlow, D. H. (2002). *Anxiety and its disorders* (2nd ed.). New York: Guilford Press.

Barlow, D. H. (2004). Psychological treatments. *American Psychologist, 59*, 869–878.

Barlow, D. H., Allen, L. B., & Choate, M. L. (2004). Toward a unified treatment for emotional disorders. *Behavior Therapy, 35*, 205–230.

Barlow, D. H., & Craske, M. G. (2000). *Mastery of Your Anxiety and Panic (MAP-3): Client workbook for anxiety and panic* (3rd ed.). San Antonio, TX: Psychological Corporation.

Beck, A. T. (1970). Cognitive therapy: Nature and relation to behavior therapy. *Behavior Therapy, 1*, 184–200.

Beck, A. T. (1993). Cognitive therapy: Past, present, and future. *Journal of Consulting and Clinical Psychology, 61*, 194–198.

Beck, A. T., Freeman, A., & Davis, D. D. (Eds.). (2004). *Cognitive therapy of personality disorders* (2nd ed.). New York: Guilford Press.

Beck, A. T., Rush, A. J., Shaw, B. F., & Emery, G. (1979). *Cognitive therapy of depression.* New York: Guilford Press.

Beck, A. T., & Steer, R. A. (1988). *Beck Hopelessness Scale.* San Antonio, TX: Psychological Corporation.

Beck, A. T., & Steer, R. A. (1993). *Manual for the Beck Anxiety Inventory.* San Antonio, TX: Psychological Corporation.

Beck, A. T., Steer, R. A., & Brown, G. K. (1996). *Beck Depression Inventory Manual* (2nd ed.). San Antonio, TX: Psychological Corporation.

Beck, J. S. (1995). *Cognitive therapy: Basics and beyond.* New York: Guilford Press.

Beck, J. S. (2005). *Cognitive therapy for challenging problems: What to do when the basics don't work.* New York: Guilford Press.

Bennett-Levy, J., & Beedie, A. (2007). The ups and downs of cognitive therapy training: What happens to trainees' perception of their competence during a cognitive therapy training course? *Behavioural and Cognitive Psychotherapy, 35*, 61–75.

Berking, M., Grosse Holtforth, M., Jacobi, C., & Kroner-Herwig, B. (2005). Empirically based guidelines for goal-finding procedures in psychotherapy: Are some goals easier to attain than others? *Psychotherapy Research, 15*, 316–324.

Bieling, P., & Kuyken, W. (2003). Is cognitive case formulation science or science fiction? *Clinical Psychology: Science and Practice, 10*(1), 52–69.

Bieling, P. J., & Antony, M. M. (2003). *Ending the depression cycle*. Oakland, CA: New Harbinger Press.

Bieling, P. J., Beck, A. T., & Brown, G. K. (2000). The Sociotropy–Autonomy Scale: Structure and implications. *Cognitive Therapy and Research, 24,* 763–780.

Bisson, J., & Andrew, M. (2007). Psychological treatment of post-traumatic stress disorder. *Cochrane Database System Review, 3,* CD00338.

Bledsoe, S. E., & Grote, N. K. (2006). Treating depression during pregnancy and the postpartum: A preliminary meta-analysis. *Research on Social Work Practice, 16,* 109–120.

Bockting, C., Schene, A., Spinhoven, P., Koeter, M., Wouters, L., Huyser, J., et al. (2005). Preventing relapse/recurrence in recurrent depression with cognitive therapy: A randomized controlled trial. *Journal of Consulting and Clinical Psychology, 73*(4), 647–657.

Borden, E. (1979). The generalizability of the psychoanalytic concept of the working alliance. *Psychotherapy: Theory, Research, Practice and Training, 16*(3), 252–260.

Borkovec, T. D., & Whisman, M. A. (1996). Psychosocial treatment for generalized anxiety disorder. In M. R. Mavissakalian & R. F. Prien (Eds.), *Long-term treatments of anxiety disorders* (pp. 171–199). Washington, DC: American Psychiatric Association Press.

Breslau, N., Davis, G. C., Andreski, P., Peterson, E. L., & Schultz, L. R. (1997). Sex differences in posttraumatic stress disorder. *Archives of General Psychiatry, 54,* 1044–1048.

Bright, J. I., Baker, K. D., & Neimeyer, R. A. (1999). Professional and paraprofessional group treatments for depression: A comparison of cognitive behavioral and mutual support interventions. *Journal of Consulting and Clinical Psychology, 67,* 491–501.

Brown, T., DiNardo, P., & Barlow, D. (1994). *Anxiety Disorders Interview Schedule for DSM-IV (ADIS-IV)*. San Antonio, TX: Psychological Corporation.

Bryceland, C., & Stam, H. J. (2005). Empirical validation and professional codes of ethics: Description or prescription? *Journal of Constructivist Psychology, 18,* 131–155.

Burns, D. D. (1989). *The feeling good handbook: Using the new mood therapy in everyday life*. New York: Morrow.

Burns, D. D. (1999). *Feeling good: The new mood therapy (revised and updated)*. New York: Avon Books.

Burns, D. D., & Nolen-Hoeksema, S. (1991). Coping styles, homework assignments, and the effectiveness of cognitive-behavioral therapy. *Journal of Consulting and Clinical Psychology, 59,* 305–311.

Burns, D. D., & Nolen-Hoeksema, S. (1992). Therapeutic empathy and recovery from depression in cognitive-behavioral therapy: A structural equation model. *Journal of Consulting and Clinical Psychology, 60,* 441–449.

Burns, D. D., & Spangler, D. L. (2000). Does psychotherapy homework lead to improvements in depression in cognitive-behavioral therapy or does improvement lead to increased homework compliance? *Journal of Consulting and Clinical Psychology, 68,* 46–56.

Butler, A. C., Chapman, J. E., Forman, E. M., & Beck, A. T. (2006). The empirical status of cognitive-behavioral therapy: A review of meta-analyses. *Clinical Psychology Review, 26,* 17–31.

Carr, E., & Durand, C. (1985). The social-communicative basis of severe behavior problems in children. In S. Reiss & R. Bootzin (Eds.), *Theoretical issues in behaviour therapy* (pp. 219–254). New York: Academic Press.

Castonguay, L. G., & Beutler, L. E. (2006). *Principles of therapeutic change that work.* New York: Oxford University Press.

Castonguay, L. G., Goldfried, M. R., Wiser, S., Raue, P. J., & Hayes, A. M. (1996). Predicting the effect of cognitive therapy for depression: A study of unique and common factors. *Journal of Consulting and Clinical Psychology, 64,* 497–504.

Castonguay, L., & Grosse Holtforth, M. (2005). Change in psychotherapy: A plea for no more "nonspecific" and false dichotomies. *Clinical Psychology: Science and Practice, 12*(2), 198–201.

Chambless, D., Caputo, G., Gracely, S., Jasin, E., & Williams, C. (1985). The Mobility Inventory for Agoraphobia. *Behaviour Research and Therapy, 23,* 35–44.

Chambless, D. L., & Ollendick, T. H. (2001). Empirically supported psychological interventions: Controversies and evidence. *Annual Review of Psychology, 52,* 685–716.

Chang, E. C., D'Zurilla, T. J., & Sanna, L. J. (Eds.). (2004). *Social problem solving: Theory, research, and training.* Washington, DC: American Psychological Association Press.

Choy, Y., Fyer, A. J., & Lipsitz, J. D. (2007). Treatment of specific phobia in adults. *Clinical Psychology Review, 27,* 266–286.

Clark, D. A., & Beck, A. T. (1991). Personality factors in dysphoria: A psychometric refinement of Beck's Sociotropy–Autonomy Scale. *Journal of Psychopathology and Behavioral Assessment, 13,* 369–388.

Clark, D. A., Beck, A. T., & Alford, B. A. (1999). *Scientific foundations of cognitive theory and therapy of depression.* Hoboken, NJ: Wiley.

Clark, D. M., Salkovskis, P. M., Hackmann, A., Middleton, H., Anastasiades, P., & Gelder, M. (1994). A comparison of cognitive therapy, applied relaxation and imipramine in the treatment of panic disorder. *British Journal of Psychiatry, 164,* 759–769.

Craighead, W. E., Sheets, E. S., Bjornsson, A. S., & Arnarson, E. (2005). Specificity and nonspecificity in psychotherapy. *Clinical Psychology: Science and Practice, 12*(2), 189–193.

Dattilio, R., & Freeman, A. (Eds.). (2000). *Cognitive-behavioral strategies in crisis intervention* (2nd ed.). New York: Guilford Press.

Davidson, P. O. (1970). Graduate training and research funding for clinical psychology in Canada: Review and recommendations. *Canadian Psychologist, 11,* 101–127.

Davis, M., Eshelman, E. R., & McKay, M. (2000). *The relaxation and stress reduction workbook* (5th ed.). New Harbinger Press.

Derogatis, L. (1994). *SCL-90-R: Administration, scoring and procedures manual* (3rd ed.) Minneapolis: National Computer Systems.

DeRubeis, R., Hollon, S., Amsterdam, J., Shelton, R., Young, P., Salomon, R., et al. (2005). Cognitive therapy versus medication in the treatment of moderate to severe depression. *Archives of General Psychiatry*, 62, 409–416.

DeRubeis, R. J., Brotman, M. A., & Gibbons, C. J. (2005). A conceptual and methodological analysis of the nonspecifics argument. *Clinical Psychology: Science and Practice*, 12, 174–193.

DeRubeis, R. J., & Feeley, M. (1990). Determinants of change in cognitive therapy for depression. *Cognitive Therapy and Research*, 14, 469–482.

Dimidjian, S., Hollon, S. D., Dobson, K. S., Schmaling, K. B., Kohlenberg, R. J., Addis, M. E., et al. (2006). Randomized trial of behavioral activation, cognitive therapy, and antidepressant medication in the acute treatment of adults with major depression. *Journal of Consulting and Clinical Psychology*, 74, 658–670.

Dobson, K. S., Beck, J. S., & Beck, A. T. (2005). The Academy of Cognitive Therapy: Purpose, history, and future prospects. *Cognitive and Behavioral Practice*, 12, 263–266.

Dobson, K. S., & Dobson, D. J. G. (2006). Empirically supported treatments: Recent developments in the cognitive-behavioural therapies, and implications for evidence-based psychotherapy. In D. Loewenthall & D. Winter (Eds.), *What is psychotherapeutic research?* (pp. 259–276). London: Karnac Books.

Dobson, K. S., & Dozois, D. (2001). Historical and philosophical bases of the cognitive-behavioral therapies. In K. S. Dobson (Ed.), *Handbook of cognitive-behavioral therapies* (2nd ed., pp. 3–39). New York: Guilford Press.

Dobson, K. S., Hollon, S. D., Dimidjian, S., Schmaling, K. B., Kohlenberg, R. J., Gallop, R., et al. (2008). Randomized trial of behavioral activation, cognitive therapy, and antidepressant medication in the prevention of relapse and recurrence of major depression. *Journal of Consulting and Clinical Psychology*, 76(3), 468–477.

Dobson, K. S., Shaw, B. F., & Vallis, T. M. (1987). Reliability of a measure of the quality of cognitive therapy. *British Journal of Clinical Psychology*, 24, 295–300.

Dugas, M., Radomsky, A., & Brillon, P. (2004). Tertiary intervention for anxiety and prevention of relapse. In D. Dozois & K. S. Dobson (Eds.), *The prevention of anxiety and depression: Theory, research, and practice* (pp. 161–184). Washington, DC: American Psychological Association.

D'Zurilla, T. J., & Nezu, A. M. (2006). *Problem-solving therapy: A positive approach to clinical intervention* (3rd ed.). New York: Springer.

Eells, T. D. (Ed.). (1997). *Handbook of psychotherapy case formulation.* New York: Guilford Press.

Elkin, I., Shea, M., Watkins, J., Imber, S., et al. (1989). National Institute of Mental Health Treatment of Depression Collaborative Research Program: General effectiveness of treatments. *Archives of General Psychiatry*, 46(11), 971–982.

Ellman, S. J. (2008). Termination and long-term treatments. In W. T. O'Donohue & M. A. Cucciare (Eds.), *Terminating psychotherapy: A clinician's guide* (pp. 205–228). New York: Routledge.

Emmelkamp, P. M., & Wessels, H. (1975). Flooding in imagination vs. flooding *in vivo*: A comparison with agoraphobics. *Behaviour Research and Therapy, 13*, 7–15.

Endicott, J., & Spitzer, R. (1978). A diagnostic interview: The Schedule for Affective Disorders and Schizophrenia. *Archives of General Psychiatry, 35*, 837–844.

Farmer, R. F., & Chapman, A. L. (2008). *Behavioral interventions in cognitive behavior therapy: Practical guidance for putting theory into action*. Washington, DC: American Psychological Association Press.

Fedoroff, I. C., & Taylor, S. (2001). Psychological and pharmacological treatments of social phobia: A meta-analysis. *Journal of Clinical Psychopharmacology, 21*, 311–324.

Feeley, M., DeRubeis, R. J., & Gelfand, L. A. (1999). The temporal relation of adherence and alliance to symptom change in cognitive therapy for depression. *Journal of Consulting and Clinical Psychology, 67*, 578–582.

Feldman, G. (2007). Cognitive and behavioral therapies for depression: Overview, new directions, and practical recommendations for dissemination. *Psychiatric Clinics of North America, 30*, 39–50.

Fennell, M. J. V., & Teasdale, J. D. (1987). Cognitive therapy for depression: Individual differences and the process of change. *Cognitive Therapy and Research, 11*, 253–271.

Ferster, C. B. (1973). A functional analysis of depression. *American Psychologist, 28*, 857–870.

First, M., Spitzer, R., Gibbon, M., & Williams, J. B. (1997). *Structured Clinical Interview for DSM-IV Axis I Disorders (SCID-I), Clinician Version*. Washington, DC: American Psychiatric Press.

Foa, E. B., Dancu, C. V., Hembree, E. A., Jaycox, L. H., Meadows, E. A., & Street, G. P. (1999). The efficacy of exposure therapy, stress inoculation training and their combination in ameliorating PTSD for female victims of assault. *Journal of Consulting and Clinical Psychology, 67*, 194–200.

Foa, E. B., Jameson, J. S., Turner, R. M., & Payne, L. L. (1980). Massed versus spaced exposure sessions in the treatment of agoraphobia. *Behaviour Research and Therapy, 18*, 333–338.

Freeman, A., & Leaf, R. C. (1989). Cognitive therapy applied to personality disorders. In A. Freeman, K. Simon, L. Beutler, & H. Arkowitz (Eds.), *Comprehensive handbook of cognitive therapy* (pp. 403–433). New York: Plenum Press.

Freeston, M. H., Ladouceur, R., Provencher, M., & Blais, F. (1995). Strategies used with intrusive thoughts: Context, appraisal, mood, and efficacy. *Journal of Anxiety Disorders, 9*, 201–215.

Freiheit, S. R., Vye, C., Swan, R., & Cady, M. (2004). Cognitive-behavioral therapy for anxiety: Is dissemination working? *Behavior Therapist, 27*, 25–32.

Gelder, M. (1997). The scientific foundations of cognitive behaviour therapy. In D. Clark & C. Fairburn (Eds.), *Science and practice of cognitive behaviour therapy* (pp. 27–46). Oxford, UK: Oxford University Press.

Gelso, C. J., & Hayes, J. A. (2002). The management of countertransference. In J. C. Norcross (Ed.), *Psychotherapy relationships that work: Therapist con-*

tributions and responsiveness to patient needs (pp. 267–284). New York: Oxford University Press.

Giesen-Bloo, J., van Dyck, R., Spinhoven, P., van Tilburg, W., Dirksen, C., van Asselt, T., et al. (2006). Outpatient psychotherapy for borderline personality disorder: A randomized trial of schema focused therapy versus transference focused therapy. *Archives of General Psychiatry, 63,* 649–658.

Goldfried, M. R., Burckell, L. A., & Eubanks-Carter, C. (2003). Therapist self-disclosure in cognitive-behavior therapy. *Journal of Clinical Psychology, 59,* 555–568.

Goodman, W., Price, L., Rasmussen, S., Mazure, C., Delgado, P., Heninger, G., et al. (1989a). The Yale–Brown Obsessive Compulsive Scale: II. Validity. *Archives of General Psychiatry, 46,* 1012–1016.

Goodman, W., Price, L., Rasmussen, S., Mazure, C., Fleishmann, R., Hill, C., et al. (1989b). The Yale–Brown Obsessive Compulsive Scale: I. Development, use, and reliability. *Archives of General Psychiatry, 46,* 1006–1011.

Gortner, E. T., Gollan, J. K., Dobson, K. S., & Jacobson, N. S. (1998). Cognitive-behavioral treatment for depression: Relapse prevention. *Journal of Consulting and Clinical Psychology, 66,* 377–384.

Greenberger, D., & Padesky, C. A. (1995). *Mind over mood: Change how you feel by changing the way you think.* New York: Guilford Press.

Groth-Marnat, G. (2003). *Handbook of psychological assessment* (4th ed.). New York: Wiley.

Haby, M. M., Donnelly, M., Corry, J., & Vos, T. (2006). Cognitive behavioral therapy for depression, panic disorder and generalized anxiety disorder: A meta-regression of factors that may predict outcome. *Australian and New Zealand Journal of Psychiatry, 40,* 9–19.

Hamilton, K. E., & Dobson, K. S. (2001). Empirically supported treatments in psychology. Implications for international dissemination. *Revista Internacional de Psicologia Clinica y de la Salad/International Journal of Clinical and Health Psychology, 1*(1), 35–51.

Hamilton, K. E., & Dobson, K. S. (2002). Cognitive therapy of depression: Pretreatment patient predictors of outcome. *Clinical Psychology Review, 22,* 875–894.

Hansen, N. B., Lambert, M. J., & Forman, E. M. (2002). The psychotherapy dose–response effect and its implications for treatment delivery services. *Clinical Psychology: Science and Practice, 9*(3), 329–343.

Haynes, S. (1984). Behavioral assessment of adults. In G. Goldstein & M. Hersen (Eds.), *Handbook of psychological assessment* (pp. 369–401). New York: Pergamon Press.

Hayes, S., Nelson, R., & Jarrett, R. (1987). The treatment utility of assessment: A functional approach to evaluating assessment quality. *American Psychologist, 42,* 963–974.

Haynes, S., & O'Brien, W. (2000). *Principles and practice of behavioral assessment.* Dordrecht, Netherlands: Kluwer Academic Press.

Hayes, S. C., Follette, V., & Linehan, M. M. (Eds.). (2004). *Mindfulness and acceptance: Expanding the cognitive-behavioral tradition.* New York: Guilford Press.

Heery, M. (2001). An interview with Albert Ellis, PhD: Rational emotive behavioral therapy. Retrieved July 4, 2008, from *www.psychotherapy.net/interview/AlbertEllis*.

Heimberg, R., & Becker, R. (2002). *Cognitive-behavioral group therapy for social phobia: Basic mechanisms and clinical strategies*. New York: Guilford Press.

Heimberg, R., Dodge, C., Hope, D., Kennedy, C., Zollo, L., & Becker, R. (1990). Cognitive behavioral group treatment for social phobia: Comparison with a credible placebo control. *Cognitive Therapy and Research, 14*, 1–23.

Helbig, S., & Fehm, L. (2004). Problems with homework in CBT: Rare exception or rather frequent? *Behavioural and Cognitive Psychotherapy, 32*, 291–301.

Held, B. S. (1995). *Back to reality: A critique of postmodern theory in psychotherapy*. New York: Norton.

Hembree, E. A., & Cahill, S. P. (2007). Obstacles to successful implementation of exposure therapy. In D. C. Richard & D. Luterbach (Eds.), *Handbook of exposure therapies* (pp. 389–408). London: Elsevier Press.

Hill, C. E., & Knox, S. (2002). Self-disclosure. In J. C. Norcross (Ed.), *Psychotherapy relationships that work: Therapist contributions and responsiveness to patient needs* (pp. 255–265). New York: Oxford University Press.

Hofmann, S. G., & Smits, J. A. J. (2008). Cognitive-behavioral therapy for adult anxiety disorders: A meta-analysis of randomized placebo-controlled trials. *Journal of Clinical Psychiatry, 68*(5), 669–676.

Hollon, S., Stewart, M., & Strunk, D. (2006). Enduring effects of cognitive behavior therapy in the treatment of depression and anxiety. *Annual Review of Psychology, 57*, 285–315.

Hollon, S. D., Thase, M. E., & Markowitz, J. C. (2005). Treatment and prevention of depression. *Psychological Science in the Public Interest, 3*, 39–77.

Horowitz, L., Rosenberg, S., Baer, B., Ureno, G., & Villasenor, V. (1988). Inventory of interpersonal problems: Psychometric properties and clinical applications. *Journal of Consulting and Clinical Psychology, 56*, 885–892.

Horvath, A., & Greenberg, L. (1986). The development of the Working Alliance Inventory. In L. Greenberg & W. Pinsof (Eds.), *The psychotherapeutic process: A research handbook* (pp. 527–556). New York: Guilford Press.

Hunot, V., Churchill, R., Teixeira, V., & Silva de Lima, M. (2007). Psychological therapies for generalised anxiety disorder. *Cochrane Database System Review, 1*, CD001848.

Hunsley, J. (2002). Psychological testing and psychological assessment: A closer examination. *American Psychologist, 57*, 139–140.

Hunsley, J., Crabb, R., & Mash, E. (2004). Evidence-based clinical assessment. *Clinical Psychologist, 57*(3), 25–32.

Hunsley, J., & Mash, E. (2005). Introduction to the special section on developing guidelines for the evidence based assessment of adult disorders. *Psychological Assessment, 17*, 251–255.

Huppert, J. D., Bufka, L. F., Barlow, D. H., Gorman, J. M., Shear, M. K., & Woods, S. W. (2001). Therapists, therapist variables, and cognitive-behavioural therapy outcome in a multicenter trial for panic disorder. *Journal of Consulting and Clinical Psychology, 69*, 747–755.

Hurn, J., Kneebone, I., & Cropley, M. (2006). Goal setting as an outcome measure: A systematic review. *Clinical Rehabilitation, 20*, 756–772.

Jackson, D. N. (1967). *Personality Research Form*. Goshen, NY: Research Psychologists Press.

Jacobson, N. S., Dobson, K. S., Truax, P. A., Addis, M. E., Koerner, K., Gollan, J. K., et al. (1996). A component analysis of cognitive behavioral treatment for depression. *Journal of Consulting and Clinical Psychology, 64*, 295–304.

Jacobson, N. S., & Truax, P. (1991). Clinical significance: A statistical approach to defining meaningful change in psychotherapy research. *Journal of Consulting and Clinical Psychology, 59*, 12–19.

Joiner, T., Walker, R., Rudd, M., & Jobes, D. (1999). Scientizing and routinizing the assessment of suicidality in outpatient practice. *Professional Psychology: Research and Practice, 30*(5), 447–453.

Josefowitz, N., & Myran, D. (2005). Towards a person-centred cognitive-behavior therapy. *Counselling Psychology Quarterly, 18*, 329–336.

Kabat-Zinn, J. (1994). *Wherever you go, there you are: Mindfulness meditation in everyday life*. New York: Hyperion.

Karpiak, C., & Smith Benjamin, L. (2004). Therapist affirmation and the process and outcome of psychotherapy: Two sequential analytic studies. *Journal of Clinical Psychology, 60*(6), 659–676.

Kazantzis, N., & Dattilio, F. N. (2007). Beyond basics: Using homework in cognitive behavior therapy with challenging clients. *Cognitive and Behavioral Practice, 14*(3), 249–251.

Kazantsis, N., Deane, F. P., & Ronan, K. R. (2000). Homework assignments in cognitive and behavioral therapies: A meta-analysis. *Clinical Psychology: Science and Practice, 7*, 189–202.

Kazantsis, N., & L'Abate, L. (Eds.). (2007). *Handbook of homework assignments in psychotherapy: Research, practice and prevention*. New York: Springer.

Keijsers, G. P. J., Hoogduin, C. A. L., & Schaap, C. P. D. R. (1994). Predictors of treatment outcome in the behavioural treatment of obsessive–compulsive disorder. *British Journal of Psychiatry, 165*, 781–786.

Keijsers, G. P. J., Schaap, C. P. D. R., & Hoogduin, C. A. L. (2000). The impact of interpersonal patient and therapist behavior on outcome in cognitive-behavioral therapy. *Behavior Modification, 24*, 264–297.

Keller, M. B. (1994). Depression: A long term illness. *British Journal of Psychiatry, 165*(Suppl. 26), 9–15.

Kendjelic, E. M., & Eells, T. D. (2007). Generic psychotherapy case formulation training improves formulation quality. *Psychotherapy: Theory, Research, Practice and Training, 44*, 66–77.

Kessler, R. C. (2002). Epidemiology of depression. In I. H. Gotlib & C. L. Hammen (Eds.), *Handbook of depression* (pp. 23–42). New York: Guilford Press.

Kessler, R. C., Berglund, P., Dernier, O., Jin, R., Koretz, D., Merikangas, K., et al. (2003). The epidemiology of major depressive disorder: Results from the National Comorbidity Survey Replication (NCS-R). *Journal of the American Medical Association, 289*, 3095–3105.

Kiresuk, T. J., Stelmachers, Z. T., & Schultz, S. K. (1982). Quality assurance and goal attainment scaling. *Professional Psychology, 13*, 145–152.

Kleespies, P., Deleppo, J., Gallagher, P., & Niles, B. (1999). Managing suicidal emergencies: Recommendations for the practitioner. *Professional Psychology: Research and Practice, 30*, 454–463.

Klein, D., Schwartz, J., Santiago, N., Vocisano, C., Castonguay, L., Arnow, B., et al. (2003). Therapeutic alliance in depression treatment: Controlling for prior change and patient characteristics. *Journal of Consulting and Clinical Psychology, 71*, 997–1006.

Koss, M. P., & Shiang, J. (1994). Research on brief psychotherapy. In A. E. Bergin & S. L. Garfield (Eds.), *Handbook of psychotherapy and behavior change: An empirical analysis* (4th ed., pp. 664–700). New York: Wiley.

Kottler, J. A. (1986). *On being a therapist.* San Francisco: Jossey-Bass.

Kovacs, M., & Beck, A. T. (1978). Maladaptive cognitive structures in depression. *American Journal of Psychiatry, 135*, 525–533.

Kuyken, W., Fothergill, C. D., Musa, M., & Chadwick, P. (2005). The reliability and quality of cognitive case formulation. *Behaviour Research and Therapy, 43*, 1187–1201.

Lambert, M. J. (2005). Early response in psychotherapy: Further evidence for the importance of common factors rather than "placebo effects." *Journal of Clinical Psychology, 61*, 855–869.

Lambert, M. J., & Barley, D. E. (2002). Research summary on the therapeutic relationship and psychotherapy outcome. In J. C. Norcross (Ed.), *Psychotherapy relationships that work: Therapist contributions and responsiveness to patient needs* (pp. 17–36). New York: Oxford University Press.

Landon, T. M., & Barlow, D. H. (2004). Cognitive-behavioral treatment for panic disorder: Current status. *Journal of Psychiatric Practice, 10*, 211–226.

Leahy, R. L. (2001). *Overcoming resistance in cognitive therapy.* New York: Guilford Press.

Leahy, R. L. (Ed.). (2003). *Roadblocks in cognitive-behavioral therapy: Transforming challenges into opportunities for change.* New York: Guilford Press.

Leahy, R. L., & Holland, S. (2000). *Treatment plans and interventions for depression and anxiety disorders.* New York: Guilford Press.

Ledley, D. R., & Heimberg, R. G. (2005). Social anxiety disorder. In M. Antony, D. R. Ledley, & R. G. Heimberg (Eds.), *Improving outcomes and preventing relapse in cognitive-behavioral therapy* (pp. 38–76). New York: Guilford Press.

Lee, C. W., Taylor, G., & Dunn, J. (1999). Factor structure of the Schema Questionnaire in a large clinical sample. *Cognitive Therapy and Research, 23*, 441–451.

Leong, F. T. L., & Zachar, P. (1999). Gender and opinions about mental illness as predictors of attitudes toward seeking professional psychological help. *British Journal of Guidance and Counselling, 27*, 123–132.

Lewinsohn, P. M., Sullivan, J. M., & Grosscup, S. J. (1980). Changing reinforcing events: An approach to the treatment of depression. *Psychotherapy: Theory, Research, Practice and Training, 17*(3), 322–334.

Liberman, R., DeRisi, W., & Mueser, K. (1989). *Social skills training for psychiatric patients.* New York: Pergamon Press.

Lilienfeld, S. O. (2007). Psychological treatments that cause harm. *Perspectives on Psychological Science, 2,* 54–70.

Linehan, M. M. (1993). *Cognitive-behavioral treatment of borderline personality disorder.* New York: Guilford Press.

Lohr, J., Olatumji, B., Parker, L., & DeMaio, C. (2005). Experimental analysis of specific treatment factors: Efficacy and practice implications. *Journal of Clinical Psychology, 61*(7), 819–834.

Luborsky, L., & Crits-Christoph, P. (1998). *Understanding transference: The core conflictual relationship theme method* (2nd ed.). New York: Basic Books.

Luborsky, L., & DeRubeis, R. J. (1984). The use of psychotherapy treatment manuals: A small revolution in psychotherapy research style. *Clinical Psychology Review, 4,* 5–14.

Ma, S. H., & Teasdale, J. (2004). Mindfulness-based cognitive therapy for depression: Replication and exploration of differential relapse prevention effects. *Journal of Consulting and Clinical Psychology, 72,* 31–40.

MacPhillamy, D. J., & Lewinsohn, P. M. (1982). The Pleasant Events Schedule: Studies on reliability, validity, and scale intercorrelation. *Journal of Consulting and Clinical Psychology, 50,* 363–380.

Mahoney, M. J. (1991). *Human change processes: The scientific foundations of psychotherapy.* New York: Basic Books.

March, J., Frances, A., Carpenter, D., & Kahn, D. (1997). The Expert Consensus Guidelines: Treatment of obsessive–compulsive disorder. *Journal of Clinical Psychiatry, 58*(Supp 4).

Marks, I., & Mathews, A. (1979). Brief standard self-rating scale for phobic patients. *Behaviour Research and Therapy, 17,* 263–267.

Martell, C., Addis, M., & Jacobson, N. (2001). *Depression in context: Strategies for guided action.* New York: Norton.

Mattick, R., & Clarke, J. (1998). Development and validation of measures of social phobia scrutiny fear and social interaction anxiety. *Behaviour Research and Therapy, 36,* 455–470.

McAlpine, D., & Mechanic, D. (2000). Utilization of specialty mental health care among persons with severe mental illness: The roles of demographics, need, insurance, and risk. *Health Services Research, 35,* 277–292.

McFarlane, T., Carter, J., & Olmsted, M. (2005). Eating disorders. In M. Antony, D. R. Ledley, & R. G. Heimberg (Eds.), *Improving outcomes and preventing relapse in cognitive-behavioral therapy* (pp. 268–305). New York: Guilford Press.

McGlinchey, J., & Dobson, K. S. (2003). Treatment integrity concerns in cognitive therapy for depression. *Journal of Cognitive Psychotherapy: An International Quarterly, 17,* 299–318.

McKay, M., Davis, M., & Fanning, P. (1995). *Messages: The communication skills book* (2nd ed.). Oakland, CA: New Harbinger Press.

McMullin, R. E. (2000). *The new handbook of cognitive therapy techniques.* New York: Norton.

McWilliams, N. (2005). Preserving our humanity as therapists. *Psychotherapy: Theory, Research, Practice and Training, 42,* 139–151.

Meyer, G., Finn, S., Eyde, L., Kay, G., Moreland, K., Dies, R., et al. (2001). Psychological testing and psychological assessment: A review of evidence and issues. *American Psychologist, 56*(2), 128–165.

Miller, W., & Rollnick, S. (2002). *Motivational interviewing: Preparing people for change* (2nd ed.). New York: Guilford Press.

Mitte, K. (2005a). Meta-analysis of cognitive–behavioral treatments for generalized anxiety disorder: A comparison with pharmacotherapy. *Psychological Bulletin, 131,* 785–795.

Mitte, K. (2005b). A meta-analysis of the efficacy of psycho- and pharmacotherapy in panic disorder with and without agoraphobia. *Journal of Affective Disorders, 88,* 27–45.

Mumma, G. (2004). Validation of idiosyncratic cognitive schema in cognitive case formulations: An intraindividual idiographic approach. *Psychological Assessment, 16,* 211–230.

Mumma, G., & Smith, J. (2001). Cognitive-behavioral–interpersonal scenarios: Interformulator reliability and convergent validity. *Journal of Psychopathology and Behavioral Assessment, 23,* 203–221.

Murray, H. A. (1938). *Explorations in personality.* New York: Oxford University Press.

Mussell, M., Mitchell, J., Crosby, R., Fulkerson, J., Hoberman, H., & Romano, J. (2000). Commitment to treatment goals in prediction of group cognitive-behavioral therapy treatment outcome for women with bulimia nervosa. *Journal of Consulting and Clinical Psychology, 68,* 432–437.

Nelson-Gray, R. (2003). Treatment utility of psychological assessment. *Psychological Assessment, 15*(4), 521–531.

Nezu, A., Nezu, C., & Lombardo, E. (2004). *Cognitive-behavioral case formulation and treatment design: A problem-solving approach.* New York: Springer.

Nezu, A. M., Ronan, G. F., Meadows, E. A., & McClure, K. S. (Eds.). (2000). *Practitioner's guide to empirically based measures of depression.* Dordrecht, Netherlands: Kluwer Academic.

Norcross, J. C. (Ed.). (2002). *Psychotherapy relationships that work: Therapist contributions and responsiveness to patient needs.* New York: Oxford University Press.

Norcross, J. C., Koocher, G. P., & Garofalo, A. (2006). Discredited psychological treatments and tests: A Delphi Poll. *Professional Psychology: Research and Practice, 37,* 515–522.

Norcross, J. C., Santrock, J. W., Campbell, L. F., Smith, T. P., Sommer, R., & Zuckerman, E. L. (2000). *Authoritative guide to self-help resources in mental health.* New York: Guilford Press.

Norris, F. H. (1992). Epidemiology of trauma: Frequency and impact of different potentially traumatic events on different demographic groups. *Journal of Consulting and Clinical Psychology, 60,* 409–418.

O'Donohue, W. T., & Cucciare, M. A. (2008). *Terminating psychotherapy: A clinician's guide.* New York: Routledge.

Ost, L. G. (1989). A maintenance program for behavioural treatment of anxiety disorders. *Behaviour Research and Therapy, 27,* 123–130.

Othmer, E., & Othmer, S. (1994). *The clinical interview using DSM-IV. Vol. I: Fundamentals.* Washington, DC: American Psychiatric Association Press.

Ottenbreit, N. D., & Dobson, K. S. (2004). Avoidance and depression: The construction of the Cognitive-Behavioral Avoidance Scale. *Behaviour Research and Therapy, 42,* 293–313.

Otto, M., Reilly-Harrington, N., Kogan, J., & Winett, C. (2003). Treatment contracting in cognitive behavior therapy. *Cognitive and Behavioral Practice, 10,* 199–203.

Pampallona, S., Bollini, P., Tibaldi, G., Kupelnick, B., & Munizza, C. (2004). Combined pharmacotherapy and psychological treatment for depression: A systematic review. *Archives of General Psychiatry, 61,* 714–719.

Paterson, R. (2000). *The Assertiveness Workbook: How to express your ideas and stand up for yourself at work and in relationships.* Oakland, CA: New Harbinger Press.

Paykel, E. S. (2007). Cognitive therapy in relapse prevention in depression. *International Journal of Neuropsychopharmacology, 10,* 131–136.

Pekarik, G., & Wolff, C. (1996). Relationship of satisfaction to symptom change, follow-up adjustment and clinical significance. *Professional Psychology: Research and Practice, 27*(2), 202–208.

Perepletchikova, R., & Kazdin, A. (2005). Treatment integrity and therapeutic change: Issues and research recommendations. *Clinical Psychology: Science and Practice, 12,* 365–378.

Persons, J. B. (1989). *Cognitive therapy in practice: A case formulation approach.* New York: Norton.

Persons, J. B., & Bertagnolli, A. E. (1999). Inter-rater reliability of cognitive-behavioral case formulations for depression: A replication. *Cognitive Therapy and Research, 23,* 271–284.

Persons, J. B., Mooney, K., & Padesky, C. (1995). Interrater reliability of cognitive behavioral case formulation. *Cognitive Therapy and Research, 19,* 21–34.

Persons, J. B., Roberts, N. A., Zalecki, C. A., & Brechwald, W. A. G. (2006). Naturalistic outcome of case formulation-driven cognitive-behavior therapy for anxious depressed outpatients. *Behaviour Research and Therapy, 44,* 1041–1051.

Reddin Long, J. (2001). Goal agreement and early therapeutic change. *Psychotherapy, 38,* 219–232.

Rees, C., McEvoy, P., & Nathan, P. (2005). Relationship between homework completion and outcome in cognitive behaviour therapy. *Cognitive Behaviour Therapy, 34*(4), 242–247.

Reik, T. (1948). *Listening with the third ear: The inner experience of a psychoanalyst.* New York: Farrar.

Richard, D. C., & Lauterbach, D. (Eds.). (2007). *Handbook of exposure therapies.* London: Elsevier Press.

Riso, L. P., du Toit, P. L., Stein, D. J., & Young, J. E. (Eds.). (2007). *Cognitive schemas and core beliefs in psychological problems: A scientist-practitioner guide.* Washington, DC: American Psychological Association Press.

Robins, L., Cottler, L., Bucholz, K., & Compton, W. (1995). *The Diagnostic Interview Schedule, Version IV.* St. Louis, MO: Washington University Medical School.

Rodebaugh, T. L., Holaway, R. M., & Heimberg, R. G. (2004). The treatment of social anxiety disorder. *Clinical Psychology Review, 24,* 883–908.

Rotgers, F., & Sharp, L. (2005). Alcohol use disorders. In M. Antony, D. R. Ledley, & R. G. Heimberg (Eds.), *Improving outcomes and preventing relapse in cognitive-behavioral therapy* (pp. 348–379). New York: Guilford Press.

Rowa, K., Bieling, P. J., & Segal, Z. V. (2005). Depression. In M. Antony, D. R. Ledley, & R. Heimberg (Eds.), *Improving outcomes and preventing relapse in cognitive-behavioral therapy* (pp. 204–245). New York: Guilford Press.

Rudd, M. D., & Joiner, T. (1998). The assessment, management and treatment of suicidality: Toward clinical informed and balanced standards of care. *Clinical Psychology: Science and Practice, 5*, 135–150.

Rudd, M. D., Joiner, T., Jobes, D., & King, C. (1999). The outpatient treatment of suicidality: An integration of science and recognition of its limitations. *Professional Psychology: Research and Practice, 30*(5), 437–446.

Saatsi, S., Hardy, G. E., & Cahill, J. (2007). Predictors of outcome and completion status in cognitive therapy for depression. *Psychotherapy Research, 17*, 185–195.

Safran, J., & Segal, Z. (1990). *Interpersonal process in cognitive therapy.* New York: Basic Books.

Safran, J., & Wallner, L. (1991). The relative predictive validity of two therapeutic alliance measures in cognitive therapy. *Psychological Assessment, 3*, 188–195.

Salkovskis, P., Clark, D., & Gelder, M. (1996). Cognition–behaviour links in the persistence of panic. *Behaviour Research and Therapy, 34*, 453–458.

Segal, Z. V., Williams, J. M. G., & Teasdale, J. D. (2001). *Mindfulness-based cognitive therapy for depression: A new approach to preventing relapse.* New York: Guilford Press.

Seidler, G. H., & Wagner, F. E. (2006). Comparing the efficacy of EMDR and trauma-focused cognitive-behavioral therapy in the treatment of PTSD: A meta-analytic study. *Psychological Medicine, 36*, 1515–1522.

Shaw, B. F., & Dobson, K. S. (1988). Competency judgments in the training and evaluation of psychotherapists. *Journal of Consulting and Clinical Psychology, 56*, 666–672.

Sheehan, D., Lecrubier, Y., Sheehan, K., Amorim, P., Janavs, J., Weiller, E., et al. (1998). The Mini-International Neuropsychiatric Interview (M.I.N.I.): The development and validation of a structured diagnostic psychiatric interview for DSM-IV and ICD-10. *Journal of Clinical Psychiatry, 59*(Suppl. 20), 22–33.

Simon, R. I., & Hales, R. E. (Eds.). (2006). *Textbook of suicide assessment and management.* Arlington, VA: American Psychiatric Publishing.

Smith, M. L., & Glass, G. V. (1977). Meta-analysis of psychotherapy outcome studies. *American Psychologist, 32*, 752–760.

Sobell, L., & Sobell, M. (2003). Using motivational interviewing techniques to talk with clients about their alcohol use. *Cognitive and Behavioral Practice, 10*, 214–221.

Spielberger, C., Gorsuch, R., Lushene, R., Vagg, P., & Jacobs, G. (1983). *Manual for the State–Trait Anxiety Inventory.* Palo Alto, CA: Consulting Psychologists Press.

Spies, R., & Plake, B. (Eds.). (2005). *The sixteenth mental measurements yearbook.* Lincoln: University of Nebraska Press.

Spitzer, R., Williams, J., Kroenke, K., Linzer, M., deGruy, R., Hahn, S., et al. (1994). Utility of a new procedure for diagnosing mental disorders in primary care: The PRIME-MD 1000 Study. *Journal of the American Medical Association, 272,* 1749–1756.

Stoppard, J. (1989). An evaluation of the adequacy of cognitive behavioural theories for understanding depression in women. *Canadian Psychology, 30,* 39–47.

Strachey, J. (1957). *Studies on hysteria* (edited from the original by J. Breuer & S. Freud, *Studien über Hysterie*; 1895). New York: Basic Books.

Strunk, D. R., DeRubeis, R. J., Chiu, A. W., & Alvarez, J. (2007). Patients' competence and performance of cognitive therapy skills: Relation to the reduction of relapse risk following treatment for depression. *Journal of Consulting and Clinical Psychology, 74*(4), 523–530.

Tang, T. Z., & DeRubeis, R. J. (1999). Sudden gains and critical sessions in cognitive-behavioral therapy for depression. *Journal of Consulting and Clinical Psychology, 67,* 894–904.

Tang, T. Z., DeRubeis, R. J., Beberman, R., & Pham, T. (2005). Cognitive changes, critical sessions, and sudden gains in cognitive-behavioral therapy for depression. *Journal of Consulting and Clinical Psychology, 73,* 168–172.

Tang, T. Z., DeRubeis, R. J., Hollon, S. D., Amsterdam, J., & Shelton, R. (2007). Sudden gains in cognitive therapy of depression and depression relapse/recurrence. *Journal of Consulting and Clinical Psychology, 75,* 404–408.

Teasdale, J. D., Segal, Z. V., Williams, J. M., Ridgeway, V. A., Soulsby, J. M., & Lau, M. A. (2000). Prevention of relapse/recurrence in major depression by mindfulness-based cognitive therapy. *Journal of Consulting and Clinical Psychology, 68,* 615–623.

Teyber, E. (2000). *Interpersonal process in psychotherapy: A relational approach.* Belmont, CA: Wadsworth.

Tryon, G. S., & Winograd, G. (2001). Goal consensus and collaboration. *Psychotherapy, 38,* 385–389.

Vallis, T. M., Shaw, B. F., & Dobson, K. S. (1986). The Cognitive Therapy Scale: Psychometric properties. *Journal of Consulting and Clinical Psychology, 54,* 381–385.

Wade, W. A., Treat, T. A., & Stuart, G. L. (1998). Transporting an empirically supported treatment for panic disorder to a service clinic setting: A benchmarking strategy. *Journal of Consulting and Clinical Psychology, 66,* 231–239.

Wampold, B. E. (2005). Establishing specificity in psychotherapy scientifically: Design and evidence issues. *Clinical Psychology: Science and Practice, 12,* 194–197.

Wang, J. (2007). *Mental health literacy in Alberta.* Presentation at Department of Psychiatry, Calgary, Alberta, Canada.

Waters, A. M., & Craske, M. G. (2005). Generalized anxiety disorder. In M. Antony, D. R. Ledley, & R. G. Heimberg (Eds.), *Improving outcomes and preventing relapse in cognitive-behavioral therapy* (pp. 77–127). New York: Guilford Press.

Watson, J., & Geller, S. (2005). The relation among the relationship conditions, working alliance, and outcome in both process–experiential and cognitive-behavioral psychotherapy. *Psychotherapy Research*, *15*(1–2), 25–33.

Weissman, A. N., & Beck, A. T. (1980). *The Dysfunctional Attitude Scale*. Unpublished manuscript, University of Pennsylvania, Philadelphia.

Weissman, M. M., Verdeli, H., Gameroff, M. J., Bledsoe, S. E., Betts, K., Mufson, L., et al. (2006). National Survey of Psychotherapy Training in Psychiatry, Psychology, and Social Work. *Archives of General Psychiatry*, *63*, 925–934.

Wells, A. (2002). Worry, metacognition, and GAD: Nature, consequences, and treatment. *Journal of Cognitive Psychotherapy: An International Quarterly*, *16*, 179–192.

Wells, A., Clark, D., Salkovskis, P., Ludgate, J., Hackmann, A., & Gelder, M. (1995). Social phobia: The role of in-situation safety behaviors in maintaining anxiety and negative beliefs. *Behavior Therapy*, *26*, 153–161.

Westen, D., Novotny, C. M., & Thompson-Brenner, H. (2004). The empirical status of empirically supported psychotherapies: Assumptions, findings, and reporting in controlled clinical trials. *Psychological Bulletin*, *130*(4), 631–663.

Whisman, M. A. (1993). Mediators and moderators of change in cognitive therapy of depression. *Psychological Bulletin*, *114*, 248–265.

Whisman, M. A. (2008). *Adapting cognitive therapy for depression: Managing complexity and comorbidity*. New York: Guilford Press.

Widiger, T. A., & Frances, A. J. (1994). Toward a dimensional model for the personality disorders. In P. T. Costa, Jr. & T. A. Widiger (Eds.), *Personality disorders and the five-factor model of personality* (pp. 19–39). Washington, DC: American Psychological Association Press.

Widiger, T. A., & Simonsen, E. (2005). Alternative dimensional models of personality disorder: Finding a common ground. *Journal of Personality Disorders*, *19*, 110–130.

Wright, J. H., Wright, A. S., Salmon, P., Beck, A. T., Kuykendall, J., Goldsmith, J., et al. (2002). Development and initial testing on a multimedia program for computer-assisted cognitive therapy. *American Journal of Psychotherapy*, *56*, 76–86.

Yalom, I., & Leszcz, M. (2005). *The theory and practice of group psychotherapy* (5th ed.). New York: Basic Books.

Yates, A. (1958). Symptoms and symptom substitution. *Psychological Review*, *65*(6), 371–374.

Young, J. E., & Beck, A. T. (1980). *Cognitive Therapy Scale rating manual*. Unpublished manuscript, University of Pennsylvania, Philadelphia.

Young, J. E., & Brown, G. (2001). *Young Schema Questionnaire: Special Edition*. New York: Schema Therapy Institute.

Young, J. E., & Klosko, J. S. (1994). *Reinventing your life*. New York: Plume.

Young, J. E., Klosko, J. S., & Weishaar, M. E. (2003). *Schema therapy: A practitioner's guide*. New York: Guilford Press.

Zubin, J., & Spring, B. (1977). Vulnerability: A new view of schizophrenia. *Journal of Abnormal Psychology*, *86*, 103–126.

Index

Page numbers followed by an *f*, *n*, or *t* indicate figures, notes, or tables.

ABAB experiment, 208
Abusive clients, 206
Academy of Cognitive Therapy, 277–278
Acceptance-based interventions, 144, 171–173
Access hypothesis, 4
Acronym use, 61
Acting "as if" technique, 164–165
Activity Log, 204
Activity scheduling, 80, 91–93, 93*f*, 204
Adherence to the treatment, 198–203, 201*t*, 202*t*, 231, 276–278
Affect
　goal setting and, 60–61
　identifying emotions and, 119–121
　reactions to, 20–21
　therapeutic relationship and, 69–70
Affirmations, positive, 140
Aggression, 205–206
All-or-nothing thinking. *see also* Cognitive distortions
　interventions for, 134–135
　overview, 129*t*
　stress and anxiety in the therapist and, 220
Alternative thought generation, 135–139, 138*f*
Ambivalence, 64
American Psychiatric Association, 5–6
Anger, 205–206
Anorexia nervosa, 239*t*, 294
Anxiety
　deciding how much therapy is enough, 183

exposure treatment and, 103–111, 105*t*, 110*f*, 112*t*
　motivation and, 63–65
　relaxation training and, 102–103
　in the therapist, 220
　therapy completion and, 194
　treatment adherence and, 202*t*
Anxiety disorder. *see* Generalized anxiety disorder
Anxiety Disorders Interview Schedule for DSM-IV (ADIS-IV), 17
Anxiety neutralization behaviors, 109–111, 110*f*
Appraisals, 242
Approach–avoidance patterns
　assessment and, 21
　motivational interviewing methods and, 64
　unrealistic expectations and, 132
Asperger syndrome, 97
Assessment
　case formulation and, 39–42, 41*f*
　empirically based, 14–16
　first aid for the therapist and, 218*t*
　goal setting and, 56–58
　interviews, 17–25, 19*f*–20*f*, 24*t*–25*t*
　observation, 27
　as an ongoing process, 29–31
　overview, 13–14
　relapse prevention and, 192–193
　schemas and, 157–158
　self-monitoring, 27–28
　self-report measures, 25–27

Assessment (*continued*)
    sequencing and length of treatment and,
        75–76
    suicide risk and, 213–216, 215*t*, 217*t*
    tools for, 16–29, 19*f*–20*f*, 24*t*–25*t*
Assumptions, 123, 151. *see also* Schemas
Attitudes, 151, 259–260. *see also* Schemas
Attributional biases, 133
Attributions
    change models and, 208–209
    dependence and, 179*t*
    relapse prevention and, 191*t*
Autogenic relaxation, 101–102, 102–
        103
Automatic thoughts. *see also* Negative
        thoughts
    behavioral activation and, 92
    downward arrow technique and,
        141–142, 142*t*
    identifying, 121–124, 122*t*
    "imposter syndrome" of the therapist
        and, 219–220
    interpersonal styles of clients and,
        207–208
Autonomy, 157–158
Avoidance
    assessment and, 21
    behavioral interventions to decrease,
        103–111, 105*t*, 110*f*, 112*t*, 114*f*
    depression and, 113
    negative thinking and, 146
    research and, 242
    schemas and, 152–153
    therapeutic relationship and, 222
    unrealistic expectations and, 132
Axis I problems, 177, 188, 269*t*
Axis II problems, 204*t*, 213, 260, 269

B

Beck Anxiety Inventory (BAI), 26
Beck Depression Inventory–II (BDI-II), 26
Beck Hopelessness Scale, 15
Beck Hopelessness Scale (BHS), 26
Behavioral activation methods
    avoidance and, 104
    exposure treatment and, 103–111, 105*t*,
        110*f*, 112*t*
    guidelines for, 93–96
    overview, 91–93, 93*f*, 112–113
    schemas and, 159–160
Behavioral Activity Schedule, 28
Behavioral assignments, 155–156,
        163–164
Behavioral Avoidance Scale, 27

Behavioral elements of treatment
    behavioral activation and, 93–96,
        112–113
    to decrease avoidance, 103–111, 105*t*,
        110*f*, 112*t*
    overview, 75–76, 90–91
    relaxation training, 101–102
    skills training and, 97–101, 98*t*, 100*t*
    traditional methods, 91–93, 93*f*
Behavioral experimentation
    change models and, 208
    problem-solving interventions and,
        84–85
    social skills training and, 100*t*
Behavioral factors, 21, 60–61
Behavioral functional analysis, 15–16
Beliefs. *see also* Schemas
    cognitive distortions and, 129–130
    confusing thoughts with, 123
    identification of, 153–158
    myths about CBT and, 246–262
    overview, 151
    relapse prevention and, 178
    therapy completion and, 189
Bern Inventory of Treatment Goals, 57
Bias, confronting the past and, 166–167
Biopsychosocial model. *see* Vulnerability
        model, case formulation and
Bipolar disorder, 239*t*, 269*t*, 294
Black-and-white thinking. *see* All-or-
        nothing thinking
Booster sessions, 180–182
Breaks from therapy, 179*t*
Breathing retraining, 101–102, 102–103
Bulimia nervosa, 239*t*, 294
Burnout, 220–221
"Buy in" from clients, 61–63, 259–260

C

Cancellation of appointments, 199
Case conceptualization
    assessment and, 13–14
    behavioral activation and, 94–95
    schemas and, 155
    sharing with the client, 155
Case formulation
    adherence to the CBT model and,
        218–219
    "buy in" from clients and, 61–62
    efficacy of treatment and, 35–39, 48,
        53*f*–54*f*
    example of, 49*f*–54*f*
    interpersonal styles of clients and,
        207–208

myths about CBT and, 247–248
    overview, 32–39
    sequencing and length of treatment and,
        75–76
    steps in, 39–49, 41*f*, 44*f*
    treatment planning and, 55–56
Caseloads, 271–273
Catastrophization, 129*t*. *see also* Cognitive
    distortions
CBT practice
    communication with potential clients
        and, 270–273
    overview, 265–266
    referrals, 266–270, 269*t*
    ways to increase, 273–275
Challenges in CBT
    angry and aggressive clients, 205–206
    change models and, 208–211
    clients and, 198–216, 201*t*, 202*t*, 204*t*,
        215*t*, 217*t*
    compliance and, 203–205, 204*t*
    crises and emergencies and, 213–216,
        215*t*, 217*t*
    entertaining clients, 207
    first aid for the therapist and, 218*t*
    interpersonal styles and, 207–208
    multiple problems and, 211–212
    outside of therapy, 223
    overview, 197
    therapeutic relationship and, 221–222
    treatment adherence and, 199–203,
        201*t*, 202*t*
Change hypothesis, 4–5
Change talk, 65
Change techniques. *see also* Interventions
    challenges related to, 208–211
    myths about CBT and, 256
    outcome and, 234
    overview, 116–117
Clients
    angry and aggressive clients, 205–206
    challenges related to, 198–216, 201*t*,
        202*t*, 204*t*, 215*t*, 217*t*
    compliance and, 203–205, 204*t*
    crises and emergencies and, 213–216,
        215*t*, 217*t*
    entertaining, 207
    first aid for the therapist and, 218*t*
    interpersonal styles and, 207–208
    multiple problems and, 211–212
    negative beliefs regarding, 257–260
    outcome and, 225–228, 226*f*, 228*t*
    treatment adherence and, 199–203,
        201*t*, 202*t*

Clinical myths. *see* Myths about CBT
Clinical significance testing, 237
Cognitions, reactions to, 20–21
Cognitive distortions. *see also* Negative
        thoughts
    examining the evidence technique and,
        128–135, 129*t*, 134*f*
    list of, 129*t*
    myths about CBT and, 245–246
    stress and anxiety in the therapist and,
        220
Cognitive factors, 60–61
Cognitive interventions, 75–76
Cognitive problems, 199
Cognitive reappraisals, 242
Cognitive restructuring
    identifying negative thoughts, 117–124,
        119*f*, 122*t*
    overview, 71–72, 116–117, 144–146
    schemas and, 159–160
Cognitive Therapy Adherence and
        Competence Scale (CTACS), 277
Cognitive Therapy Scale (CTS)
    complete, 285–290
    myths about CBT and, 257
    overview, 219, 230, 277–278
Cognitive-behavioral therapy in general,
        4–11, 11–12, 282–284, 283*t*
Collaboration with other professionals,
        46–49
Collaborative empiricism, 72–73, 232
Collaborative stance with clients
    myths about CBT and, 251
    problem-solving interventions and,
        82–83
    therapy completion and, 176
    treatment adherence and, 202*t*
    treatment planning and, 59
Common factors, 253
Communication, motivational interviewing
        methods and, 64
Communication skills training, 97–101,
        98*t*, 101*t*
Communication with other professionals,
        46–49
Comorbidity, 183
Compensation behaviors, 172. *see also*
        Schema compensation behaviors
Competence. *see also* Expertise in CBT
    communication with potential clients
        and, 270–273
    maximizing, 276–282, 280*t*
    overview, 231, 268, 276–282, 280*t*
    therapeutic relationship and, 66–67

Completion of treatment, 31
Compliance, treatment adherence and, 203–205, 204*t*
Confrontation, schemas and, 163
Confronting the past technique, 166–167
Consequences, assessment and, 18, 20
Consumer movement, 10
Contingency contracting, 95–96
Continua, schemas and, 161
Contracts, therapeutic. *see* Therapeutic contract
Contradictory thinking, 138–139
Coping
    assessment and, 21
    behavioral treatments and, 92, 114*f*
    overview, 88*t*, 143
    relapse prevention and, 192
Coping model, therapeutic relationship and, 67
Core beliefs. *see also* Beliefs
    cognitive distortions and, 129–130
    downward arrow technique and, 141–142, 142*t*
    overview, 149–150
Core conflictual relationship theme (CCRT), 36. *see also* Case formulation
Cost considerations, 10–11
Cost–benefit analysis, 138, 168–169
Countertransference, 233. *see also* Therapeutic alliance
Course of the problem, assessment and, 22–23
Credentialing, 282
Crises, 213–216, 215*t*, 217*t*, 218*t*
Critical incident stress debriefing, 241
Crutches in exposures, 111
Cultural factors, 8–11

D

Defense mechanisms, exposure treatment and, 109–111, 110*f*
Demand and supply of CBT, 6–8
Demanding clients, 205–206
Dependence, 178, 178–180, 179*t*
Depression
    deciding how much therapy is enough, 183
    demand of CBT and, 6
    exclusion criteria for treatment and, 269*t*
    motivation and, 63–65
    review of the literature and, 239*t*, 293

"third-wave" behavioral activation and, 112–113
    treatment outcome and, 227
Developmental factors, 22–23
Diagnosis
    assessment and, 14–15
    Axis II problems, 204*t*, 213, 260, 269
    case formulation and, 40–42, 41*f*
    communication skills training and, 97
    exclusion criteria for treatment and, 269*t*
    overview, 2–3
    relapse prevention and, 177
    review of the literature and, 239*t*–240*t*
    schemas and, 152
    suicide risk and, 213
    therapy completion and, 188
    treatment adherence and, 199
Diagnostic interviews. *see* Interviews in assessment
Diagnostic utility, 15
Diathesis–stress model. *see* Vulnerability model, case formulation and
Dichotomous thinking, 256–257. *see* All-or-nothing thinking
Discouragement, 71–72
Discrepancy, 64–65
Disqualifying the positive, 129*t*. *see also* Cognitive distortions
Distorted thinking. *see* Cognitive distortions
Distraction, negative thinking and, 143–144
Dobson Adapted Thought Record, 137, 138*f*
Dose–response effect, 248
Downward arrow technique, 141–142, 142*t*, 155
DSM
    Axis I symptoms, 177, 188, 269*t*
    Axis II problems, 204*t*, 213, 260, 269
    evaluation of treatments, 235–236
    exclusion criteria for treatment and, 269*t*
Duration of therapy
    myths about CBT and, 246, 248–249
    overview, 75–76
    psychological diagnosis and, 260
Dysfunctional Attitude Scale (DAS), 157–158
Dysfunctional Thoughts Record. *see also* Thought Record forms
    "imposter syndrome" of the therapist and, 219–220

interpersonal styles of clients and,
207–208
myths about CBT and, 252
overview, 28, 80, 124–125
Dysphoric disorders, 228

E

Eclectic therapy, 278–279
Emergencies, 213–216, 215t, 217t, 218t
Emotional prime, 156–157
Emotional reasoning, 129t, 139. see also
Cognitive distortions
Emotional self-expression, 119–120
Emotion-focused coping skills, 88t
Emotions, 119–121. see also Affect
Empathy, 64
Encouragement, therapeutic relationship
and, 70
Entertaining clients, 207
Environmental factors, goal setting and,
60–61
Equality, therapeutic relationship and,
66–67
Evidence for and against negative thoughts.
see also Examining the evidence
technique
generating alternative thoughts and,
135–139, 138f
overview, 128–135, 129t, 134f
schemas and, 162
Evidence-based psychotherapy. see also
Research evidence
case formulation and, 35–39
current context of, 5–8
outcome and, 231–234
overview, 242–243
schemas and, 161–167
Examining the evidence technique,
128–135, 129t, 134f, 162. see also
Evidence for and against negative
thoughts
Exclusion criteria, 268–270, 269t,
270–273
Exercise habits, 99
Expectations, 71–72, 131–133
Experiences, recurrent, 154–155
Expertise in CBT
communication with potential clients
and, 270–273
overview, 7, 267–268
therapeutic relationship and, 66–67
Exposure treatment
avoidance and, 103–111, 105t, 110f,
112t

CBT practice and, 266–267
myths about CBT and, 249–250
planning for, 77–78
relaxation training and, 102–103

F

Family, in assessment, 28
Family conflict, behavioral activation and,
92
Family factors, assessment and, 22
Family practice model, 182
Fear Questionnaire, 26–27
Feedback
angry and aggressive clients, 206
relapse prevention and, 191t
schemas and, 168
social skills training and, 100t
therapy completion and, 194
Feelings. see Affect
Financial considerations, 10–11, 228, 249
First-aid, 218t
Flexibility, therapeutic relationship and,
70–71
Follow-up assessments, 31
Fortune telling, 129t. see also Cognitive
distortions
Frequency of sessions, 191t
Frequency Record form, 125–126
Functional analysis, 15–16, 18

G

Gender, myths about CBT and, 251
Generalized anxiety disorder, 239t,
254–255, 292, 293
Global Assessment of Functioning (GAF),
186
Goal Attainment Scaling (GAS), 30, 59–60
Goal setting
"buy in" from clients and, 61–63
overview, 56–65, 58f
steps in, 59–61
Goals in therapy
assessment and, 30
reevaluation of, 30
therapy completion and, 185–187, 186t,
188–189
Graduated thinking, 134–135
Group treatment, 99, 266–267

H

Handouts in therapy, 191t
Health care systems, 10–11
Health habits, 99

Health maintenance organizations
    (HMOs), 7, 10–11, 249
Helplessness, 84–85
Hierarchies in exposure, 105t
Historical perspective, 156
History of treatment, 23
Homework assignments
    adherence to, 198–203, 201t, 202t
    generating alternative thoughts and,
        136–137, 138f
    outcome and, 233
    overview, 80–82, 82f
    relapse prevention and, 191t
    schemas and, 155–156
    social skills training and, 100t
    unrealistic expectations and, 132–133
Hope, therapeutic relationship and, 71–72
Humor use, 137–138, 207
Hypothesis testing, 130
Hypothetical situations, 156

I

Idiographic case formulation, 37
"If–then" statements, 151
Imaginal exposure, 106
"Imposter syndrome", 219–220, 276
In vivo exposure, 106, 107, 266–267
Individualized treatments, 37
Insight, myths about CBT and, 250
Insurance, 10–11, 249
Integration, 32–33
Integrity, treatment, 231, 278–279
Intentional specific treatment, 255–256
International Center for Clubhouse
    Development, 95
Interoceptive exposure, 107
Interpersonal model, 254
Interpersonal problems
    assessment and, 22
    behavioral activation and, 92
    challenges related to, 207–208
    goal setting and, 60–61
Interventions. see also Change techniques
    acceptance-based interventions and,
        172–173
    effectiveness of, 234–237
    evaluation of, 235–237
    examining the evidence technique,
        128–135, 129t, 134f
    for negative thinking, 127–146, 129t,
        134f, 138f, 142t
    outcome and, 226f, 231–234
    research and, 234–237
    schemas and, 158–170, 159t, 170t

Interventions, problem-solving, 82–83,
    83f, 84f
Interviews in assessment, 15, 17–25,
    19f–20f, 24t–25t. see also Assessment

L

Labeling, 129t, 134. see also Cognitive
    distortions
Lapse, 177, 191t
Length of treatment
    myths about CBT and, 246, 248–249
    overview, 75–76
    psychological diagnosis and, 260
Logical change methods, 167–170, 170t

M

Magnification/minimization, 129t. see also
    Cognitive distortions
Maintenance behaviors, 109–111, 110f.
    see also Schema maintenance
    behaviors
Maintenance sessions, 180–182
Manuals, treatment
    case formulation and, 33–34, 37
    evaluation of treatments and, 235–236
    myths about CBT and, 246, 247–248
    overview, 2
    research and, 242–243
    sequencing and length of treatment and,
        75–76
Mastery activities, 94–95
Mastery model, 67
Mediation hypothesis, 4
Medication, 184, 209–211
Meta-analysis, 235, 236–237
Metacognition
    identifying negative thoughts and,
        117–124, 119f, 122t
    schemas and, 173
    therapeutic relationship and, 69
Mind reading, 129t. see also Cognitive
    distortions
Mindfulness, 172–173, 194
Mini-International Neuropsychiatric
    Interview (MINI), 17
Minimization, unrealistic expectations and,
    132
Misattribution, 129t, 133–134, 134f. see
    also Cognitive distortions
Mobility Inventory for Agoraphobia, 26
Modeling, social skills training and, 100t
Mood, "third-wave" behavioral activation
    and, 112–113

Motivation, 61–63, 63–65, 199
Motivational interviewing methods, 64
Myths about CBT
    negative beliefs and, 246–262
    overview, 244–246
    positive beliefs and, 262–264
    presence of emotion and, 69–70
    therapeutic relationship and, 69–70

N

Negative beliefs, 246–262, 257–260,
    261–262
Negative thoughts. *see also* Automatic
        thoughts
    behavioral activation and, 92
    examining the evidence technique and,
        128–135, 129*t*, 134*f*
    identifying, 117–124, 119*f*, 122*t*
    interventions for, 127–146, 129*t*, 134*f*,
        138*f*, 142*t*
    methods for collecting, 124–127, 126*f*
    myths about CBT and, 251–252
Negativity, therapeutic relationship and,
    71–72
Neurotic paradox, 109
New age therapies, 241
Nonspecific factors, 253
Nonverbal communication, 97–98
Normalization, self-disclosure and, 68
Notes during sessions, 191*t*

O

Observational assessment, 27
Obsessional thinking, 143–144
Obsessive–compulsive disorder (OCD),
    146, 239*t*, 292
Occupational problems, 228
Onset, assessment and, 22–23
Orientation, 76–78
Outcome
    assessment and, 30–31
    case formulation and, 35–39, 48,
        53*f*–54*f*
    client factors and, 225–228, 226*f*, 228*t*
    interventions and, 226*f*
    myths about CBT and, 246
    relapse rates and, 184
    relationship factors and, 226*f*, 229–231,
        232*t*
    research and, 226*f*, 228*t*, 232*t*,
        239*t*–240*t*
    self-disclosure and, 257
    therapist factors and, 226*f*, 228–229

    treatments that do not work, 241–242
Out-of-office exposure, 108
Overgeneralization, 129*t*. *see also*
        Cognitive distortions

P

Panic Attack Log, 28
Panic attacks, relaxation training and,
    102–103
Panic disorder, 239*t*, 292
Passiveness, 84–85
Past, confronting, 166–167
Patterns of beliefs and behaviors, 153–154,
    240–245
Perfectionism, 100*t*, 169, 201
Personality disorders, treatment outcome
    and, 228
Personality traits, schemas and, 151–152
Personalization, 129*t*, 220. *see also*
        Cognitive distortions
Phobias, 239*t*, 291
Placebo, myths about CBT and, 253
Pleasant events, behavioral activation and,
    94–95
Pleasant Events Schedule, 94
Point–counterpoint response strategy, 136
Positive beliefs, myths about CBT and,
    262–264
Positive Data Log, 161–162
Positive thoughts, encouraging, 139–140
Positivity, therapeutic relationship and,
    71–72
Posttraumatic stress disorder, 239*t*, 293
Praise, homework assignments and,
    200–201
Precipitating situations, 189
Predictions, schemas and, 156
Predictive validity, case formulation and,
    37–38
Prescription for Change form, 83*f*, 200,
    202*t*
Presenting problem
    assessment and, 18, 22–23
    case formulation and, 39–42, 41*f*
    multiple problems and, 211–212
    therapy completion and, 187–188
Primary Care Evaluation of Mental
    Disorders (PRIME-MD), 17
Prior documentation, in assessment, 28–
    29
Problem list
    goal attainment scaling and, 59–60
    goal setting and, 59
    overview, 39–42, 41*f*

Problem-solving interventions
    example of, 88–89
    overview, 82–88, 83f, 84f, 88t
    skills training and, 99
    unrealistic expectations and, 132
Problem-solving model, 83–85, 84f
Process-oriented self-disclosure, 68–69
Progressive muscle relaxation, 101–102,
    102–103
Psychoeducation
    change models and, 209–210
    exposure treatment and, 107–108
    myths about CBT and, 247, 250
    overview, 78–80, 81t
    schemas and, 157, 167–168
Psychological assessment, 14–15. see also
    Assessment
Psychological Assessment Work Group
    (PAWG), 14–15
Psychological disorders, 199. see also Axis
    I problems; Axis II problems; specific
    disorders
Psychosis, 239t, 269t, 294–295
Public awareness campaigns, 9–10

Q

Questioning, 62–63, 87

R

Rational Role Play intervention, 136
Reactions, assessment and, 20–21
Reading materials, 157, 167–168. see also
    Psychoeducation
Realist assumption, 5
Reassurance-seeking behavior, 179t
Reattribution of causes, 133–134, 134f
Recovery, 177
Recurrence, 177
Recurrent experiences, 154–155
Referrals
    communication with potential clients
        and, 270, 271
    increasing your CBT practice and,
        273–275
    overview, 266–270, 269t
Relapse, 177, 184, 250–251
Relapse prevention. see also Therapy
    completion
    challenges related to, 222
    overview, 175–176, 176–183, 179t,
        190–194, 191t
Relapse Prevention Plan, 193
Relationship factors, outcome and, 226f,
    229–231, 232t

Relaxation training, 101–102, 102–103,
    241
Reliability, of case formulations, 36
Remission, 177
Repetitive thinking, 143–144
Research evidence. see also Evidence-based
        psychotherapy
    effective treatments, 234–237
    myths about CBT and, 246, 254
    outcome and, 225–243, 226f, 228t,
        232t, 239t–240t
    overview, 224–225
    review of the literature, 237–243,
        239t–240t, 291–295
    treatments that do not work, 241–242
Resistance, 65, 198–199, 254. see also
    Adherence to the treatment
Resources
    dependence and, 179t
    myths about CBT and, 263–264
    psychoeducation and, 78–80
    therapy completion and, 185, 186t
Responsibility, 179t, 191t
Responsiveness, 70–71
Risk assessment, 213–216, 215t, 217t,
    218t
Risk taking, 100t
Role play, 100t, 162–163
Ruminative thinking, 143–144

S

Safety behaviors, 109–111, 110f
Satisfaction with treatment, 186–187
Schedule for Affective Disorders and
        Schizophrenia (SADS), 17
Schema avoidance behavior, 152–153
Schema change interventions
    evidence-based change methods,
        161–167
    logical change methods and, 167–170,
        170t
    overview, 158–170, 159t, 170t
Schema compensation behaviors, 152–153
Schema maintenance behaviors, 152–153.
    see also Maintenance behaviors
Schema therapy, 149–150
Schemas. see also Beliefs
    acceptance-based interventions,
        171–173
    changing, 158–170, 159t, 170t
    cognitive distortions and, 129–130
    confusing thoughts with, 123
    downward arrow technique and,
        141–142, 142t

identification of, 153–158
  overview, 149–150, 151–153
  therapy completion and, 189
Schizophrenia, 97
Science, 1, 3–4
Selective abstraction, 129t. *see also*
  Cognitive distortions
Self-assessments, relapse prevention and,
  192–193
Self-care, 220
Self-diagnosis, 9
Self-disclosure, 68–69, 257
Self-efficacy, 65
Self-esteem, 164–165
Self-harm behaviors, suicide risk and, 214
Self-help groups, 194
Self-monitoring, 27–28
Self-report measures, 25–27. *see also*
  Assessment
Self-statements, 140
Semistructured interviews, 17–18. *see also*
  Interviews in assessment
Sequence of treatment, 75–76
Session structure, 76–78, 211–212
Sexual problems, 22
Simple Frequency Record, 28
Situation–thought–response pattern, 118,
  119f
Skills deficits, 21–22, 97–101, 98t
Skills training
  avoidance and, 104
  communication, 97–101, 98t, 101t
  overview, 96–97
Sleep disorders, 239t, 294
Sleep hygiene, 99
"Slip", 177
SMART acronym, 61
Social acceptance, 10
Social factors, 8–11, 113
Social phobia, 239t
Social skills, 21–22, 97–101, 98t
Social skills training, 97–101, 98t, 100t
Social support, 22, 168, 194
Sociotropy, 157
Sociotropy–Autonomy Scale (SAS), 157–158
Somatization disorder, 240t, 295
Specialty credentialing, 282
Specialty clinic model
  CBT practice and, 267–268
  communication with potential clients
    and, 270–273
  therapy completion and, 182–183
  training and competence and, 276–282,
    280t

Specific phobias, 239t, 291
Standards, 5–6
State–Trait Anxiety Inventory (STAI), 26
Stepped approach, 6, 79, 281
Stigma, 9–10
Stress, in the therapist, 220
Structure, therapeutic relationship and,
  70–71
Structured Clinical Interview for DSM-IV
  Axis I Disorders (SCID), 17
Structured interviews, 17–18, 23, 24t–25t.
  see also Interviews in assessment
Substance use disorders, 239t, 269, 295
Sudden changes, 234, 256
Suicide risk
  exclusion criteria for treatment and,
    269t
  first aid for the therapist and, 218t
  overview, 213–216, 215t, 217t
Supply and demand of CBT, 6–8
Support groups, 194
Symptom List, 42
Symptom substitution, 250–251
Symptoms, 188–189. *see also* Axis I
  problems
System factors, 176–183, 179t

T

Tape recording of sessions, 202t
Task-Interfering Cognitions–Task-
  Orienting Cognitions (TIC–TOC)
  intervention, 139
Termination, 178, 180–181, 222. *see also*
  Therapy completion
Themes in beliefs and behaviors, 153–154
Therapeutic alliance
  angry and aggressive clients, 206
  case formulation and, 37–38, 46
  challenges related to, 221–222
  cognitive restructuring and, 145
  entertaining clients, 207
  myths about CBT and, 252–257,
    253–254, 255, 263
  outcome and, 226t, 229–231, 232, 232t
  overview, 65–73
  research and, 243
  therapy completion and, 176
  treatment adherence and, 199
Therapeutic contract, 56–65, 58f
Therapeutic rupture, 190
Therapist factors
  adherence to the CBT model, 218–219
  burnout and, 220–221
  CBT practice and, 276–282, 280t

Therapist factors (*continued*)
    challenges related to, 216, 218–221
    exposure treatment and, 106–108
    first aid and, 218*t*
    "imposter syndrome", 219–220
    outcome and, 226*f*, 228–229
    referrals and, 266–270
    role of the therapist, 66–70
    stress and anxiety and, 220
    therapeutic relationship and, 65–73
Therapist's Schema Questionnaire, 220
Therapy binder, relapse prevention and,
    191*t*
Therapy completion. *see also* Relapse
        prevention
    challenges related to, 222
    deciding how much therapy is enough,
        183–185
    decisions regarding, 187–190
    factors in, 175–183, 179*t*
    outcome and, 226*f*
    overview, 183–190, 186*t*
    realities regarding treatment and,
        185–187
Therapy notebooks, treatment adherence
        and, 200
"Third-wave" behavioral activation,
    112–113
Thought Record forms. *see also*
        Dysfunctional Thoughts Record
    cognitive distortions and, 130
    generating alternative thoughts and,
        137, 138*f*
    overview, 124–127, 126*f*
    for the therapist, 272
Thoughts, 121–124, 122–123, 122*t*, 123–
    124. *see also* Automatic thoughts;
    Negative thoughts
TIC–TOC intervention, 139
Time management, 99
Time projection technique, 169–170
Time-limited dynamic psychotherapy,
    254–255
TRACS model, 113, 114*f*
Training
    case formulation and, 35–36, 38–39
    CBT practice and, 268
    interviews in assessment and, 17–18
    myths about CBT and, 261–262
    overview, 276–282, 280*t*
    standards of, 5–6

supply and demand of CBT and, 6–7
    treatment integrity and, 279, 280*t*
Transference, 233. *see also* Therapeutic
        alliance
Transparency, 72–73
TRAPS model, 113, 114*f*
Treatment contracts. *see* Therapeutic
        contract
Treatment integrity, 231, 278–279
Treatment manuals. *see* Manuals,
        treatment
Treatment planning
    assessment and, 13–14
    exposure treatment and, 104–108, 105*t*
    overview, 55–65, 58*f*
    review of the literature and, 239*t*–240*t*
    steps in, 59–61
Treatment teams, case formulation and,
    47–48
Treatment utility, 15
Triggers
    anxiety and, 102–103
    assessment and, 18–19
    behavioral treatments and, 113, 114*f*
    identifying negative thoughts and,
        118–120
    relapse prevention and, 192

U

Unrealistic expectations, 131–133. *see also*
        Expectations

V

Validity, 14–15, 37–38
Values, 151. *see also* Schemas
Visualization exercises, 101–102, 102–103
Vulnerability model, case formulation and,
    43–44, 44*f*

W

Warning signs, 192. *see also* Triggers
Working Alliance Inventory, 56–57, 254
Worry, 143
Worry time technique, 143

Y

Yale–Brown Obsessive–Compulsive Scale
(Y-BOCS), 26
Young Schema Questionnaire (YSQ), 158,
    159*t*